MW01474222

Assessing Literacy in Deaf Individuals

Donna A. Morere • Thomas Allen
Editors

Assessing Literacy in Deaf Individuals

Neurocognitive Measurement and Predictors

Springer

Editors
Donna A. Morere
Department of Psychology
Gallaudet University
Washington, DC, USA

Thomas Allen
Science of Learning Center
Gallaudet University
Washington, DC, USA

ISBN 978-1-4614-5268-3   ISBN 978-1-4614-5269-0 (eBook)
DOI 10.1007/978-1-4614-5269-0
Springer New York Heidelberg Dordrecht London

Library of Congress Control Number: 2012951414

© Springer Science+Business Media New York 2012
This work is subject to copyright. All rights are reserved by the Publisher, whether the whole or part of the material is concerned, specifically the rights of translation, reprinting, reuse of illustrations, recitation, broadcasting, reproduction on microfilms or in any other physical way, and transmission or information storage and retrieval, electronic adaptation, computer software, or by similar or dissimilar methodology now known or hereafter developed. Exempted from this legal reservation are brief excerpts in connection with reviews or scholarly analysis or material supplied specifically for the purpose of being entered and executed on a computer system, for exclusive use by the purchaser of the work. Duplication of this publication or parts thereof is permitted only under the provisions of the Copyright Law of the Publisher's location, in its current version, and permission for use must always be obtained from Springer. Permissions for use may be obtained through RightsLink at the Copyright Clearance Center. Violations are liable to prosecution under the respective Copyright Law.
The use of general descriptive names, registered names, trademarks, service marks, etc. in this publication does not imply, even in the absence of a specific statement, that such names are exempt from the relevant protective laws and regulations and therefore free for general use.
While the advice and information in this book are believed to be true and accurate at the date of publication, neither the authors nor the editors nor the publisher can accept any legal responsibility for any errors or omissions that may be made. The publisher makes no warranty, express or implied, with respect to the material contained herein.

Printed on acid-free paper

Springer is part of Springer Science+Business Media (www.springer.com)

Preface

Construction requires tools. Whether we are constructing a house, an educated citizen, or a scientific theory, we will be stymied if we do not have the right tools. However rich our raw materials are, they are mere bits and scraps of unrealized potential if we lack the means of assembling them into the products we envision. Imagine a carpenter arriving at Home Depot, her truck already full of lumber, and finding an empty tool counter. Her house will go unbuilt.

The building that we are seeking to construct is a strong foundation of knowledge regarding the cognitive underpinnings of how deaf individuals learn, especially how they acquire literacy. Our truck is indeed full of raw materials: reading researchers have, in recent years, made great strides in describing how literacy is acquired in hearing individuals; neuroscientists have made considerable progress in identifying the neural networks involved in reading and cognition; cognitive scientists have greatly increased our understanding of the underlying mechanisms of memory, executive functioning, visuospatial reasoning, and other processes.

Yet, we strongly suspect that the applicability of this burgeoning knowledge to the very unique population of deaf individuals has limitations. When an individual's primary source of information about the world is through vision, the processes through which he navigates the world, learns to read, and acquires knowledge are quite different from those of individuals who hear as well as see their world. How do we understand those differences? How do we come to understand how visual knowledge, in the absence (or near absence) of auditory knowledge, affects the development of cognitive functions and the acquisition of language? How do visual languages contribute to literacy?

These questions are important, not only for improving the lives of deaf individuals but for enriching our understanding of learning for all individuals. But, of course, we need the right tools to answer these questions. Unfortunately, the myriad of assessments that have contributed remarkably to the growing knowledge base for understanding cognitive development for hearing individuals cannot simply be administered to deaf individuals (either in research, clinical, or educational settings) with confidence in the validity of the scores. The uniqueness of deaf individuals' perceptual experiences, their linguistic histories, and their social and cultural backgrounds mandates an intensive effort to reengineer many commonly utilized assessment practices so that they will yield information that can be accepted and interpreted without hesitation. Additionally, a battery of new assessments will also be necessary to measure visual language skills, since these skills play a critical role in the lives of many deaf individuals.

The Toolkit project described and presented in this book represents a step in pursuit of effective and valid cognitive, linguistic, and achievement assessments for deaf individuals. This project was undertaken at the Science of Learning Center in Visual Language and Visual Learning (VL2) at Gallaudet University. VL2 is one of six national centers funded by the National Science Foundation to address questions that are of critical concern for the Science of Learning. VL2 was funded (in 2006) to pursue answers to the questions posed above; i.e., to contribute to our knowledge of how visual languages and the unique sensory and perceptual experiences of deaf individuals contribute to their brain development, their cognitive capacities, their language development, and their acquisition of literacy.

From the beginning days of VL2, it was evident that we would need to devote our energies to the development of tools for our scientific work. We also knew that there were critical needs for better assessments among practitioners in fields of deaf education and clinical practice. As well, we understood that there was considerable overlap between the needs for assessments that would serve the needs of researchers and those that would serve the needs of practitioners. Center scientists representing different disciplines met to discuss the different assessment needs of the Center and to suggest existing instruments, discuss tests that could be modified or adapted for use for this population, and outline needs for new visual language assessments.

The result of these discussions was the VL2 Toolkit Project. In this project, we assembled a variety of assessments into a comprehensive battery and designed a project wherein we would administer the entire battery to the same group of project participants. This design would allow us to evaluate the underlying systems of correlations among measures of general cognitive functioning, including executive functioning, visuospatial abilities, short-term and working memory, reading comprehension, math and writing fluency and general academic knowledge, and expressive and receptive language skill. The data would allow us to speak to the issues of reliability and both concurrent and construct validity, and also give us an opportunity to examine the underlying covariance structure of a broad set of measures.

This book presents the findings from the VL2 Toolkit project. In these chapters, each Toolkit measure is described, and a statistical analysis is presented that speaks to the psychometric properties of the measure. Thus, the descriptions should be useful both for readers interested in a compendium of measures that have been used and studied successfully with this population, and for readers interested in understanding some of the technical properties of these tools when administered to this population. Chapters 1 and 2 present a more detailed discussion of the rationale for the project, describe the procedures used in conducting the project, and display the background characteristics of the individuals who participated in the project. Chapter 3 presents the findings for Toolkit measures of general cognitive functioning. Chapter 4 discusses the measures selected for assessing visuospatial ability.

Chapter 5 offers the analyses and descriptions for measures of short-term memory, working memory, and signed verbal learning. Chapter 6 discusses the findings for four separate measures of reading. Chapter 7 presents the results of other areas of academic achievement, including writing and math fluency and general academic knowledge. Chapter 8 discusses measures of expressive language, while Chapter 9 discusses measures of receptive language. Chapters 10–12 delve more deeply into a variety of issues having to do with visual languages and visual representations of English: Chapter 10 discusses fingerspelling and presents some descriptive data based on an analysis of the error patterns of Toolkit participants on the fingerspelling test. Chapter 11 presents a discussion of considerations in the development of tests of American Sign Language and provides short descriptions of existing measures that are currently in use and under development. Chapter 12 describes an innovative strategy for using the written responses of participants to the speechreading test as a window on deaf students' writing strategies. In Chapter 13, we present the results of a factor analysis of the toolkit measures in an effort to identify underlying cognitive structures for this population, and we use the resulting factor scores combined with data from the project background questionnaire to explore the interrelationships among selected background characteristics and performance on the derived neurocognitive factors.

We acknowledge the support and participation of many in both conducting the Toolkit Project and in producing this manuscript. We especially thank the National Science Foundation for their significant support in establishing the VL2 Center (under Cooperative Agreement SBE -0541953). We are indebted to the scientists from the Center who contributed to the selection of instruments and the design and execution of the project, especially Dr. Peter Hauser and Dr. Diane Clark. VL2's data assistant Selina Agyen expertly organized all project recruitment and scheduling. We bow deeply to the hard working group who helped prepare the testing materials, particularly former student, Dr. Christen Szymanski, and the team of student and postdoc assessors, which included Assessment Coordinator Leah Murphy, Postdoctoral Fellow Dr. Shilpa Hanumantha, Predoctoral Fellow Wyatte Hall, and graduate assistants Yunjae Hwang, Millicent Musyoka, and Greg Witkin. Finally, we are deeply grateful to the 90 Gallaudet student participants, many of whom endured over 9 h of testing spread out over 3 days. Their contributions to this project are in evidence on every page of this book.

Washington, DC, USA	Donna A. Morere
Washington, DC, USA	Thomas Allen

About the Editors

Donna A. Morere, Ph.D., has been involved in the field of deafness since 1986. She has been a faculty member in the Clinical Psychology Program at Gallaudet since August, 1990. She is the Neuropsychological Assessment Director for the VL2 Psychometric Toolkit Study and Early Education Longitudinal Study (VL2EELS). Dr. Morere also maintains a private practice in Clinical Neuropsychology providing services to individuals who are deaf or hard of hearing using ASL, Cued Speech, or Oral communication. Since the early 1990s, the focus of this practice has been children with complex special needs, primarily those affecting language development. Dr. Morere's research interests include primary language disorders in deaf children, adaptation of neuropsychological assessment instruments for use with deaf and hard of hearing individuals, cognition and memory, executive functioning and attention disorders, and reading and language development in deaf children.

Thomas Allen, Ph.D., is the Founding Director of the VL2 Center and currently serves as its Co-Principal Investigator. He holds a faculty appointment in the Department of Educational Foundations and Research, where he has taught courses in statistics and research design. Dr. Allen formerly served a 9-year term as Dean of the Graduate School at Gallaudet. Prior to becoming Dean, Dr. Allen was the Director of the Gallaudet Research Institute, where he conducted or supervised many large-scale statistical studies of the deaf population in the USA. These included an annual survey of deaf and hard of hearing children and youth and two national efforts to develop norms for standardized achievement tests for the population of deaf and hard of hearing students. He designed and conducted studies of national patterns of classroom communication strategies for deaf and hard of hearing students, and a longitudinal study of school-to-work transition for students who are deaf. As the Dean of the Graduate School, Dr. Allen has implemented Ph.D. programs in Linguistics and Audiology, an Au.D. professional doctorate in Audiology, a Master of Arts in Teaching that focuses on preparing teachers to work in bilingual ASL-English environments, a Master of Arts degree in International Development, and a Master of Arts degree in Deaf Studies. He is currently the lead investigator for a several ongoing research projects at the Visual Language and Visual Learning (VL2) Center at Gallaudet University.

Contents

Part I Rationale and Participant Characteristics

1. **The "Toolkit Project": Introduction** 3
   Elizabeth Halper, Thomas Allen, and Donna A. Morere

2. **The VL2 Toolkit Psychometric Study: Summary of Procedures and Description of Sample Characteristics** 21
   Thomas Allen and Donna A. Morere

Part II Cognitive Functioning

3. **Measures of General Cognitive Functioning** 39
   Donna A. Morere, Evan Goodman, Shilpa Hanumantha, and Thomas Allen

4. **Measures of Visuospatial Ability** 59
   Donna A. Morere, Wyatte C. Hall, and Thomas Allen

5. **Measures of Memory and Learning** 75
   Donna A. Morere

Part III Academic Achievement

6. **Measures of Reading Achievement** 107
   Donna A. Morere

7. **Measures of Writing, Math, and General Academic Knowledge** 127
   Donna A. Morere

Part IV Linguistic Functioning

8. **Measures of Expressive Language** 141
   Donna A. Morere, Gregory Witkin, and Leah Murphy

9	Measures of Receptive Language	159
	Donna A. Morere and Daniel S. Koo	
10	Fingerspelling	179
	Donna A. Morere and Rachel Roberts	
11	Issues and Trends in Sign Language Assessment	191
	Raylene Paludneviciene, Peter C. Hauser, Dorri J. Daggett, and Kim B. Kurz	
12	Analysis of Responses to Lipreading Prompts as a Window to Deaf Students' Writing Strategies	209
	Corine Bickley, Mary June Moseley, and Anna Stansky	

Part V Further Analyses and Translational Implications

13	Underlying Neurocognitive and Achievement Factors and Their Relationship to Student Background Characteristics	231
	Thomas Allen and Donna A. Morere	

Index 263

Contributors

Thomas Allen Science of Learning Center on Visual Language and Visual Learning, Gallaudet University, Washington, DC, USA

Corine Bickley Department of Hearing, Speech, and Language Sciences, Gallaudet University, Washington, DC, USA

Dorri J. Daggett Department of Psychology, Gallaudet University, Washington, DC, USA

Evan Goodman Department of Psychology, Gallaudet University, Washington, DC, USA

Wyatte C. Hall Department of Psychology, Gallaudet University, Washington, DC, USA

Elizabeth Halper Doctor Halper & Associates, Fairfax, VA, USA

Shilpa Hanumantha Science of Learning Center on Visual Language and Visual Learning, Gallaudet University, Washington, DC, USA

Peter C. Hauser Deaf Studies Laboratory, National Technical Institute for the Deaf, Rochester Institute of Technology, Rochester, NY, USA

Daniel S. Koo Department of Psychology, Gallaudet University, Washington, DC, USA

Kim B. Kurz American Sign Language and Interpreting, National Technical Institute for the Deaf, Rochester Institute of Technology, Rochester, NY, USA

Donna A. Morere Department of Psychology, Gallaudet University, Washington, DC, USA

Mary June Moseley Department of Hearing, Speech & Language Sciences, Gallaudet University, Washington, DC, USA

Leah Murphy Department of Psychology, Gallaudet University, Washington, DC, USA

Raylene Paludneviciene Department of Psychology, Gallaudet University, Washington, DC, USA

Rachel Roberts Department of Psychology, Gallaudet University, Washington, DC, USA

Anna Stansky Department of Hearing, Speech, and Language Sciences, Gallaudet University, Washington, DC, USA

Gregory Witkin Department of Psychology, Gallaudet University, Washington, DC, USA

Lists of Tests and Abbreviations

VL2	Science of Learning Center in Visual Language & Visual Learning
D/HOH	Deaf and Hard of Hearing

Tests of Cognitive abilities:

KBIT-2	Kaufman Brief Intelligence Test (2nd ed.) Matrices.

Tests of Executive Functioning:

WCST	Wisconsin Card Sorting Test
TOH	Towers of Hanoi
TOL	Tower of London
BMVT	Brief Visuospatial Memory Test-Revised
MRT	Mental Rotation Test
	Print Digit Span
	Print Letter Span
	ASL Digit Span
	ASL Letter Span
	Corsi Blocks (manual version)
	Corsi Blocks (computer version)
SVLT	Morere Signed Verbal Learning Test
WJ-III Achievement	Woodcock Johnson Tests of Academic Achievement (3rd ed.)
	WJ-III Reading Fluency
	WJ-III Passage Comprehension
PIAT-R	Peabody Individual Achievement Test-Revised, Reading Comprehension
TOSWRF	Test of Silent Word Reading Fluency
	WJ-III Writing Fluency
	WJ-III Math Fluency
	WJ-III Academic Knowledge
	Phonemic Fluency Measures
	F-A-S
	5-1-U--
	Semantic Fluency Measures

	Animals
	Food
ASL-SRT	American Sign Language Sentence Reproduction Test
	Finger Spelling Test
Koo PDT	Koo Phoneme Detection Test
TSA	Test of Syntactic Ability
LST	Lipreading Screening Test

Part I
Rationale and Participant Characteristics

This part introduces the wide-ranging Psychometric Toolkit project undertaken at the Science of Learning Center in Visual Language and Visual Learning (VL2) at Gallaudet University. This part includes two chapters. Chapter 1 introduces the project and explains the rationale behind the study. The Toolkit Project was designed to investigate a wide range of cognitive, linguistic, and academic factors and their interrelationships and a set of background characteristics in a sample of deaf individuals for whom American Sign Language (ASL) is the primary mode of communication. The constructs investigated and the instruments used to evaluate them are introduced in the first chapter. Chapter 2 expands upon this with details of the experimental procedures used in the study, such as the distribution of tests across multiple assessment sessions and the recruitment of participants and development of the database. Chapter 2 also presents the background characteristics of the participants in the study, including not only the typical demographic data but also data specific to this population, such as factors associated with deafness, parental hearing status, and linguistic background and usage. These two chapters provide the foundation on which the discussions presented in the remaining parts of the book are based.

Chapter 1
The "Toolkit Project": Introduction

Elizabeth Halper, Thomas Allen, and Donna A. Morere

Psychometric testing provides valuable information for a wide variety of purposes: test scores can (a) give clinicians valuable information for diagnosing the strengths and weaknesses in the cognitive functioning of their clients; (b) facilitate an understanding of individual differences in achievement, cognition, and psychological well-being which will have relevance in building effective learning environments designed for individual learners; (c) give researchers behavioral data to test hypotheses that can lead to a better understanding of the underlying cognitive structures of individuals (and of the groups to whom they belong); (d) help to identify environmental precursors to cognitive development; and (e) in aggregate, provide policy makers with information from which to make informed decisions about providing instructional and other human services.

Unfortunately, psychometric testing has played a less than ideal role in serving the needs of deaf individuals. There are three primary reasons for this. First, many tests are written in English and rely on spoken or written prompts or items. The difficulties that many deaf individuals face in mastering the reading skills necessary for the successful administration of these tests have been well documented in the

---

E. Halper
Doctor Halper & Associates, 10560 Main Street, Suite 201,
Fairfax, VA 22030, USA
e-mail: ehalper@drhalper.com

T. Allen (✉)
Science of Learning Center on Visual Language and Visual Learning, Gallaudet University,
SLCC 1223, 800 Florida Avenue, NE, Washington, DC 20002, USA
e-mail: thomas.allen@gallaudet.edu

D.A. Morere
Department of Psychology, Gallaudet University,
800 Florida Avenue, NE, Washington, DC 20002, USA
e-mail: Donna.Morere@Gallaudet.edu

literature (Allen 1986; Allen et al. 1983; Furth 1966; Gallaudet Research Institute 1996; Holt 1993; Holt et al. 1997; Karchmer et al. 1979; Karchmer and Mitchell 2003; Marschark 2001; Traxler 2000). Thus, deaf test-takers may have limited access to or understanding of test content or item response requirements, preventing valid score interpretation. Second, test developers have most likely not considered the specific needs of deaf individuals in developing tools. For example, they may not have adequately evaluated the potential biasing influences of particular item formats or content (those that rely on the experience of sound, for example). This issue is present even on many tests intended for use with deaf individuals, such as "nonverbal" intelligence tests which have multiple items involving sound devices such as musical instruments. Such bias can lead to differential item functioning,[1] a topic that has received considerable attention in the psychometric literature (see Osterlind 1983 for a concise discussion of test item bias). Also, developers may not have adequately included deaf individuals in their standardization samples, limiting the usefulness of "hearing" norms for deaf examinees. Third, given the considerable importance of visual language and the processing of visual information for a population having limited, if any, access to auditory information, it is possible that the underlying cognitive processes manifested for these individuals are quite different than those for hearing individuals, whose realm of perceptual engagement with the world (and, indeed the regions of brain functioning) are influenced by their auditory experience (Hauser and Marschark 2009). Thus, the interpretations applied to test scores of deaf individuals may not be valid.

Despite considerable effort at establishing appropriate, non-biased, testing standards for all individuals, the reliability and validity of many instruments used to measure cognition and learning among deaf individuals remain elusive. The current volume, and the research study that it presents in detail, is hopefully a step in the right direction. At the outset, we note that the "Toolkit Project" presented here does not entail a full-blown norming project for any of the instruments or measurement strategies that are presented and analyzed. The sample of examinees that are the focus of the analyses presented in this book is comprised of a relatively small number of deaf college students. Our purpose in conducting this project was to field test a large number of achievement, cognitive, and language measures *with the same group* of examinees. In so doing, we are able to address a number of critical measurement issues:

First, we are able to address issues of test reliability for a group of tests that are scored with correct and incorrect test items and are therefore conducive to an assessment of their internal consistency. (While this is true for many of the tests that will be discussed here, some rely on clinical judgment using well-established protocols for scoring, and the reliabilities for these will not be presented.) For many of tests

---

[1] Differential item functioning (DIF) occurs when a test item is rendered systematically more difficult (or easy), for a particular group of examinees due to some biasing aspect of its format or content. For example, reading a comprehension passage about the joys of listening to a Bach concerto may render higher levels of difficulty for comprehension items directed to the passage for individuals with no musical experience, yielding DIF.

included in the project, this effort represents the first time that internal consistency data are reported for deaf examinees.

Second, we are able to assess whether the tests perform as anticipated in terms of their "fit" with the levels of abilities of the examinees. Through Rasch analyses (on selected Toolkit measures) and an examination of the distributional characteristics of the derived scores (for all measures), we can report on the viability of these tools (as well as their limitations) when used with deaf examinees.

Third, we can report on a wide array of concurrent and construct validity indicators for the tools that are presented. Given the administration of a large number of instruments to the same group of examinees, we now have extensive correlational data that can be summarized in support of the validity of the tools included in the Toolkit.

Fourth, we can evaluate selected adaptation procedures that we have employed (for example, the translation of some tests into American Sign Language, ASL) to ensure the valid assessment of selected neuropsychological constructs presented in a visual language.

Fifth, we are able to present and analyze data on some new tests that are being developed for deaf examinees that measure ASL language (signs and fingerspelling) and verbal learning and memory skills.

Sixth, we are able to begin to study, through factor analysis of Toolkit measures, the underlying cognitive constructs that may represent the underlying factors involved in cognition among deaf individuals similar to those in the present sample.

Seventh, by combining Toolkit data with retrospective background data on the examinees' early language experiences, we can assess the impacts of individual differences in reported early experiences and family backgrounds on cognitive development and literacy growth.

Brief History of Psychometric Testing of Deaf Individuals

The arrival of intelligence testing in the early 1900s provided an opportunity for researchers to test the intelligence of deaf individuals. The first to do so were Pintner and Patterson (1915, 1916, 1917), who tested deaf children on measures of intelligence. When the results yielded levels of intelligence far below hearing cohorts, Pintner and Patterson recognized that language deprivation was moderating the outcome, and so they developed the Pintner Non-language Test (Pintner and Patterson 1924). Although this test yielded higher IQ on average than the traditional tests of intelligence initially used, results still indicated that deaf individuals were significantly less intelligent than hearing individuals.

Several other studies in the early 1920s revealed similar results using "non-language tests" (Vernon 2005), resulting in the belief that deaf individuals were, on average, 2 years behind their hearing peers in intellectual development. However, in 1928, Drever and Collins administered a performance test to 200 deaf and 200 hearing children, revealing that when the Drever–Collins test was used, deaf children yielded intelligence levels equal to their hearing peers (Drever and Collins 1928). A review of intelligence testing on deaf children from 1930 to 1967 exposed similar discrepancies depending on the testing method used; approximately half the tests revealed IQ levels significantly lower than hearing cohorts, while the other half showed intelligence levels equal or even superior to hearing cohorts (Vernon 2005).

Helmer Myklebust wrote, in *The Psychology of Deafness* (1960), that "when one type of sensation is lacking, it alters the integration and function of all others. Experience is now constituted differently; the world of perception, conception, imagination and thought has an altered foundation. (p. 1)" Myklebust is credited with being one of the first practitioners to claim that deaf children interact and learn in ways that are functionally different from hearing children, and that deafness may impact psychological development (Andrews et al. 2004; Braden 1994; Hauser and Marschark 2009; Marschark and Clark 1993). The implications of this claim are profound when considering the entire psychometric enterprise. To the extent that a deaf individual's cognitive development proceeds along a different trajectory when the perceptual inputs are primarily visual, we must be extremely cautious in using and interpreting test score data that employ standards that convey information derived from norming studies of individuals with a different developmental trajectory, i.e., studies of those who have both auditory and visual inputs. Despite the theoretical advances in recognizing that deaf individuals may not test the same as their hearing peers, researchers are just beginning to explore these differences in depth. Ultimately, a greater understanding of the underlying cognitive domains that contribute to academic growth and success in society for deaf individuals may radically alter assessment practices for deaf individuals. Until we develop this understanding, we must fully articulate both the benefits and limitations of current practice, as we develop new tools. We have both a legal and an ethical mandate to do so, as we discuss in the next section.

Legal Implications and Ethical Standards

In 1975, Public Law 94–142 (PL 94–142, or the Education of All Handicapped Children Act) was passed, for the first time mandating a free and appropriate public education (often referred to by its acronym, FAPE) for all children with disabilities (Smith 2005). In 1990, the Americans with Disabilities Act (ADA) was signed into law. The ADA guarantees equal access to psychological services for all individuals (Raifman and Vernon 1996). Other federal laws, including Section 504 of the Vocational Rehabilitation Act of 1973, Title I of the Elementary and Secondary Education Act (ESEA), and an update of PL94-142, the Individuals with Disabilities Education Act of 2004 (IDEA 2004), require assessments to include all students with disabilities (Case 2005).

Current demographic research estimates that there are between 400,000 and 700,000 deaf or hard of hearing individuals in the United States between the ages of 6 and 19 (National Health and Nutrition Examination Survey (NHANES) in Mitchell 2005) and that 70,000 school aged children are currently receiving special education services due to a hearing loss of educational significance (Implementation of the Individuals with Disabilities Education Act (IDEA) in Mitchell 2005). Because psychological tests often are used to determine educational placement for deaf children, providing "appropriate" public education and "equal" access to psychological services becomes both a practical and ethical concern for practitioners working in these areas. Few measures have been designed for evaluating deaf children, and many are outdated or poorly designed. Thus, based on the author's clinical experience, practitioners evaluating deaf children typically use tests which are designed for hearing children and (if they are aware of the concerns related to appropriateness) include caveats about interpretation in their reports.

In addition to the mandates put forth by the ADA, The American Psychological Association (APA) holds psychologists to ethical standards regarding clinical work, research, and educational conduct. These guidelines state that, "Psychologists use assessment instruments whose validity and reliability have been established for use with members of the population tested. When such validity or reliability has not been established, psychologists describe the strengths and limitations of test results and interpretation." (American Psychological Association 2002, section 9.02 (b)). Without data to support the validity of test results, practitioners walk a fine line between the obligation to provide services to deaf individuals and the limitation of only offering services for which the practitioner has established competence. With extensive training in the assessment of deaf individuals, a practitioner may adapt testing measures to accommodate deaf clients; however, they are then faced with the task of defending both a break from testing protocol and the accuracy of the resulting outcome. Without solid research to support the use of these tests within the deaf population, it is difficult to defend testing results under these conditions.

The APA's ethical standards also state, "Psychologists use assessment methods that are appropriate to an individual's language preference and competence, unless the use of an alternative language is relevant to the assessment issues." (American Psychological Association 2002, section 9.02 (c)). It is difficult to estimate the exact number of deaf individuals in the United States who communicate primarily using ASL; the last study to ask this question, which was conducted in 1972, estimated that there were approximately 375,000 deaf signing Americans at that time (Mitchell et al. 2006). Nonetheless, many deaf individuals prefer to use sign language either exclusively, or in combination with oral and written communication, and assessment measures should, according to the APA, accommodate these individuals. However, because ASL is a visual language, the structure and grammar are communicated in a way that is functionally different from any spoken language. Therefore, adapting assessment measures to accommodate sign language runs the risk of fundamentally changing the measure itself.

In 2005, Pearson Assessments, the publisher of many widely used standardized tests of intelligence and achievement, published a policy report entitled "Accommodations to Improve Instruction and Assessment of Students Who are

Deaf or Hard of Hearing" (Case 2005). Here, they provide a detailed explanation of the difference between *accommodations*, where changes are made in the presentation or response method on a test but the construct of the measure stays the same, and *modifications*, which alter the construct of the test so that it is no longer considered standardized. According to this policy report, the use of sign language (e.g., ASL or manually coded English) and interpreters is considered an accommodation on high stakes educational tests if used *only* while providing the test directions. After reviewing the available research, Pearson deemed that these accommodations are "incidental to the construct intended to be measured by the test" (AERA et al. 1999; Case 2005, p. 101). However, it should be noted that these accommodations are judged by the perceived change in the construct of the test materials themselves, not on the deaf individual's testing outcome. Research investigating the accuracy of the testing *results* for the deaf population, with or without the use of accommodations, is still needed, as is similar to research targeting psychometric testing with deaf populations.

Literacy and Cognitive Development in Deaf Individuals

Assembling a set of tools covering a broad array of cognitive, literacy, and language skills among individuals who are deaf is long overdue. In recent years, there has been an upsurge of research activity aimed at more fully understanding the processes of learning in the visual modality. Indeed, much of this research challenges commonly held assumptions about learning and cognition in deaf individuals. Current theories of literacy development have emphasized the role of speech and audition for extracting meaning from printed text. The role of vision in this learning process has largely been neglected. Yet some individuals who rely primarily on vision (deaf individuals) appear to acquire naturally occurring visual languages (signed language) following typical developmental trajectories (Bonvillian and Folven 1993) and are able to learn how to read and write fluently. The multiple pathways used to derive meaning from visual symbols and print have yet to be fully understood. Hence, a better understanding of visual language and visual learning is essential for enhancing educational, sociocultural, and vocational outcomes. If it is true that deaf individuals acquire literacy skills through unique perceptual and cognitive pathways, then it is important that a set of tools be assembled and studied that help shed light on these pathways and provide a means for diagnosing the underlying cognitive factors of deaf students who may have difficulty reading.

Unlike spoken language, sign language is received primarily through visual pathways and activates both visual and motor regions of the brain, as well as the language centers (Petitto et al. 2000). Research has demonstrated several robust differences between deaf and hearing populations regarding visuospatial abilities and cognition. Notably, both hearing and deaf native signers demonstrate a left hemisphere advantage for processing motion; indicating that the acquisition of ASL alters brain laterality and may impact the functional organization of dorsal stream processing (Bosworth and Dobkins 1999; Neville and Lawson 1987). In addition, research has established a functional reorganization in the dorsal stream for selective visual attention in adult visual learners (Bavelier et al. 2006; Bosworth and Dobkins 2002; Dye et al. 2008). The dorsal stream provides the mechanism by which we recognize object location in space, interpret spatial relationships, and detect and analyze movement. These processes are inherent to the comprehension of ASL, indicating that visual spatial pathways used to process sign language likely play an important role in the acquisition and comprehension of the language itself.

Research investigating literacy in deaf ASL signers has demonstrated that sound-based phonological processing skills, which play a key role in literacy for hearing populations, may not significantly contribute to literacy rates in the deaf population (Mayberry et al. 2011). At the same time, it has also been demonstrated (Petitto et al. 2000) that the regions of the brain that are activated in the processing of sound-based phonology in hearing individuals are activated in the processing of sign-based linguistic phonology in deaf signers. This finding challenges a commonly held assumption that the language centers of the brain are specifically wired to process sounds. As Petitto et al. (2000) note, "Contrary to prevailing wisdom, the planum temporale may not be exclusively dedicated to processing speech sounds, but may be specialized for processing more abstract properties essential to language that can engage multiple modalities (p. 13961)." Thus, the brain is wired for the processing of temporally segmented sublexical units of language, independent of the modality, signed, or spoken. This finding has significant implications for both understanding the development of reading, and, on a more practical level, for interpreting results of psychometric tests.

Currently, researchers are investigating the roles of visual spatial processing, visual attention, and phonological and orthographical processing of written language in the acquisition of English literacy. To date, research has demonstrated that early language acquisition, prior to age 3, best predicts English language literacy (Mayberry and Eichen 1991). Additionally, enrollment in early intervention programs prior to the age of 11 months correlates with better vocabulary and verbal reasoning skills at age 5 (Moeller 2000). While it makes sense that a child would need a primary language in order to learn a secondary written language, evidence indicating that native signers process morphological information about signs differently from children who learn sign language after age 4 (Galvan 1999) suggests underlying cognitive differences in those that acquire sign language early. These cognitive differences appear to play a role in access to literacy development that is not completely explained by adequacy of later language access.

Deaf children are typically "visual learners". This means that unlike their hearing peers, they may not utilize a combined audio-visual mechanism to understand printed language. Harm and Seidenberg (2004) present a conceptual framework that describes reading in terms of a "triangle" of learning mechanisms that include orthography, sound-based phonology, and semantics. Within this connectionist triangle, the visual learner who is not able to associate sound with symbol must use other intermediary cognitive mechanisms to effectively map print onto meaning. Current research is underway by our colleagues at the VL2 Center that is examining computational models of reading among deaf children that build in intermediary mapping mechanisms (such as fingerspelling) that provide for these translations. One of the goals of the Toolkit Project (and of this book) is to provide much needed empirical data for researchers, educators, and clinicians who are struggling to untangle the complex interactions among the visual, cognitive, and linguistic processing factors for deaf individuals.

Constructs and Instruments Selected for the Toolkit: A Preview

To investigate the cognitive structures underlying literacy in the deaf population, specific constructs were selected for investigation. These included: General Cognitive Functioning, Visuospatial Ability, Short-Term/Working Memory and Learning, Academic Achievement, and Expressive and Receptive Linguistic Ability.

General Cognitive Functioning

Tests of General Cognitive Functioning evaluate overall intellectual and executive functioning. The Kaufman Brief Intelligence Test, 2nd Edition (KBIT-2) Matrices subtest (Kaufman and Kaufman 2004) was administered in order to estimate the impact of intelligence on the parameters studied. Executive functioning involves a set of higher order control processes, including planning, organization, maintaining and shifting cognitive sets, attention, and inhibitory control. It has broad impacts on academic and vocational performance as well as daily living (Biederman et al. 2004; Meltzer 2007). Research has supported a bilingual advantage for working memory and some aspects of executive functioning tasks (Feng et al. 2009). In addition, numerous studies have demonstrated that bilingual children show advantages in cognitive flexibility and inhibitory control, two core executive functions (Bialystok 2001; Bialystok and Martin 2004; Bialystok and Shapero 2005; Kovács 2009; Martin-Rhee and Bialystok 2008; Mezzacappa 2004). As executive functioning is a multifactorial process, several measures were employed, including the Wisconsin Card Sorting Test (WCST), the Towers of Hanoi (TOH) and the Tower of London (TOL). All of these measures involved nonverbal stimuli and required nonverbal responses. Thus, the impact of language on task performance was minimized.

The Matrices subtest of the KBIT-2 produces the KBIT-2 Fluid Intelligence Scale (Kaufman and Kaufman 2004). It provides an estimate of general intelligence using visuospatial stimuli, thus avoiding the impact of language on participant's performance. It has been used to estimate overall cognitive functioning in deaf individuals (Schorr et al. 2008).

The WCST (Heaton et al. 1993) is a widely used measure of executive functioning. This test reflects abstract reasoning, as well as the ability to use and sustain a strategy while it is effective, and then alter that strategy in response to changing task demands. The TOH (Simon 1975) and the TOL (Culbertson and Eric 2005) are measures of executive functioning that require abstract reasoning, and that have been found to be significantly affected by the ability to shift cognitive sets (Bull et al. 2004).

Visuospatial Ability

Because sign language is a visual–spatial method of communication, cognitive ability in visual–spatial tasks plays a fundamental role in the comprehension of language. Furthermore, there is evidence to suggest that in deaf signers, visuospatial skills correlate with verbal ability (Halper 2009) in deaf individuals.

To measure ability in this area the Brief Visuospatial Memory Test-Revised (Benedict et al. 1996) and the Mental Rotation Test (MRT; Vandenberg and Kuse 1978) were selected. The BMVT-R is a measure of visuospatial memory. It is affected by visual perception, visual memory (for both content and location), the graphomotor skills required for drawing, and, to a lesser extent, the organization of visuospatial information. The MRT used is a variation of the Vandenberg MRT (Vandenberg and Kuse 1978), one of the most widely used measures of visuospatial ability and higher order abstract reasoning. The MRT reflects spatial organization and the ability to mentally visualize and rotate three-dimensional shapes. Because ASL is a spatial language that incorporates mental rotation and spatial relationships into its linguistic structure, measurement of this ability is critical for understanding the complex role that mental rotation plays in learning and in language for deaf individuals.

Measures of Short-Term/Working Memory and Learning

Short-term memory was investigated in relation to reading and linguistic ability in deaf individuals. Research has shown that short-term recall is affected by the modality of stimulus encoding (visual, auditory, etc.) and that short-term memory is related to overall performance in deaf readers (MacSweeney 1998). Native language and communication mode have also been shown to affect short-term recall of lexical items in deaf samples (Koo et al. 2008). Given this, several measures of short-term memory appropriate for use with deaf individuals were used. These included the forward and backward span versions of a Digit Span task presented in English via print and ASL via video clips. A letter span equivalent was also presented in each modality, as well as a visuospatial span task, the Corsi blocks (Kessels et al. 2010), presented both manually and via computer.

Linguistic immediate recall and working memory are commonly measured using the ability to recall a string of numbers; either in the order given or in reversed order.

Historically the forward span, or longest string of digits recalled in the correct order for the forward recall task, is seven plus or minus two (7±2) for spoken English (Miller 1956). However, research with deaf signers has indicated a span of five, plus or minus one (5±1) to be a more typical span for this population (see Brownfeld 2010 for a review).

Some studies investigating this effect used a series of signed letters instead of numbers, arguing that the visual similarity of the numbers could affect recall (e.g., Bavelier et al. 2008). However, as discussed in Chap. 5, this adjustment did not result in a significant gain in the length of the sequence recalled. Furthermore, previous research suggests that hearing individuals between the ages of 20 and 30 have a letter span consistent with their digit span, with a mean of 6.7 (Lezak et al. 2004) To evaluate this area the print digit and letter and ASL digit and letter span tasks were administered.

Visual (or spatial) Span has been used as a visual equivalent of digit span tests (Lezak et al. 2004). On the Corsi Block task, the individual is asked to repeat a sequence of locations touched variably on an array of blocks, squares on paper, or locations on a computer screen. The current assessment administered identical arrays on blocks and computer. Lezak and colleagues note that previous research indicates a one to two unit lower recall for these types of tasks compared to digit spans; however, clinical experience has suggested that deaf individuals may have spatial spans that are more consistent with their linguistic spans.

The M-SVLT (Morere et al. 1992) is a list learning task similar to the California Verbal Learning Test (Delis et al. 1987). The M-SVLT was developed to evaluate linguistic list memory in deaf users of ASL. The impact of formational characteristics of ASL as well as the phonology and orthography of English were taken into consideration in the development of the sign lists and for the types of potential errors on the recognition trial.

Academic Achievement

Often, due to differences in educational access, deaf individuals fall behind their hearing counterparts on academic tasks, despite comparable intellectual abilities. Measures of achievement evaluate how well an individual can learn in educational settings. In other words, unlike intellectual tests that measure one's capacity to learn both incidentally and through instruction, achievement tests look specifically at how well one is able to retain and apply information has been taught. As reading is a critical area of functioning and scores can vary depending on the type of reading task administered, multiple measures of reading were used.

To investigate the performance of deaf individuals compared to normative standards, a range of achievement measures were selected. These included a variety of subtests from the Woodcock Johnson Test of Academic Achievement, 3rd ed. (WJ-III; Woodcock et al. 2001), the Reading Comprehension subtest of the Peabody

Individual Achievement Test-Revised (PIAT-R; Markwardt 1998) and the Test of Silent Word Reading Fluency (TOSWRF; Mather et al. 2004).

The WJ-III tests are a widely used standard measure of academic achievement. This test is constructed such that subtests can be used individually or as a battery. The following subtests were selected: Reading Fluency, Writing Fluency, Academic Knowledge, Passage Completion, and Math Fluency.

Reading assessments include the WJ-III Reading Fluency subtest, which measures basic sentence level reading comprehension performed under time constraints, reflecting adequacy of both cognitive fluency and basic reading skills. WJ-III Passage Comprehension measures reading comprehension at the paragraph level by requiring the participant to produce a specific word to fill in a blank late in the paragraph. The PIAT-R Reading Comprehension is an untimed measure of reading comprehension at the sentence level using a pictorial response; participants are required to indicate their answer by selecting one out of four pictures. This method of response avoids the impact of expressive limitations in English on the participant's ability to demonstrate understanding of print. The TOSWRF evaluates an individual's ability to recognize words quickly and accurately. This test presents a series of words as a string of letters without spaces between words. The participant must identify individual words by drawing lines between the final letter of one word and initial letter of the next word in the sequence.

Collectively, these measures assess the various aspects of literacy that are typically learned through instruction and by reading. In the general hearing population, the ability to differentiate between words, comprehend paragraph content, pick the appropriate response to fill in the blank, and utilize an academic knowledge base all contribute to literacy success.

Other aspects of academic skills measured included math, writing, and general academic knowledge. The WJ-III Writing Fluency measures the ability of the participant to quickly write a series of short, simple sentences, each of which uses a set of three words and describes a drawing. The WJ-III Math Fluency measures the ability of the participant to perform simple calculations quickly and accurately. The WJ-III Academic Knowledge measures knowledge of subject specific information and reflects subject-related vocabulary in addition to general knowledge of the topic. These tasks reflect basic academic skills and knowledge required to function in both academic and nonacademic settings.

Linguistic Ability

Limitations in language functioning affect long-term academic outcomes (Young et al. 2002). For this study, both ASL and English skills were measured in order to investigate the relative impacts of skill levels in the two languages on academic performance. As no standardized measures of ASL skills are currently available, the ASL Sentence Repetition Test (ASL-SRT), a measure of ASL skills currently under development, was adopted for the project. Measures of verbal fluency that included the F-A-S and a sign-based analog developed for this study, the 5–1–U, were used to reflect English and sign-based searches. A measure of fingerspelling reception was used to reflect the ability of the participants to receive English words through the manual alphabet and to use their knowledge of English vocabulary to support such reception. Facility with English phonology, typically considered critical for reading decoding, was measured using the Koo Phoneme Detection Test (PDT). The Test of Syntactic Ability (TSA) was used to estimate basic knowledge of English syntax, while a speechreading test was used to measure the participant's ability to receive spoken English in the absence of sound. While incomplete, information from lipreading provides information about the phonology of the language of print as well as English syntax and vocabulary (Auer and Bernstein 2007; Leybaert 2005).

Although linguistic fluency tasks are also reflective of executive functioning due to the cognitive search strategies required for performance, they were included in the section on linguistic functioning and reflect the expressive language portion of this section. The F-A-S is the most commonly used measure of verbal fluency (Lezak et al. 2004) and was therefore selected for the Toolkit. Additionally, a sign-based analog, the 5–1–U, was developed for this project to reflect sign-based linguistic fluency. This task requires the participant to generate signs that use specific handshapes rather than words beginning with a specific letter, as is the case with F-A-S. The 5–1–U is anticipated to recruit sign-based strategies comparable to those used on the letter-based task. Although the prompt for the F-A-S task is English-based, the participants signed all responses. Implications of this dual-language task are discussed in Chap. 8. Performance on these tasks is measured by the number of words/signs that the participant is able to produce within a 1-min time frame. While affected by vocabulary, performance is also influenced by the cognitive search strategy used and efficacy of word/sign retrieval. Typically, there are two types of verbal fluency tasks; those requiring participants to produce words starting with a specific letter, and those requiring participants to produce words from a specific category. For the current study, the F-A-S/5–1–U measures were used for the letter and sign analogue tasks, while categorical fluency was measured using animal and food categories.

Receptive language was assessed using a wide range of tasks. The primary measure of ASL skills was the VL2 funded experimental measure modeled after the *Speaking Grammar* subtest of the *Test of Adolescent and Adult Language, 3rd ed.* (Hammill et al. 1994); the *American Sign Language—Sentence Reproduction Test* (ASL-SRT; Hauser et al. 2008), which is continuing to undergo refinement. In this test, participants watch video clips of deaf native signers presenting ASL sentences of increasing length and complexity. The participants are required to repeat the sentences exactly as they had been signed and their responses are recorded by a webcam. The responses are then transmitted back to a centralized server where they are scored for accuracy. The original version of the ASL-SRT had 32 items, and the scoring protocol required perfect fidelity to the original in order to register a correct response. This version of the test demonstrated good inter-rater reliability and adequately discriminated native versus nonnative signers. The version of the test used in the current study contained only 20 items, but retained a strict scoring protocol. The test authors are currently evaluating alternative scoring rubrics that are more flexible with respect to syntactic and phonological accuracy and rely more heavily on semantic accuracy.

The fingerspelling test (Morere 2008) presented the participants with fingerspelled words that the participants are asked to either write or fingerspell (in which case the response is recorded for later scoring) verbatim. The test included both real words and pseudo (fake) words. As deaf individuals are exposed to English vocabulary through fingerspelling in addition to print, the accuracy of their reception of such input would be expected to affect their English vocabulary skills. Additionally, the relative performance on real words compared to the pseudo-words may reflect the ability of participants to use vocabulary knowledge to support reception.

The Koo PDT (Koo et al. 2008) reflects the participants' awareness of English sound-based phonology using a print-based format. Phonological awareness is thought to be a key component of reading and writing ability, although its association with reading in the deaf population is controversial. This measure was developed specifically to measure the phonological awareness of deaf individuals.

The TSA (Quigley et al. 1978) evaluates syntactic knowledge of written English. The Screening Test component of the TSA is a 120-question multiple choice test which provides a relatively quick and reliable assessment of a participant's general knowledge of written English syntax and pinpoints overall strengths and weaknesses in individual syntactic structures. The individual structures of syntax include: Negation, Determiners, Question Formation, Nominalization, Verb Processes, Complementation, Pronominalization, Conjunction, and Relativization (Bickley 2010).

The Lipreading Screening Test, a measure of speechreading skills developed by Auer and Bernstein (2007), measures the individual's ability to accurately perceive a spoken sentence based on visual reception, without auditory support. Two scores are generated: the number of words that are correct in each sentence and the number of sentences that are semantically correct (Bickley 2010).

The constructs and the corresponding assessments that make up the battery of tools to be analyzed and described in the remainder of this are listed at the beginning of this volume.

Intended Uses for This Book

To date, there is no single resource providing psychometric data for deaf individuals on a variety of neurocognitive measures. This work is intended as a resource for clinicians, educators, and researchers tasked with assessing deaf and hard of hearing individuals. We have included individuals from a wide range of educational and linguistic backgrounds to provide the community with a greater understanding of the biological, cognitive, linguistic, sociocultural, and pedagogical conditions that influence the acquisition of language and knowledge via visual modes.

Furthermore, since the goal of this publication is to provide background and research based information on language and literacy development in signing deaf individuals, if applied, the knowledge gained from this text may help improve education for deaf students and contribute to the understanding of how learning occurs through the visual pathway for all individuals, deaf and hearing.

The main aim of the book is to provide empirical data concerning learning in signing deaf students. Both psychometric data for a variety of measures and a detailed and statistically sophisticated explanation of the relationships between test measures are provided. The preliminary data presented here represent a collection of new data designed for use with signing deaf individuals. The book is primarily intended for researchers, clinicians, teachers, and other professionals such as psychologists, audiologists and linguists working in the field of deafness and deaf education. The information herein is intended to help clinicians working with deaf and hard of hearing clients with their interpretive process. Educated parents might want to use this book as a reference while navigating the educational system and educational testing that will pave the way for where and how their child is educated. Finally, the book can become a valuable resource for students in psychology, education, deaf studies, and pedagogy, both in the US and abroad.

References

Allen, T. E. (1986). Patterns of academic achievement among hearing impaired students: 1974 and 1983. In A. N. Schildroth & M. A. Karchmer (Eds.), *Deaf children in America* (pp. 161–206). San Diego, CA: College Hill Press.

Allen, T. E., White, C. S., & Karchmer, M. A. (1983). Issues in the development of a special edition for hearing impaired students of the seventh edition of the Stanford Achievement Test. *American Annals of the Deaf, 128*(1), 34–39.

American Educational Research Association (AERA), American Psychological Association (APA), & National Council on Measurement in Education (NCME). (1999). *Standards for educational and psychological testing*. Washington, DC: AERA, APA, NCME.

American Psychological Association. (2002). Ethical principles of psychologists and code of conduct. *American Psychologist, 57*, 1060–1073.

Andrews, J. F., Leigh, I. W., & Weiner, M. T. (2004). *Deaf people: Evolving perspectives from psychology, education, and sociology*. Boston, MA: Pearson Education, Inc.

Auer, E. T., & Bernstein, L. E. (2007). Enhanced visual speech perception in individuals with early-onset hearing impairment. *Journal of Speech, Language, and Hearing Research, 50*(5), 1157–1165.

Bavelier, D., Dye, M. W., & Hauser, P. C. (2006). Do deaf individuals see better? *Trends in Cognitive Science, 10*(11), 512–518.

Bavelier, D., Newport, E. L., Hall, M. L., Supalla, T., & Boutla, M. (2008). Ordered short-term memory differs in signers and speakers: Implications for models of short-term memory. *Cognition, 10*, 433–459.

Benedict, R., Schretlen, D., Groninger, L., Dobraski, M., & Shpritz, B. (1996). Revision of the Brief Visuospatial Memory Test of normal performance, reliability, and validity. *Psychological Assessment, 8*(2), 145–153.

Bialystok, E. (2001). *Bilingualism in development: Language, literacy, and cognition*. New York: Cambridge University Press.

Bialystok, E., & Martin, M. (2004). Attention and inhibition in bilingual children: Evidence from the dimensional change card sort task. *Developmental Science, 7*, 325–339.
Bialystok, E., & Shapero, D. (2005). Ambiguous benefits: The effect of bilingualism on reversing ambiguous figures. *Developmental Science, 8*, 595–604.
Bickley, C. (2010). *Visual language and visual learning*. Washington, DC: Science of Learning Center.
Biederman, J., Monuteaux, M. C., Doyle, A. E., Seidman, L. J., Wilens, T. E., Ferrero, F., et al. (2004). Impact of executive function deficits and attention-deficit/hyperactivity disorder (ADHD) on academic outcomes in children. *Journal of Consulting and Clinical Psychology, 72*(5), 757–766.
Bonvillian, J. D., & Folven, R. J. (1993). Sign language acquisition: Developmental aspects. In M. Marschark & M. D. Clark (Eds.), *Psychological perspectives on deafness* (pp. 229–265). Hillsdale, NJ: Lawrence Erlbaum Associates.
Bosworth, R. G., & Dobkins, K. R. (1999). Left-hemisphere dominance for motion processing in deaf signers. *Psychological Science, 10*(3), 256–262.
Bosworth, R. G., & Dobkins, K. R. (2002). The effects of spatial attention on motion processing in deaf signers, hearing signers, and hearing nonsigners. *Brain and Cognition, 49*(1), 152–169.
Braden, J. P. (1994). *Deafness, deprivation, and IQ*. New York, NY: Plenum.
Brownfeld, A. (2010). *Memory spans in the visual modality: A comparison between American Sign Language and print in deaf signers*. USA: Gallaudet University.
Bull, R., Espy, K. A., & Senn, T. E. (2004). A comparison of performance on the Towers of London and Hanoi in young children. *Journal of Child Psychology and Psychiatry, 45*(4), 743–754.
Case, B. (2005). *Accommodations to improve instruction and assessment of students who are deaf or hard of hearing*. Boston: Pearson Education.
Culbertson, W. Z., & Eric, A. (2005). *Tower of London—Drexal University* (2nd ed.). North Tonawanda, NY: Multi-Health Systems, Inc.
Delis, D. C., Kramer, J. H., Kaplan, E., & Ober, B. A. (1987). *The California verbal learning test*. San Antonio, TX: Psychological Corporation.
Drever, J., & Collins, M. (1928). *Performance tests of intelligence*. Edinburgh: Oliver & Boyd.
Dye, M. W. G., Hauser, P. C., & Bavelier, D. (2008). Visual attention in deaf children and adults: Implications for learning environments. In M. Marschark & P. C. Hauser (Eds.), *Deaf cognition: Foundations and outcomes* (pp. 250–263). New York, NY: Oxford University Press.
Feng, X., Bialystok, E., & Diamond, A. (2009). *Do bilingual children show an advantage in working memory?* China, Canada, Toronto, Canada: Nanjing University, York University, University of British Columbia, Canada.
Furth, H. H. (1966). A comparison of reading test norms of deaf and hearing children. *American Annals of the Deaf, 111*(2), 461–462.
Gallaudet Research Institute. (1996). *Stanford Achievement Test, 9th Edition, Form S: Norms booklet for deaf and hard of hearing students*. Washington, DC: Gallaudet University, Gallaudet Research Institute.
Galvan, D. (1999). Differences in the use of American Sign Language morphology by deaf children: Implications for parents and teachers. *American Annals of the Deaf, 144*, 320–324.
Halper, E. (2009). *The nature of relationships between mental rotation, Math and English in deaf signers*. Unpublished dissertation, Gallaudet University, Washington, DC.
Hammill, D., Brown, V., Larsen, S., & Wiederholt, J. L. (1994). *Test of adolescent and adult language* (3rd ed.). Austin, TX: PRO-ED, Inc.
Harm, M. W., & Seidenberg, M. S. (2004). Computing the meanings of words in reading: Cooperative division of labor between visual and phonological processes. *Psychological Review, 111*, 662–720.
Hauser, P., & Marschark, M. (2009). What we know and what we don't know about cognition and deaf learners. In M. Marschark & P. C. Hauser (Eds.), *Deaf cognition: Foundations and outcomes* (pp. 439–457). New York, NY: Oxford University Press.
Hauser, P. C., Paludnevičienė, R., Supalla, T., & Bavelier, D. (2008). American sign language-sentence reproduction test: Development and implications. In R. M. de Quadros (Ed.), *Sign*

languages: Spinning and unraveling the past, present and future (pp. 160–172). Petrópolis, Brazil: Editora Arara Azul.

Heaton, R. K., Chelune, G. J., Talley, J. L., Kay, G. G., & Curtiss, G. (1993). *Wisconsin card sorting test manual: Revised and expanded*. Odessa, FL: Psychological Assessment Resources.

Holt, J. (1993). Stanford Achievement Test, 8th edition: Reading comprehension subgroup results. *American Annals of the Deaf, 143*(2), 172–175.

Holt, J., Traxler, C. B., & Allen, T.E. (1997). *Interpreting the scores: A user's guide to the 9th Edition Stanford Achievement Test for educators of deaf and hard-of-hearing students* (Technical Report 97-1). Washington, DC: Gallaudet University, Gallaudet Research Institute.

Karchmer, M. A., Milone, M. N., & Wolk, S. (1979). Educational significance of hearing loss at three levels of severity. *American Annals of the Deaf, 124*(2), 97–109.

Karchmer, M., & Mitchell, R. (2003). Demographic and achievement characteristics of deaf and hard of hearing students. In M. Marschark & P. Spencer (Eds.), *Oxford handbook of deaf studies, language and education* (pp. 21–37). New York: Oxford University Press.

Kaufman, A. S., & Kaufman, N. L. (2004). *Kaufman brief intelligence test* (2nd ed.). Bloomington, MN: Pearson, Inc.

Kessels, R., van Zandvort, M., Postma, A., Kapelle, L. & de Haan, E. (2010). The Corsi Block-Tapping Task: standardization and normative data. *Applied Neuropsychology 7*(4), 252–258.

Koo, D. C., Kelly, L., LaSasso, C., & Eden, G. (2008). Phonological awareness and short-term memory in hearing and deaf individuals of different communication backgrounds. *Learning, Skill, Acquisition, Reading, and Dyslexia, 1145*, 83–99.

Kovács, A. (2009). Early bilingualism enhances mechanisms of false-belief reasoning. *Developmental Science, 12*, 48–54.

Leybaert, J. (2005). Learning to read with a hearing impairment. In C. H. M. J. Snowling (Ed.), *The science of reading: A handbook* (pp. 379–396). Malden, MA: Blackwell.

Lezak, M. D., Howieson, D. B., & Loring, D. W. (2004). *Handbook of normative data for neuropsychological assessment* (2nd ed.). New York: Oxford University Press.

MacSweeney, M. (1998). *Short-term memory processes and reading by deaf children*. Paper presented at the ACFOS II.

Markwardt, F. C. (1998). *Peabody individual achievement test-revised normative update*. Minneapolis, MN: Pearson.

Marschark, M. (2001). *Language development in children who are deaf: A research synthesis*. Alexandria, VA: National Association of State Directors of Special Education. ERIC Document Reproduction Service No. ED455620.

Marschark, M., & Clark, M. (1993). *Psychological perspectives on deafness*. Hillsdale, NJ: Erlbaum.

Martin-Rhee, M. M., & Bialystok, E. (2008). The development of two types of inhibitory control in monolingual and bilingual children. *Bilingualism: Language and Cognition, 11*, 81–93.

Mather, N., Hammill, D., Allen, E. A., & Roberts, R. (2004). *TOSWRF examiner's manual*. Austin, TX: Pro-Ed.

Mayberry, R. I., & Eichen, E. B. (1991). The long-last advantage of learning sign language in childhood: Another look at the critical period for language. *Journal of Memory and Language, 30*, 486–512.

Mayberry, R. I., Giudice, A., & Lieberman, A. M. (2011). Reading achievement in relation to phonological coding and awareness in deaf readers: A meta-analysis. *Journal of Deaf Studies and Deaf Education, 16*(2), 164–188.

Meltzer, L. (Ed.). (2007). *Executive function in education: From theory to practice*. New York: Guilford.

Mezzacappa, E. (2004). Alerting, orienting, and executive attention: Developmental properties and sociodemographic correlates in an epidemiological sample of young, urban children. *Child Development, 75*, 1373–1386.

Miller, G. A. (1956). The magical number seven, plus or minus two: Some limits to our capacity for processing information. *Psychological Review, 63*, 81–97.

Mitchell, R. (2005). Can you tell me how many deaf people there are in the United States? Retrieved September 23, 2011, from Gallaudet Research Institute: http://research.gallaudet.edu/Demographics/deaf-US.php.

Mitchell, R., Young, T., Bellamie, B., & Karchmer, M. (2006). How many people use ASL in the United States? Why estimates need updating. *Sign Language Studies, 6*(3), 306–335.

Moeller, M. P. (2000). Early intervention and language development in children who are deaf and hard of hearing. *Pediatrics, 106*(3), 43.

Morere, D. (2008). *The fingerspelling test.* Washington, DC: Science of Learning Institute Visual Language and Visual Learning.

Morere, D. A., Fruge', J. G., & Rehkemper, G. M. (1992, August). *Signed Verbal Learning Test: Assessing verbal memory of deaf signers.* Poster presented at the 100th Annual Convention of the American Psychological Association, Washington, DC.

Myklebust, H. E. (1960). *The psychology of deafness.* New York: Grune and Stratton.

Neville, H. J., & Lawson, D. (1987). Attention to central and peripheral visual space in a movement detection task: An event-related potential and behavioral study. II. Congenitally deaf adults. *Brain Research, 405,* 268–283.

Osterlind, S. J. (1983). *Test item bias* (Quantitative applications in the social sciences). Beverly Hills, CA: Sage.

Petitto, L. A., Zatorre, R., Gauna, K., Nikelski, E. J., Dostie, D., & Evans, A. (2000). Speech-like cerebral activity in profoundly deaf people while processing signed languages: Implications for the neural basis of human language. *Proceedings of the National Academy of Sciences, 97*(25), 13961–13966.

Pintner, R., & Patterson, D. G. (1915). The Binet Scale and the deaf child. *Journal of Educational Psychology, 6,* 201–210.

Pintner, R., & Patterson, D. G. (1916). A measurement of the language of deaf children. *Psychological Review, 23,* 413–436.

Pintner, R., & Patterson, D. G. (1917). Psychological tests for the deaf children. *Volta Review, 19,* 661–667.

Pintner, R., & Patterson, D. G. (1924). Results obtained with the non-language group tests. *Journal of Educational Psychology, 15,* 473–483.

Quigley, S., Steinkamp, M., & Jones, B. (1978). The assessment and development of language in hearing impairment individuals. *Journal of the Academy of Rehabilitative Audiology, 11*(1), 24–41.

Raifman, L. J., & Vernon, M. (1996). Important implications for psychologists of the Americans with disabilities act: A case in point, the patient who is deaf. *Professional Psychology: Research and Practice, 27*(4), 372–377.

Schorr, E. A., Roth, F. P., & Fox, N. A. (2008). A comparison of the speech and language skills of children with cochlear implants and children with normal hearing. *Communication Disorders Quarterly, 29*(4), 195–210.

Simon, H. A. (1975). The functional equivalence of problem solving skills. *Cognitive Psychology, 7,* 268–288.

Smith, T. E. C. (2005). IDEA 2004: Another round in the reauthorization process. *Remedial and Special Education, 26*(6), 314–319.

Traxler, C. B. (2000). The Stanford Achievement Test, 9th edition: National norming and performance standards for deaf and hard of hearing students. *Journal of Deaf Studies and Deaf Education, 5*(4), 337–348.

Vandenberg, S. G., & Kuse, A. R. (1978). Mental rotations, a group test of three-dimensional spatial visualization. *Perceptual and Motor Skills, 47,* 599–601.

Vernon, M. (2005). Fifty years of research on the intelligence of deaf and hard-of-hearing children: A review of the literature and discussion of implications. *Journal of Deaf Studies and Deaf Education, 10*(3), 225–231.

Woodcock, R. W., McGrew, K. S., & Mather, N. (2001). *Woodcock-Johnson III tests of achievement.* Itasca, IL: Riverside Publishing.

Young, A. R., Beitchman, J. H., Johnson, C., Douglas, L., Atkinson, L., Escobar, M., et al. (2002). Young adult academic outcomes in a longitudinal sample of early identified language impaired and control children. *Journal of Child Psychology and Psychiatry, 43*(5), 635–645.

Chapter 2
The VL2 Toolkit Psychometric Study: Summary of Procedures and Description of Sample Characteristics

Thomas Allen and Donna A. Morere

The Toolkit Psychometric Study required extensive planning, discussion, and design work prior to testing, carried out by an interdisciplinary team of researchers affiliated with the Science of Learning Center on Visual Language and Visual Learning (VL2) at Gallaudet University, funded by the National Science Foundation (Cooperative Agreement #SBE0541953). As noted in Chapter 1, our goal was to field test a battery of instruments with a sample of deaf individuals from a variety of backgrounds. In this chapter, we will briefly outline our procedures and present a description of the Toolkit sample, using information from a web-based Background Questionnaire administered to all participants. In the following sections, we describe: protocol development and design, sample recruitment, scoring procedures and data base development, and sample background characteristics.

Protocol Development and Design

Given the large number of tests selected for the Toolkit, considerable attention was given to assembling protocols and organizing the testing for study participants. The Toolkit was made up of three categories of tests: (1) those published tests that were *adopted* for our use, requiring the purchasing and organizing of published protocols; (2) those that were *adapted* from published tests, requiring the preparation of special materials, such as video-taped ASL presentation of test items, and, in some

---

T. Allen (✉)
Science of Learning Center on Visual Language and Visual Learning, Gallaudet University,
SLCC 1223, 800 Florida Avenue, NE, Washington, DC 20002, USA
e-mail: thomas.allen@gallaudet.edu

D.A. Morere
Department of Psychology, Gallaudet University,
800 Florida Avenue, NE, Washington, DC 20002, USA
e-mail: Donna.Morere@Gallaudet.edu

cases, procedures for videotaping participant responses to test items; and (3) those that were developed (or were under development) for the current effort. A team of researchers worked on test selection, test procedures, protocol development, order of test administration, and the scheduling of testing.

Once the final set of tests were selected, and the protocols assembled, we estimated that the total testing time for each participant would be approximately 8–9 h. Thus, we decided to divide the testing into three testing sessions per participant. The battery was first divided into two sets of tests: those that focused on audiology, lip reading, and syntactical knowledge, and those that focused on literacy, sign comprehension, and cognition. This division placed roughly one-third of the total assessment time in the former category and two-thirds in the latter. The tests in this latter category were further divided into two sets of tests. Although the assignment of tests to grouping was largely random, care was taken to split tests of similar constructs and methods (for example the ASL and print digit span tests) into different groupings so that they would be administered to the participants on separate days. Furthermore, for each grouping, two randomized orderings of the tests were created, with the additional constraint that tests of memory (for example, the Brief Visuospatial Memory Test and the Morere Signed Verbal Learning Test) required elapsed time between the stimulus training and the recall and recognition assessments. Finally, with two groupings of tests and two randomized orders within each grouping, the orderings were further counterbalanced to ensure that test order would not systematically affect results. A counterbalancing schedule was prepared, and, as participants arrived for testing, they were assigned to the next test ordering on the schedule. The counterbalancing design is presented in Fig. 2.1.

All neuropsychological, literacy, and ASL testing were carried out by members of an assessment team comprised of clinical psychology Ph.D. students who had completed coursework in assessment and had received training in assessment procedures. Dr. Donna Morere, Professor of Psychology at Gallaudet University and a licensed Psychologist specializing in conducting neuropsychological assessments with deaf children (and the first author of this volume), trained and supervised the assessment team. Dr. Morere met regularly with the assessment team, observed the assessment sessions, and maintained the assessment quality throughout the project. The audiological, syntactical knowledge, and lipreading assessments were carried out by Au.D. and MS students at Gallaudet University under the supervision of Gallaudet's Hearing and Speech Center and were coordinated by Drs. Corine Bickley and Mary-June Moseley, Professors in Gallaudet's Department of Hearing, Speech, and Language Sciences (and coauthors of Chap. 12 in this volume).

Sample Recruitment

Study participants were recruited from the student body of Gallaudet University. Most of the participants were identified through an online volunteer participant pool that is maintained by the VL2 Center. These volunteers are solicited through a

PSYCHOMETRIC STUDY		ORDER OF ADMINISTRATION	
Session Aa	Time	**Session Ba**	Time
K-BIT 2	20	Corsi Blocks- Computer	5
BVMT-R	5	Digit Span (Fwd & Bwd)- Computer	10
Fingerspelling Test	30	Morere's SVLT	20
BVMTR- Recall, Recognition	5	WCST- 64	20
Letter Span (Fwd & Bwd)	10	Morere's SVLT- Recall	5
BREAK	10	Tower of Hanoi	10
Mental Rotation Task	20	BREAK	10
WJ-PC	10	FAS-ASL	5
Digit Span (Fwd & Bwd)	10	Academic Knowledge	15
Tower of London	10	ASL-SRT	15
Corsi Blocks- Manual	5	Letter Span (Fwd & Bwd)- Computer	10
FAS- English	5	Koo Test	3
Math Fluency	3	PIAT-R	20
TOSWRF	5		
Session Ab	Time	**Session Bb**	Time
TOSWRF	5	Academic Knowledge	15
Corsi Blocks- Manual	5	FAS-ASL	5
Letter Span (Fwd & Bwd)	10	ASL-SRT	15
FAS- English	5	PIAT-R	20
Tower of London	10	Koo Test	3
Math Fluency	3	BREAK	10
WJ-PC	10	Corsi Blocks- Computer	5
Mental Rotation	20	Morere's SVLT	20
BREAK	10	Letter Span (Fwd & Bwd)- Computer	10
K-BIT 2	20	Tower of Hanoi	10
BVMT-R	5	Morere's SVLT- Recall	5
Fingerspelling Test	30	Digit Span (Fwd & Bwd)- Computer	10
BVMTR- Recall, Recognition	5	WCST- 64	20
Digit Span (Fwd & Bwd)	10		
Counterbalance order:	Aa-Ba; Aa-Bb; Ba-Aa; Ba-Ab		
	Ba-Ab; Ba-Aa; Aa-Bb; Aa-Ba		

Fig. 2.1 Toolkit project counterbalancing design

first-year experience program at the University, through which science educators from VL2 present an introduction to research methods and to the work of the VL2 Center. At the end of the introduction, the students are asked if they would like to sign up for possible participation in a variety of Center research projects. The sample was supplemented by recruiting additional participants on campus through word-of-mouth, flyers, and notices in the daily campus online digest distributed via email to all campus community members. Participants were paid $45 for each of the three testing sessions.

Scoring Procedures and Database Development

For the published tests with norms, scoring followed the strict scoring protocols provided by the test publishers. For the adapted and newly developed tests, we employed raw scores. Each participant was assigned a unique ID number, which was transcribed onto each protocol. To protect confidentiality, student names were never written onto the protocols themselves. Members of the assessment team were responsible for scoring the protocols. Throughout the process, the scoring proceeded under close supervision of the project's assessment director, Dr. Morere. Since some of the scoring required clinical judgments, the assessment team brought all questions to its weekly meetings for discussion and resolution.

To facilitate the merging of test scores into a database for analysis, a score sheet was developed containing all score elements (included as an Appendix). Scoring was transcribed from the testing protocols to the scoring sheet and double-checked for accuracy and completeness. An online version of the scoring sheet was created for entering score data into a Microsoft Access database. This data entry program also contained data entry routines for entering individual item data for Toolkit assessments with test items that could be scored as right or wrong. All data were double entered for verification. When the data entry was complete, the database was converted to an SPSS system file and merged with data from the Background Questionnaire.

Sample Characteristics: The Background Questionnaire

The VL2 Center employs a standard Background Questionnaire in a number of its studies in order to understand the differences and similarities in characteristics of study participants, using a common set of questions. Given the diversity of the population of deaf individuals in the Unites States, as well as their low prevalence, and the relatively small sample sizes used in many studies of deaf individuals, it is critical that all empirical investigations of this population report on the characteristics of the samples studied. The VL2 Background Questionnaire resides online and is therefore available to researchers throughout the Center for use in their studies.

The Background Questionnaire includes questions in six sections: (1) demographics; (2) deafness and language/assistive device usage; (3) parents and family members; (4) language history; (5) educational history; and (6) medical information. Below, we present distributional statistics for selected variables within the first five sections. Responses to the questions in Sect. 6 will not be discussed in this chapter.

Section 1: Demographics

N. There were a total of 90 participants in the Toolkit Project. As noted, testing was scheduled in three 2.5–3 h-long sessions. One session took place in the Hearing and

Table 2.1 Mother and father's race or ethnic heritage (multiple responses allowed)

	Frequency (percent)	
	Mother	Father
African-American	23 (29.1%)	23 (29.1%)
Asian American	5 (6.3%)	3 (3.8%)
European American	40 (50.6%)	40 (50.6%)
Latino/Hispanic	9 (11.4%)	10 (12.7%)
Native American	6 (7.6%)	6 (7.6%)
Other	2 (2.5%)	0 (0.0%)

Speech Center at Gallaudet (for audiological testing, the Test of Syntactic Abilities, and the Lipreading Screening Test). The other two sessions took place in the VL2 Assessment Lab. In all, only 31 (34.4%) participants attended all three sessions; 16 (17.8%) participants attended ONLY one or both of the neuropsychological testing sessions in the VL2 Assessment Lab; 43 (47.8%) attended ONLY the audiological testing in the Hearing and Speech Center. Thus, we have fairly complete neuropsychological data on a total of 47 participants, and fairly complete audiological, syntax, and lipreading data on 74 participants. These distributions unfortunately limit our ability to perform analyses that combine scores from across all sessions. We were unable to randomly assign the full battery of Toolkit tests across all three sessions because the audiology and lipreading testing required special equipment and expertise that resides in the Hearing, Speech, and Language Department at Gallaudet. Because the testing was long, and spread out over several days, some participants decided not to attend all of their scheduled testing appointments.

Age. As noted, the sample for this was comprised of students at Gallaudet University at both the graduate and undergraduate levels. The Mean Age for study participants was 25.1 (SD=6.51). The distribution was positively skewed, with 20% of the sample over age 30 and 40% of the sample between the ages of 19 and 21.

Sex. The sample was made up of 31.8% males ($N=28$) and 68.2% females ($N=60$).

Parent's race or ethnic heritage (Table 2.1). Approximately half of the participants reported that their mother's and their father's racial heritage was European American. These figures are similar to national figures derived from a large national sample of 37,352 deaf and hard of hearing school-aged children in the United States from the 2006–2007 Annual Survey of Deaf and Hard of Hearing Children and Youth (Gallaudet Research Institute 2007), in which 47.4% were reported in the "White, non-Hispanic" category. However, the distributions of participants in the current study from non-European American heritages differed markedly from Annual Survey figures. In the current data, 29.1% of the participants reported that they were from African-American families (compared to the national figures showing 15.1% from African-American households). In the current study, 11.4% reported their mothers were of Latino/Hispanic descent; this compares to 28.3% from the Annual Survey. These differences are reflective of student demographics at Gallaudet University.

Table 2.2 The age at which the participant first became deaf or hard of hearing

Born deaf or hard of hearing	57 (67.1%)
Not born deaf, but became deaf or hard of hearing younger than age 2	7 (8.2%)
Became deaf or hard of hearing at age 2 or older	21 (24.7%)
Total	85 (100.00%)

Section 2: Deafness and Language/Assistive Device Usage

Participants' pure tone average (PTA) hearing thresholds in their better ear. Full audiograms were available for 54 participants. Among this group, five participants (9.3%) showed better ear PTA's in the Less Than Severe category (PTA<71 dBs). Ten participants (18.5%) were in the Severe category (71–89 dB). The remaining 39 participants (72.2%) were in the Profound category (90 dB or greater). The Background Questionnaire included a question asking participants to self-report their level of hearing loss. For the 36 participants who did not have audiological results, 7 self-rated their hearing loss in the Less Than Severe category; 13 self-rated their hearing loss in the Severe category; 9 self-rated their hearing loss in the Profound category; and 7 did not respond to the question. Using the self-ratings as proxies for the actual audiogram results and aggregating the frequencies yields: 12 participants Less Than Severe (14.5%); 23 participants Severe (27.7%); and 48 participants Profound (57.8%). As a point of comparison, the 2006–2007 Annual Survey reports the following distribution of hearing threshold categories: Less Than Severe (58%); Severe (14.0%); and Profound (28%). The comparison demonstrates the fact that Gallaudet serves students who are predominantly in the Severe to Profound categories, as defined by their audiological results.

Participants' age at onset of deafness (Table 2.2). Greater than two-thirds (67.1%) of the participants in the Toolkit sample reported that they had been born deaf or hard of hearing. Another 8.2% reported that they had become deaf or hard of hearing before their second birthday. In the national figures from the 2006–2007 Annual Survey, these numbers are 40.9% and 15.5%, respectively. Thus, the Toolkit sample was comprised of individuals with much earlier ages of onset than the national sample. This can be attributed to the fact that Gallaudet University more often attracts deaf students with longer histories of deafness than those with later onsets. This is a critical aspect of the Toolkit sample, as deaf individuals who are either born deaf or who become deaf in their first 2 years of life will have little or no exposure to spoken language in their earliest months, during a sensitive developmental period for language acquisition.

Participants' language preference (Table 2.3). Over 90% of the participants reported a preference for ASL, and close to 14% reported a preference for English with Sign Support. (Multiple responses were allowed for this variable, so participants could select more than one preference.) These results are consistent with Gallaudet's mission as a bilingual ASL-English University. The Annual Survey reports on the primary mode (not language) of communication used in instruction. In the 2006–2007 school year, only 11.2% of deaf and hard of hearing students

Table 2.3 Participants' language preferences

Language preferences	Frequency (%)
ASL	79 (90.8%)
Spoken English	19 (21.8%)
English with Sign Support	12 (13.8%)
Other	5 (5.7%)
Total Respondents	87

Table 2.4 If participants had ever used a hearing aid and/or cochlear implant

	Hearing aid	Cochlear implant
Yes	80 (93.0%)	4 (4.7%)
No	6 (7.0%)	82 (95.3%)
Total	86 (100.00%)	86 (100.00%)

Table 2.5 If participants currently use a hearing aid or cochlear implant

	Hearing aid	Cochlear implant
Yes, regularly	22 (27.5%)	3 (75.0%)
Yes, but only occasionally	13 (16.2)	
No	45 (56.2%)	1 (25.0%)
Total	80 (100.00%)	4 (100.00%)

nationwide were reported in "Sign Only" classrooms; 35.5% were reported from "Sign with Speech"; and 51.6% were reported in "Speech Only" classrooms. Thus, the Toolkit sample contained a far higher proportion of individuals with a preference for using ASL (and a high percentage of Gallaudet's classes are "sign only"). Again, the comparisons of our participant characteristics with national student data demonstrate Gallaudet University's mission and its student demographics.

Hearing aid and cochlear implant usage (Tables 2.4 and 2.5). A large majority of Toolkit participants (93.0%) reported that they had, at some point in their lives, used a hearing aid. However, among those that had previously used a hearing aid, over half (56.2%) reported that they were no longer using one, and only 27.5% reported regular hearing aid use. These 22 individuals (noted in Table 2.4) who reported regular hearing aid use comprised only 25.5% of the full participant sample. The modal reasons given for why participants had stopped using their hearing aids were: no perceived benefit ($N=18$); pain, headache, or discomfort ($N=9$); social factors ($N=7$); too noisy ($N=7$); and lost or broken ($N=6$). The Annual Survey does not report on whether the children reported to the survey had ever used a hearing aid, but it does report whether students are currently using a hearing aid in instruction. In 2006–2007, 58.7% were reported as using a hearing aid in instruction. Thus, Toolkit participants were considerably less likely to be regular current hearing aid users than those from the national Annual Survey data.

Regarding the use of cochlear implants, only four Toolkit participants reported that they had ever used a cochlear implant, and three of these four reported that they

Table 2.6 Participants' reporting of which parents had raised them

Both a mother and father	62 (70.5%)
Only by the mother or a female guardian	23 (26.1%)
Only by the father or a male guardian	1 (1.1%)
Other	2 (2.3)
Total	88 (100.00%)

Table 2.7 Deaf/hearing status of mother and father

	Mother	Father
Deaf	22 (25.6%)	18 (28.1%)
Hard of hearing	3 (3.5%)	5 (7.8%)
Hearing	61 (70.9%)	41 (64.1%)
Total	86 (100.00%)	64 (100.00%)

Both parents hearing: ($N=38$, 60.3%)
Both parents deaf or hard of hearing: ($N=18$, 28.6%)
One parent deaf or hard of hearing: ($N=7$, 11.1%)
(These percentages based on the 63 participants reporting deaf/hearing status for BOTH parents)

were current, regular users of their implant. In the 2006–2007 Annual Survey, 12.6% were reported as having ever had an implant, 92.2% of whom were currently using their implant in instructional settings.

Section 3: Parents and Family Members

Which parents had raised the participants (Table 2.6). Over two-thirds (70.5%) of the participants in the Toolkit project reported that both a mother and a father had raised them, while over a quarter (26.1%) reported being raised by only a mother or a female guardian. While there are no comparable figures from the Annual Survey for deaf and hard of hearing youth nationwide, comparisons to U.S. National Census data reveal that the Toolkit participant sample is highly similar to the US population at large. The US Census reports that, in 1995, 69% of children under age 18 lived with two parents and 27% lived with only one parent (U.S. Department of Commerce 1997). As noted by the Census, being raised by a single mother can be associated with lower socioeconomic status (though only for never-married mothers and not for divorced or widowed mothers).

Parents' deaf/hearing status (Table 2.7). While 70.9% of the participants reported having a hearing mother, and 64.1% reported a hearing father, only 60.3% reported having both a hearing mother and a hearing father. Thus, near 40% of the participants had at least one deaf or hard of hearing parent. It should be noted that only 63 participants reported data on both parents. Quite obviously, this is due to the fact that 23 participants reported being raised by only a mother, as noted in Table 2.6, and is likely that they were unaware of the deaf/hearing status of their fathers. An examination of

2 The VL2 Toolkit Psychometric Study: Summary of Procedures and Description...

Table 2.8 Reported levels of parents' highest educational levels

	Mother	Father
Some high school, but no diploma	9 (11.7%)	9 (15.8%)
High school diploma	25 (32.5%)	23 (40.4%)
Some college, but no BA/BS	15 (19.5%)	9 (15.8%)
BA/BS	15 (19.5%)	11 (19.3)
Some graduate school, but no MA/MS	1 (1.3%)	0 (0.0%)
MA/MS	7 (9.1%)	2 (3.5%)
Some post-masters courses, but no Ph.D.	1 (1.3%)	0 (0.0%)
Doctorate (Ph.D., MD, Ed.D, etc.)	4 (5.2%)	3 (5.3%)
Total	77 (100.0%)	57 (100.0%)

Table 2.9 Reported sign use while participants were growing up

Parents sign use while respondent was growing up	Mother	Father
Yes, well enough to communicate with me fully and effectively	49 (56.3%)	25 (39.1%)
Yes, but only basic signs	18 (20.7%)	17 (26.6%)
No	20 (23.0%)	22 (34.4%)
Total	87 (100.00%)	64 (100.00%)

these 23 participants reporting single mothers had raised them reveals that 17 of them (73.9%) reported that their mothers were hearing.

Comparisons to Annual Survey numbers reveal that the Toolkit participants were more likely to have one or both deaf or hard of hearing parents than those reported in the national data. In the 2006–2007 Annual Survey, 83.4% of the children were reported from families where both parents are hearing, but only 3.8% are reported from families where both parents are deaf or hard of hearing. (The remaining were reported as: one deaf or hard of hearing and one hearing, 4.4%; one deaf or hard of hearing and the other unknown, 1.0%; and one hearing and the other unknown, 7.4%.)

Parents' highest levels of education (Table 2.8). There was wide variability in educational attainment levels reported for the participants' parents. More than 71% of the fathers and more than 63% of the mothers were reported as having achieved only a high school diploma or below (including those with some college, but no college degree). At the same time, 28.1% of the fathers and 36.4% of the mothers had had attained a BA degree or above. These figures compare well to U.S. Census data that reports, for 2010, 70% of the United States population aged 25 or older attaining, at most, a high school diploma, and 30% attaining a college degree.

Parents' knowledge of and use of signs while respondents were growing up (Table 2.9). As noted in the above sections, 85% of the participants had levels of hearing loss in the severe to profound range, 75% reported that they were born deaf or became deaf before the age of 2, and 91% reported ASL as a language preference. Nonetheless, over half of the participants reported that their parents either did not know or use signs with them while they were growing up or that they only used basic signs but were unable to communicate in signs "fully or effectively." We have no national-level comparisons for this finding, but note that these data suggest considerable variation in the early language experiences for study participants. We will return

Table 2.10 Self-reported knowledge of selected languages and modalities

	ASL	Signed English	Spoken English	Lip reading	Cued English
Yes	86 (97.7%)	57 (64.8%)	58 (65.9%)	72 (81.8%)	4 (5.0%)
No	2 (2.3%)	31 (35.2%)	30 (34.1%)	16 (18.2%)	76 (95.0%)
Total	88 (100.00%)	88 (100%)	88 (100%)	88 (100%)	80 (100%)

Table 2.11 Reported sources of acquisition for languages and modalities

	ASL	Signed English	Spoken English	Lip reading	Cued English	Written English
Parents	37 (42.5%)	16 (26.7%)	46 (79.3%)	49 (68.1%)	1 (25.0%)	63 (71.6%)
Siblings	19 (21.8%)	8 (13.3%)	36 (62.1%)	31 (42.1%)	1 (25.0%)	32 (36.4%)
Friends	62 (71.3%)	23 (38.3%)	33 (56.9%)	32 (44.4%)	2 (50.0%)	43 (48.9%)
Teachers	76 (87.4%)	45 (77.0%)	46 (79.3%)	44 (61.1%)	1 (25.0%)	85 (96.6%)
Other	21 (24.1%)	11 (18.3%)	17 (29.3%)	24 (33.3%)	1 (25.0%)	9 (10.2%)
Total	87 (100%)	60 (100%)	58 (100%)	72 (100.0%)	4 (100.0%)	88 (100.0%)

to these differences in the final chapter of this book, where we present an analysis of test performance, and its relationship to reported early communication experience.

Section 4: Current Language Use and Language Histories

Knowledge of languages and modalities (Table 2.10). With the exception of Cued English, Toolkit Study participants rated themselves highly as knowing ASL (97.7%) and English in signed (64.8%), spoken (65.9%), and lipreading (81.8%) modalities. Only four participants rated themselves as having competence in Cued English. We emphasize that these are self-reports provided by the study participants and are not based on objective measures.

Sources of language acquisition (Table 2.11). While 79.3% of the participants reported their parents as a one of the sources of their knowledge of spoken English (among those 58 participants who indicated competence in spoken English), and 71.6% reported their parents as one of the sources of their knowledge of written English, only 42.5% reported that their parents were a source of ASL acquisition. As the data show, friends and teachers were most often reported as the source of ASL acquisition (71.3% and 87.4%, respectively). Teachers were most often reported as one of the sources for signed English acquisition (77% of those 60 participants who reported competence in signed English), spoken English acquisition (79.3% of those 58 participants reporting competence in spoken English), and written English acquisition (96.6% of those 88 participants reporting competence in written English).

Frequency of language use (Table 2.12). Overwhelmingly, Toolkit participants reported either "All the time" or "daily" use of both ASL (96.5%) and written English (97.8%). Interestingly, for those participants reporting competence in signed

Table 2.12 Frequency of use for different languages and modalities

	ASL	Signed English	Spoken English	Lip reading	Cued English	Written English
All the time	67 (77.9%)	5 (8.6%)	18 (31.0%)	18 (25.0%)	0 (0.0%)	57 (64.8%)
Daily	16 (18.6%)	13 (22.4%)	19 (32.8%)	20 (27.8%)	2 (50.0%)	29 (33.0%)
Few times a week	2 (2.3%)	11 (19.0%)	10 (17.2%)	12 (16.7%)	0 (0.0%)	1 (7.1%)
Once a week	0 (0.0%)	0 (0.0%)	1 (1.7%)	4 (5.6%)	1 (25.0%)	0 (0.0%)
Once a month	0 (0.0%)	1 (1.7%)	2 (3.4%)	4 (5.6%)	0 (0.0%)	0 (0.0%)
<Once a month	0 (0.0%)	15 (25.9%)	1 (1.7%)	4 (5.6%)	1 (25.0%)	0 (0.0%)
Special occasions	1 (1.2%)	13 (22.4%)	7 (12.1%)	10 (13.9%)	0 (0.0%)	1 (1.1%)
Total	86 (100.0%)	58 (100.0%)	58 (100.0%)	72 (100.0%)	4 (100.0%)	88 (100.0%)

Table 2.13 When participants began using different languages and modalities

	ASL	Signed English	Spoken English	Lip reading	Cued English	Written English
Before school	34 (39.1%)	17 (30.4%)	35 (60.3%)	22 (31.0%)	0 (0.0%)	32 (36.4%)
Elementary	24 (27.6%)	29 (51.8%)	21 (36.2%)	33 (46.5%)	1 (25.0%)	51 (58.0%)
Middle/Jr. HS	8 (9.2%)	4 (7.1%)	1 (1.7%)	12 (16.9%)	3 (75.0%)	4 (4.5%)
HS	14 (16.1%)	3 (5.4%)	1 (1.7%)	2 (2.8%)	0 (0.0%)	1 (1.1%)
After HS	7 (8.0%)	3 (5.4%)	0 (0.0%)	2 (2.8%)	0 (0.0%)	0 (0.0%)
Total	87 (100%)	56 (100%)	58 (100.0%)	71 (100.0%)	4 (100.0%)	88 (100.0%)

English, spoken English, and lipreading, usage was far less frequent. Only 31% of those reporting competence in signed English reported using it all the time or daily; 63.8% of those reporting competence in spoken English reported all the time or daily use; 52.8% of those reporting competence in lipreading reported all the time or daily use. Thus, in the Toolkit sample, ASL and Written English are the predominant languages and modes of communication, with other modalities of spoken English used considerably less often.

Ages when different languages and modalities were first used (Table 2.13). Even among those participants reporting competence in ASL, only 39.1% reported that they had begun using ASL before starting elementary school. Among those reporting competence in written English, only 36.4% reported that they began using written English before starting school. As noted, these two groups essentially comprise the entire Toolkit sample. Thus, a majority of the participants in the Toolkit sample did not begin using the languages that they report currently using "all the time" or "on a daily basis" until after starting school. Among those 58 participants who self-reported competence in spoken English, 60.3% reported that they began using spoken English before starting school. While this is a higher percentage than that reported for ASL use, it should be kept in mind that the 58 participants in this group comprise 64% of the participant pool. In general, the prevalence of all language use before elementary school is low for participants in the Toolkit sample.

Section 5: School and Instructional Mode of Communication History

Types of schools attended (Table 2.14). Participants exhibited considerable mobility among different educational programming options throughout their schooling. Across the school range from preschool to college, 74.1% reported that they had attended a mainstream program at some point in their educational lives, 55.1% had attended a deaf education classroom in a public school, 28.1% had attended a day school for the deaf, and 59.6% had attended a residential school for the deaf.

Table 2.14 Types of schools participants report attending at different educational levels

	Mainstream	Deaf ed. classroom in public school	Day SFD	Deaf residential school
Preschool	39 (43.8%)	23 (25.8%)	15 (16.9%)	12 (13.5%)
Elementary	45 (50.6%)	34 (38.2%)	14 (15.7%)	24 (27.0%)
Middle/Jr.	46 (51.7%)	22 (24.7%)	10 (11.2%)	34 (38.2%)
HS	44 (49.4%)	17 (19.1%)	8 (9.0%)	49 (55.1%)
College	19 (21.3%)	6 (6.7%)	10 (11.2%)	44 (49.4%)
Total respondents	66 (74.1%)	49 (55.1%)	25 (28.1%)	53 (59.6%)

Note: All percentages are based on the 89 participants who responded to this set of questions

Table 2.15 Languages used in instruction

	ASL	Signed English	Spoken English	Non-English spoken Language	Sign Language Not ASL	Cued speech
Preschool	34 (38.2%)	27 (30.3%)	39 (43.8%)	0 (0.0%)	1 (1.1%)	3 (3.4%)
Elementary	46 (51.7%)	39 (43.8%)	39 (43.8%)	4 (4.5%)	4 (4.5%)	3 (3.4%)
Middle/Jr.	61 (68.5%)	24 (27.0%)	35 (39.3%)	3 (3.4%)	2 (2.2%)	1 (1.1%)
HS	74 (83.1%)	21 (23.6%)	35 (39.3%)	3 (3.4%)	3 (3.4%)	1 (1.1%)
College	81 (91.0%)	15 (16.9%)	30 (33.7%)	2 (2.2%)	3 (3.4%)	1 (1.1%)
Total	84 (94.3%)	52 (58.4%)	45 (50.6%)	6 (6.7%)	7 (7.9)%	4 (4.5%)

Note: All percentages are based on the 89 participants who responded to this set of questions

The sum of these percentages (216.9 cumulative percent points and a total of 193 different school types indicated across the range) suggests that each participant reported, on average, 2.169 different types of schools attended. Throughout the elementary to high school range, the percentage of participants who reported attending mainstream programs remains relatively constant (although this does not necessarily imply that the same participants remained in mainstream programs throughout their schooling). At the same time, the percentages of participants reporting attendance in deaf education programs in the public school and at day schools for deaf decrease systematically from elementary to high school, while the percentages of participants attending residential schools show a systematic increase across these levels. These shifts suggest greater migration among self-contained educational options, resulting in higher percentages of participants moving from day programs to residential schools in the later school years.

Languages of instruction at different educational levels (Table 2.15). Across all educational levels from preschool to college, 94% of participants report the use of ASL at some point in their schooling. The reported instructional use of ASL increased systematically for the participants: 38.2% reported the use of ASL in preschool, 51.7% in elementary, 68.5% in middle school, 83.1% in high school, and 91% in college. The prevalence of reported Signed English and Spoken

English use is lower (58.4% and 50.6% respectively). Across the school levels, the reported use of spoken English stays fairly constant throughout elementary school (43.8%), middle school (39.3%), and high school (39.3%). The use of signed English, however, decreases systematically across the school levels from elementary school (43.8%) to middle school (27.0%), to high school (23.6%), and to college (16.9%).

Summary

In this chapter, we have described the procedures we followed in conducting the Toolkit Project and presented an analysis of the sample characteristics using data from a Background Questionnaire developed for use by a number of different research projects conducted in the VL2 Center. The questionnaire includes questions about demographics, factors related to deafness and the use of languages and assistive technologies, parent and family information, and language and education histories.

When we compare the profiles of the Toolkit participants to those of a large national sample of deaf and hard of hearing children, as reported in the national summary of the 2006–2007 Annual Survey of Deaf and Hard of Hearing Children and Youth (Gallaudet Research Institute 2007), a considerable number of differences can be noted. Our sample contains a higher percentage of individuals with severe to profound levels of hearing loss than those reported to the Annual Survey. Our participants are more likely to come from families who sign. They are more likely to have one or both deaf or hard of hearing parents. They are more likely to have become deaf before the age of 2.

These differences mitigate the broad generalization of our study results to the national population of deaf and hard of hearing students. On the other hand, the greater homogeneity of our participants with respect to these variables serves the purposes of our project quite well. Our intent is to examine a set of literacy, language, and neuropsychological measures for use with individuals who have had little or no exposure to sound and who have relied to a great extent on visual processes and visual languages for learning. It is precisely these individuals for whom current assessment practices are the most risky, and for whom a systematic study of test properties would prove the most beneficial. It is also hoped that an in-depth examination of the correlational patterns and underlying cognitive factors demonstrated in our results will contribute to a greater understanding of the unique cognitive processes of deaf learners. For these varied purposes, we believe the unique nature of the participant sample assembled for this project has particular merit.

Appendix

Page 1 of 2 (revised 11/30) Birthday:			Age:						
Subject ID#: VL2 ID#:				Examiner Name:					
PARTICIPANT SCORING SUMMARY									
Session ☐				Session ☐					
Date of Testing:	Raw	Z/T/SS*	%ile	Code	Date of Testing:		Raw	Z/T/SS*	%ile	Code
VISUOSPATIAL									
BVMT-R Form ☐			>16% =50 T		Mental Rotation Task ☐				
Trial 1									
Trial 2									
Trial 3									
Total Recall									
Delayed Recall									
Discrimination Index									
ACHIEVEMENT		SS / Age Equivalent						SS / G.E.	
PIAT-R Reading Comprehension									
TOSWRF									
WJ-Test of Achievement									
Reading Fluency					Passage Comprehension				
Writing Fluency					Math Fluency				
Academic Knowledge									
GENERAL COG. FUNCTIONING	Raw	Z/T/SS*	%ile	Code			Raw	Z/T/SS*	%ile	Code
WCST - Total Correct					Tower of London				
Total Errors					Total Correct Score				
Perseverative Errors					Total Move Score				
Categories Completed					Timed Violations				
Trials to Complete 1st Cat.									
Failure to Maintain Set					FAS:	Total Score			
Tower of Hanoi						Animals		Food	
Total Score (31-119 moves =1 point)									
Total Moves									
Total Time (min:sec)									
K-BIT 2 - Matrices									
Koo Test: Total Score									
/k/ in C		/k/ in CH							
/s/ in C		/g/ in G							
/j/ in G									

References

Gallaudet Research Institute. (2007, December). *Regional and national summary report of data from the 2006–2007. Annual survey of deaf and hard of hearing children and youth*. Washington, DC: GRI, Gallaudet University.

U.S. Department of Commerce. (1997). *Census brief: Children with single parents—How they fare (Publication CENBR/97-1)*. Washington, DC: U.S. Department of Commerce, Economics and Statistics Administration, Bureau of the Census.

Part II
Cognitive Functioning

Functioning in the environment, be it academic, social, vocational, or adaptive, depends on underlying cognitive processes. The VL2 Toolkit was intended to provide an understanding of the relationships among academic achievement and a range of underlying cognitive processes. Thus, in addition to administering academic achievement measures, data were collected on a range of cognitive functions, including intelligence, executive and visuospatial functioning, and memory and learning. While standard measures were used whenever available, a number of modified measures and tasks developed specifically for the evaluation of signing deaf individuals were also included. The measures of cognitive functioning and the resulting data will be presented in the following chapters. Due to its importance, particularly with this population, language will be addressed in a separate section.

Chapter 3
Measures of General Cognitive Functioning

Donna A. Morere, Evan Goodman, Shilpa Hanumantha, and Thomas Allen

Two areas of overall cognitive functioning were evaluated. First, a nonverbal measure of intellectual functioning was administered to provide an estimate of general cognitive functioning. This can provide a benchmark to which other measures can be compared. The second area evaluated was executive functioning (EF). This area of functioning affects all aspects of the person's life and impacts efficacy of other aspects of cognitive functioning as well as academic outcomes.

Intellectual Functioning

Kaufman Brief Intelligence Test, 2nd Edition

The Matrices subtest of the Kaufman Brief Intelligence Test, 2nd Edition (K-BIT2) (Kaufman and Kaufman 2004) was selected to estimate overall cognitive functioning of the participants. The Matrices subtest produces the Nonverbal Scale of the K-BIT2 which is believed to represent fluid intelligence. The Matrices subtest is normed for individuals aged 4–90, and the Nonverbal Standard Score it produces has a mean of 100 and a standard deviation (SD) of 15, with a minimum score of 40.

D.A. Morere (✉) • E. Goodman
Department of Psychology, Gallaudet University,
800 Florida Avenue, NE, Washington, DC, 20002, USA
e-mail: Donna.Morere@Gallaudet.edu; Evan.Goodman@Gallaudet.edu

S. Hanumantha • T. Allen
Science of Learning Center on Visual Language and Visual Learning,
Gallaudet University, SLCC 1223, 800 Florida Avenue, NE,
Washington, DC 20002, USA
e-mail: shanumantha@hotmail.com; thomas.allen@gallaudet.edu

Table 3.1 Kaufman Brief Intelligence Test 2nd Edition (K-BIT2)—descriptive statistics

Test	Subtest	Range	N	Mean	Standard deviation
K-BIT2	Matrices	85–125	48	104.48	10.96

It provides an estimate of general intelligence using visuospatial stimuli, thus avoiding the impact of language on participant's performance. Both this and the original Matrices subtest from the K-BIT2 have been used in research to estimate overall cognitive functioning in deaf individuals (Emmorey et al. 2011; Emmorey and Petrich 2012; Schorr et al. 2008, 2009), the purpose for which it was used in this study. Performance on the Matrices subtest reflects nonverbal reasoning ability, including the participant's ability to solve new problems, perceive relationships, and complete visual analogies.

For the Matrices subtest, the participant is shown a design with one element missing and must select the picture (from a choice of 5–8) which is the best fit for the missing component. The Matrices subtest includes 46 items and takes approximately 20–25 min to complete. Early items include familiar objects and measure understanding of the logical relations among these objects. The later items are composed of abstract geometric forms, similar to those used on Raven's Progressive Matrices (Raven 1960) measures which have been used to measure cognitive functioning with deaf individuals during the past half century (Bishop 1983; Blennerhassett et al. 1994; Goetzinger and Houchins 1969; Goetzinger et al. 1967). Descriptive data from the current sample are presented in Table 3.1.

The mean score suggests that the performances of the 48 participants who took the K-BIT2 Matrices were consistent with the test norms. The lower end of the test range was one SD below the test mean, while the upper extreme of the participant outcomes was one- and two-thirds of a SD above the test mean. While the participants at the lower end of the range would be expected to have difficulty succeeding in college, the overall data are consistent with the cognitive functioning expected in a college population.

Table 3.2 presents the significant correlations between the K-BIT2 Matrices and the other Toolkit measures. Not surprisingly, Matrices correlated most highly with measures of EF (e.g., Towers of Hanoi and London), which also require the use of nonverbal reasoning.

Rasch Analysis

A Rasch analysis using Winsteps software (Bond and Fox 2007; Linacre 1994a, 2006) was conducted on five of the Toolkit measures: the Kaufman Brief Intelligence Test (K-BIT2), the Mental Rotation Test (MRT), the Peabody Individual Achievement Test Reading Comprehension Test-Revised (PIAT-R), the Woodcock Johnson Passage Comprehension Test, and the Woodcock Johnson Academic Knowledge Test. Here,

Table 3.2 Kaufman Brief Intelligence Test 2nd Edition (K-BIT2) Matrices—significant correlations

Test	r	N
WJ-III Academic Knowledge	0.32	47
PIAT Reading	0.43**	48
WCST Total Score	0.49**	36
WCST Total Errors	0.46**	36
WCST Categories Completed	0.41	36
WCST Trials to Complete 1st Set	−0.35	36
Towers of Hanoi	0.43**	44
ASL-SRT	0.35	32
Finger Spelling Test Total Correct	0.41**	47
TOSWRF	0.34	47
Print Letter Backward Span	0.34	35
Print Digit Forward Span	0.32	45
Corsi Blocks Computer Backward Span	0.31	46
Corsi Blocks Manual Backward Span	0.41**	47
ASL Letter Backward Span	0.29	47
ASL Digit Backward Span	0.29	47

**Significance at $p<0.01$, all others significant at $p<0.05$

we present the results of this analysis for the K-BIT2. Rasch analyses for the other tests will be presented as the tests are discussed in the chapters to follow.

Rasch analysis allows for a simultaneous estimation of test item difficulty and person ability parameters, and allows us to examine the "fit" of a test (and its range of item difficulties) to the sample participants (and their range of abilities). It is often used in test development to identify and rectify poor test items that do not contribute to the assessment of a particular trait. For our current purposes, this analysis will help us demonstrate whether individual tests perform, for our unique population, in a similar way to that of the hearing populations for whom the tests were originally developed.

The Rasch analyses that are presented in this book will include a table showing relevant Rasch statistics pertinent to the measures of person abilities (the performance levels of individuals) and test item difficulties. (Table 3.3 presents the results for the K-BIT2.) We also include a graphical depiction of the relationships of participants to test items. Figure 3.1 presents a map showing each of the items on the K-BIT2 (on the right of the vertical axis) and each of the participants (on the left). The vertical scale is presented in terms of a unit of measure called a "logit". In Fig. 3.1 the logit scale for the K-BIT2 ranges from −4 logits to +4 logits. (Note that the range of this scale can vary, depending on the range of item difficulties and person abilities in a given data set.) Logit scores are assigned to both participants (as a measure of their ability), and to items (as a measure of their difficulty). Higher logit values for items indicate those that are of greater difficulty. Higher logit values for persons indicate those that are of higher ability. The logit scales for items and for persons are aligned, such that if we know the person's logit score (ability), we can calculate the probability that he will get an item correct, given the item's logit score (its difficulty).

Table 3.3 Kaufman Brief Intelligence Test (K-BIT2) Matrices—Rasch analysis person and item reliability

Statistics	Persons	Items
Mean raw scores	16.6 (out of 24)	31.0 (out of 47)
SD of raw scores	3.5	13.0
Mean Rasch measures	1.42	0
SE of means (for measures)	0.20	0.44
Measure range	−1.54 to 3.81	−3.18 to 3.53
# with MSq out-fit >2.0	6	2
Reliability (KR-20)	0.77	–

For example, when a person's ability score equals the difficulty score for a particular item, the probability that he will answer the item correct is 50%. The probability of a correct response to a test item will increase as its item difficulty logit score deviates negatively from the examinees ability score. Conversely, the probability of a correct item response will decrease as an item's logit scale score deviates positively from the examinee's ability score.

Of course, the accuracy of these predictions depends on whether certain assumptions are met, most notably that the construct being measured consists of a single dimension and that the likelihood of a correct response to a given item can be calculated from the knowledge of the estimated person ability and item difficulty parameters.

Fortunately, Rasch analysis provides statistics to help assess the validity of these assumptions, through the calculation of "fit" statistics. The fit statistics are based on a chi-square analysis, where, for each individual, we can assess whether her ability estimate correctly predicts performance on each of the test's items, given their calculated levels of difficulty. For example, we do not expect low scorers to get difficult items correct (except through guessing or through idiosyncratic knowledge patterns), nor do we expect high scorers to get easy items wrong (except through carelessness or other idiosyncratic knowledge patterns). On the item side, we do not expect difficult items to be answered correctly by examinees of low ability, nor do we expect easy items to be answered incorrectly by examinees of high ability. This parallel and simultaneous assessment of fit for both persons and items is a characteristic of Rasch analysis.

In the current analyses, we present the number of participants (and the number of items) showing fit statistics greater than a value of 2. As a point of reference, if an individual's item-by-item performance were perfectly predicted by her logit score, her fit statistic would be equal to 1. A value of 2 or greater indicates a significant amount of deviation or "noise" in a person's item responses (i.e., she made careless mistakes on easy items, got lucky on more difficult ones, or possesses a unique pattern of knowledge that is at odds with the definition of the trait that formed the basis for test construction). Similarly for items, an item fit statistic greater than 2 indicates an item with significant noise, with respect to the performance of low versus high ability examinees on the item.

As with most statistics, the achievement of stable parameter estimates relies heavily on sample size. We note that Rasch analysis is often used in the construction

Fig. 3.1 Rasch person ability by item difficulty map: K-BIT2 matrices

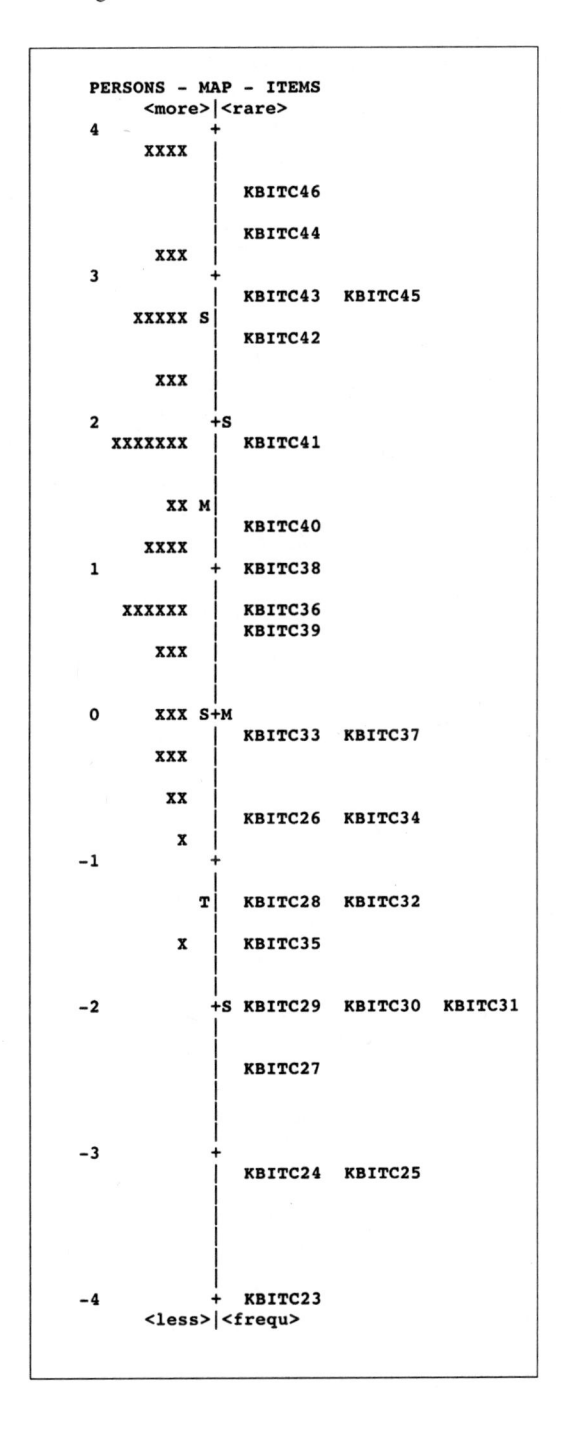

```
PERSONS - MAP - ITEMS
        <more>|<rare>
    4         +
         XXXX |
              |
              |  KBITC46
              |
              |  KBITC44
              |
         XXX  |
    3         +
              |  KBITC43    KBITC45
       XXXXX S|
              |  KBITC42
              |
              |
         XXX  |
              |
    2         +S
      XXXXXX  |  KBITC41
              |
              |
              |
           XX M|
              |  KBITC40
         XXXX |
    1         +  KBITC38
              |
       XXXXXX |  KBITC36
              |  KBITC39
         XXX  |
              |
              |
    0    XXX S+M
              |  KBITC33    KBITC37
         XXX  |
              |
           XX |
            X |  KBITC26    KBITC34
   -1         +
              |
             T|  KBITC28    KBITC32
              |
            X |  KBITC35
              |
              |
   -2         +S KBITC29 KBITC30 KBITC31
              |
              |  KBITC27
              |
              |
              |
   -3         +
              |  KBITC24    KBITC25
              |
              |
              |
              |
   -4         +  KBITC23
       <less>|<frequ>
```

of large-scale, high stakes tests that require a high level of stability (i.e., small standard errors and large sample size). Estimates computed here, because of our relatively small sample sizes, would clearly not satisfy this requirement. Nonetheless, as Linacre (1994b) notes, our sample sizes are adequate for pilot and exploratory studies, and, even with Ns as small as 30, will likely lead to the calculation of item calibrations that have 95% confidence intervals within ±1 logits.

K-BIT2 Results

Figure 3.1 shows that there is a high degree of overlap between person abilities and item difficulties and that the range of item difficulties has a fairly wide spread. Table 3.3 shows that the actual range in item difficulties extends from −3.18 to 3.53 logits, which is excellent for tests developed to fit a Rasch model. Figure 3.1 also shows the presence of a group of very easy items on the K-BIT2. The Winsteps software always sets the mean item difficulty logit value to 0 logits as an anchor for the calibrations. The mean ability measure for persons is 1.42, indicating that, in this sample, a person who scores at the mean level of ability *among these examinees* has a probability far greater than 0.5 of correctly responding to an item at the mean level of difficulty. This finding is perfectly consistent with expectations; the K-BIT2 is designed to measure abilities across an extremely wide range (as noted above, from ages 4 to 90). It is important to note that Rasch analysis uses raw scores and performances on individual items. Thus we would fully expect a sizeable number of very easy items for a sample of college students.

The standard error for the Rasch person measure is 0.20 logits. This translates to a 95% confidence interval of ±0.39 logits, also an excellent result in an exploratory study of 47 examinees. Table 3.3 shows that 6 (out of 47) examinees had significant noise in their response patterns (i.e., they had Fit statistics >2), as did 2 of the 24 test items. If we were doing further developmental work with the K-BIT2 to improve its applicability with deaf examinees, we might study the characteristics of these six students more intensively, re-run the analysis without these participants included, and look carefully at the two items showing poor fit to our model.

Finally, the KR20 reliability coefficient for this test (for these participants) is 0.77, an acceptable level of internal test item consistency. In sum, these findings attest to the appropriateness of using this test for this population.

Executive Functioning

The executive functions are considered to be a set of cognitive processes that underlie cognitive, behavioral, and emotional control, problem solving, and goal-oriented behavior and are seen as fundamental to self-regulation (Meltzer and Krishnan 2007; Powell and Voeller 2004). Component processes include attention, organization, mental flexibility, response inhibition/impulse control, and working memory. These processes ultimately involve the regulation of emotions and behavior, and coordinate the perceptual and motor functions to produce meaningful behavior

(Denckla 2007). Individuals with normally developed EF possess the ability to create structure for themselves in a variety of situations and to engage in higher order reasoning. In practical terms, these are used to respond effectively to situational demands and to respond to them in a purposeful manner.

As with all cognitive processes, EF develops during childhood; however, the various components of EF develop at differential rates and some aspects continue developing through early adulthood (De Luca and Leventer 2008; Fischer and Daley 2007). Deficits in one or more aspects of EF are implicated in both acquired disorders such as stroke (Su et al. 2008) and brain injuries (Sherer et al. 2003), developmental disorders such as attention deficit-hyperactivity disorder and learning disabilities (Denckla 2007; Meltzer and Krishnan 2007), and a range of other neurological conditions (Powell and Voeller 2004). Effective EF is critical for the development of academic skills, particularly those involving re-organizing and synthesizing information, extracting themes, and drawing inferences (e.g., reading comprehension), planning and organization (e.g., written expression), and problem solving (e.g., science and mathematics), in addition to social and vocational functioning (Meltzer and Krishnan 2007).

Assessment of the EF consists of tasks that require the individual to generate structure for themselves and independently solve novel problems. This is in contrast with many psychological assessment tools and procedures that provide the individual with an external structure; real deficits and impairments can be overlooked due to this feature of the process and tools (Lezak et al. 2004). As it is a multifaceted set of functions, EF can be measured using a range of tasks, many of which measure multiple areas of EF as well as other cognitive functions (Bull et al. 2004). EF can be evaluated using drawing (Somerville et al. 2000) and other visual and motor tasks (Powell and Voeller 2004), language-based tasks such as digit span and verbal fluency tests (Lezak et al. 2004), and reasoning tasks such as the tower and card sorting tasks used for this study. EF does not refer to discrete functions, but rather processes which underlie various functions and abilities. Examples of the manner in which EF measures evaluate two or more aspects of EF in addition to other areas of functioning include complex drawing tasks which measure organization, planning, and visual memory, and trail making tests which measure working memory and shifting. Tests that are verbal in nature by necessity reflect language skills as well as working memory, organization, and inhibition. Individuals can have areas of strengths and weaknesses within the realm of EF (Powell and Voeller 2004). In order to evaluate the various aspects of EF, Delis et al. (2001) created a battery that assesses a range of verbal and non-verbal EF processes, while clinicians and researchers may employ either a battery or several tests that are known to measure overlapping constructs and use data to pinpoint EF strengths and weaknesses.

Deaf Individuals and Executive Functioning

While a comprehensive review of EF data with deaf individuals is beyond the scope of this volume, a brief overview is provided. Please see Hauser et al. (2008) for a recent review of EF in deaf children and Corina and Singleton (2009) for a review of cognitive processes in the context of deafness. While the majority of research on EF in the deaf population has focused on children, there are some studies addressing deaf adult's EF performances. Rehkemper (1996) examined prelingually deaf adults (mean age 23 years) who were undergraduate students at a university for deaf and hard of hearing students and fluent users of ASL. The participants had varying causes of deafness and family language backgrounds. They were grouped into those with hereditary deafness and those born to hearing parents and deaf by nonhereditary causes (e.g., rubella, meningitis, and high fever). The results indicated that those in the nonhereditary group had significantly more difficulty with response inhibition than the participants with hereditary etiologies.

These results have implications for the finding by Hauser et al. (2008) that while early research suggested that deaf children were more impulsive than typical expectations, these studies included participants who were at risk for neurological dysfunction due to etiologies of deafness such as maternal rubella. They added that more recent studies have found conflicting data, particularly when the participants were deaf adults with deaf parents. Similar conflicting data have been reported related to attention tasks which are affected by impulsive responding, and it has been observed that attentional differences in deaf individuals depend on the task, with visuospatial stimuli eliciting the observed differences (Bavelier et al. 2006).

Within the research of deaf children, Rhine (2002) studied EF based on parent ratings of deaf and hard of hearing children on the Behavior Rating Inventory of Executive Function (BRIEF; Gioia et al. 2000). As with previous studies, she reported limitations in response inhibition in this population as well as issues with cognitive flexibility and working memory; however, other aspects of EF were rated as consistent with standard norms. In a later study, she found that language skills were predictive of both BRIEF ratings and performance on EF measures (Rhine Kalback 2004). These data were consistent with those of Figueras et al. (2008), who also found that performance of deaf children, regardless of whether they used hearing aids or cochlear implants, was lower than hearing peers on a range of EF measures, particularly on language-mediated tasks. These authors found that EF performance was related to language functioning for both the deaf and hearing participants, and the differences between the deaf and hearing children's EF performances appeared to be associated with the deaf children's more limited language functioning. These findings are consistent with the study by Edwards et al. (2011) which found that English vocabulary and grammar skills were predictive of verbal analogic reasoning in deaf and hard of hearing children (oral and Total Communication), but not the hearing children in the study.

Similarly, Oberg and Lukomski (2011) found that BRIEF ratings of deaf students by their parents and teachers were positively correlated with scores on EF measures, including the Wisconsin Card Sorting Test, the Children's Color Trails Test, and the Writing Fluency subtest of the Woodcock Johnson Test of Academic Achievement, Third Edition (WJ-III). As in the above studies, ratings and scores of deaf children with genetic etiologies of deafness were better than those of the children with nongenetic etiologies.

The above data suggest that deaf individuals with significant language delays are at greater risk of EF limitations than those who have adequate and timely language development. Similarly, those with nongenetic causes of deafness are at increased risk of EF weaknesses. This may be at least partially mediated by the early language access of genetically deaf children with deaf parents. Another possible source of this difference is the risk of additional conditions associated with some nongenetic causes of deafness, such as meningitis, maternal rubella, Rh incompatibility, and cytomegalovirus (Mauk and Mauk 1992, 1998; Samar et al. 1998; Spreen et al. 1995; Vernon and Andrews 1990).

Toolkit Executive Functioning Measures

As previously noted, measures of EF are multifaceted, and many tests measure other constructs in addition to one or more aspects of EF. The measures used that focus primarily on EF will be discussed in this chapter, and include the Wisconsin Card Sorting Test, Towers of Hanoi (TOH), and Tower of London (TOL). Verbal Fluency and working memory tasks, while being EF measures, will be discussed in the chapters related to linguistic and memory functioning, respectively, due to their strong associations with those constructs.

Wisconsin Card Sorting Test-64 Card Version

The Wisconsin Card Sorting Test-64 Card Version (WCST) (Kongs et al. 2000), which for convenience will be referred to as the WCST although the standard acronym is WCST-64 for this brief version, is a shortened version of the 128 card Wisconsin Card Sorting Test, a widely used measure of EF. While multiple short versions of the Wisconsin Card Sorting Test are available, the 64 card version has strong norms and is "the one to which the existing WCST literature is most likely to generalize" (Greve 2001, p. 230). According to the test manual, "Similar to other measures of executive function, the WCST requires (a) concentration, (b) planning, (c) organization, (d) cognitive flexibility in shifting set, (e) working memory, and (f) inhibition of impulsive responding" (Kongs et al. 2000, p. 1). Specifically, the WCST reflects strategy development in response to feedback, and the ability to use and sustain the strategy while it is effective and then alter the strategy in response to changing task demands.

The examinee is presented with cards with designs which have one to four circles, crosses, triangles, or stars which are yellow, green, red, or blue. They are then asked to match them to one of four model cards. No matching rules for sorting the cards are given, and the only feedback provided is whether the response is correct or incorrect. Both manual and computer versions are available. For the present research the 64-card computer version was used. Although this task is not timed, most participants took between 5 and 10 min to complete the task. Scores are derived from the number of attempts required to successfully complete the first set based on the initial strategy, how successfully they shift strategies to accommodate new task demands

Table 3.4 Wisconsin Card Sorting Test (WCST)—descriptive statistics

Test	Scale	Range	N	Mean (SD)
WCST (64 card)	Total Correct (Raw Score)	33–57	36	51.39 (6.21)
	Total Errors	58–121	36	100.72 (13.60)
	Perseverative Errors	53–127	36	98.06 (14.50)
	Categories Completed (Raw Score)	1–5	36	4.00 (1.24)
	Trials to Complete 1st Set (Raw Score)	10–53	36	15.33 (9.98)
	Failure to Maintain Set	0–2	36	0.39 (0.65)

(reflected in total number of correct responses), and how many errors are made (perseverative, total). Perseveration in the WCST describes response behavior that occurs when the participant continues to use previously successful strategies despite negative feedback provided when the rules of the task change. As with the original 128 card version, the WCST has been used extensively in research and neuropsychological assessment in clinical settings (Maddox et al. 2010; Sherer et al. 2003; Su et al. 2008). In their review of the instrument, Strauss et al. (2006) noted that while the 64 card version correlates highly with the original Wisconsin (0.70–0.91 as reported in the 64 card test manual), there may be inconsistencies between the two on a case-by-case basis. This type of task requires the participant to inhibit previously effective behaviors while shifting strategies in the face of changing task demands.

WCST Results. On the WCST, the current sample performed in a manner consistent with the test norms for both Total Errors and Perseverative Errors. Furthermore, the average group performances on the remaining WCST scores are within normal limits, suggesting that overall, deaf college students are able to perform these tasks in an appropriate manner. However, as with the academic achievement tasks, all of the scores range from clinically impaired levels to advanced performances. Table 3.4 presents the descriptive statistics for the WCST. Note that the Total Errors and Perseverative Errors are reported as standard scores with a mean of 100 and SD of 15. All other scores represent raw scores, and those data should be directly compared to normative data.

Table 3.5 presents the significant correlations between the WCST Total Correct Score, representing the total number of correct matches, and the other toolkit measures. Not unexpectedly, this score correlates significantly with other WCST scores, and a moderate to large association was observed between this score and the general cognitive estimate. Interestingly, despite a moderate correlation with the TOH, significance was not achieved between this WCST score and the TOL.

Consistent with the previously discussed research suggesting that EF outcomes, and specifically card sorting performances, correlate with language functioning in deaf individuals, moderate correlations were observed between this score and the two measures of reading comprehension, and moderate to high relationships with other measures reflecting English skills (TOSWRF and TSA). This contention is further supported by the fact that on the Fingerspelling Test, while a significant relationship was observed with the Real Words task, no significant relationship was observed with the pseudo-word task, suggesting that this relationship reflects the

Table 3.5 Wisconsin Card Sorting Test (WCST), Total Score—significant Pearson correlations

Test	r	N
WJ-III Passage Comprehension	0.40	33
PIAT Reading Comprehension	0.44**	36
WCST Total Errors	0.69**	36
WCST Perseverative Errors	0.34**	36
WCST Categories Completed	0.87**	36
WCST Trials to Complete 1st Set	−0.79**	36
Towers of Hanoi	0.41	34
K-BIT2 Matrices	0.49**	36
F-A-S Food	0.35	35
5–1–U Food	0.37	35
M-SVLT List A	0.59**	35
M-SVLT Cued Recall	0.39	34
M-SVLT Delayed Cued Recall	0.33	35
Finger Spelling Test	0.35	35
Finger Spelling Test: Real Words	0.36	35
TOSWRF	0.53**	35
TSA Percent Correct	0.49	17
Print Letter Backward Span	0.51**	26
Print Digit Backward Span	0.48*	33
Corsi Blocks Computer Backward	0.48**	35
Corsi Blocks Manual Backward	0.51**	35
ASL Letter Forward Span	0.37	35
ASL Letter Backward Span	0.34	35
ASL Digit Backward Span	0.44**	35

**Significance at $p<0.01$, all others significant at $p<0.05$

linguistic aspect of this task rather than the short-term memory component. This linguistic association is likely responsible for the associations seen with the measure of linguistic memory (M-SLVT), in the absence of significant associations with the measure of visuospatial ability and memory (BVMT). The lack of a significant correlation with the ASL-SRT may relate to the potential dependence of that task on visual memory based on the current scoring system.

Moderate to large correlations were observed with both linguistic (letter and digit backward span tasks) and visual (Corsi blocks backward span tasks) working memory tasks. As only one forward sequencing task correlated significantly with this measure, it appears likely that these relationships relate to the working memory aspects of the tasks rather than simple verbal/visual sequencing.

Interestingly, as can be seen in Tables 3.6 and 3.7, while the WCST Categories Completed score correlated with the other measures in a manner very similar to that of the WCST Total Correct Responses, a more limited set of tests correlated with the WCST Perseverative Errors. This latter score may represent a greater focus on response inhibition and cognitive flexibility/switching on this aspect of the test.

Table 3.6 Wisconsin Card Sorting Test (WCST), Perseverative Errors—significant correlations

Test	r	N
WJ-III Math Fluency	0.37	33
WCST Total Correct	0.34	36
WCST Total Errors	0.79**	36
WCST Categories Completed	0.32	36
WCST Trials to Complete 1st Set	−0.38	36
5–1–U Total Score	−0.32	36
ASL-SRT Total Correct	−0.43	23
Print Letter Backward Span	0.46	26
Print Digit Backward Span	0.39	33
ASL Letter Forward Span	0.32	35

**Significance at $p<0.01$, all others significant at $p<0.05$

Table 3.7 Wisconsin Card Sorting Test (WCST), Categories Completed—significant correlations

Test	r	N
BVMT Total Recall	0.38	36
BVMT Delayed Recall	0.33	36
BVMT Discrimination Index	0.50**	34
WJ-III Passage Comprehension	0.36	33
PIAT Reading Comprehension	0.47**	36
WCST Total Correct	0.87**	36
WCST Total Errors	0.70**	36
WCST Perseverative Errors	0.32	36
WCST Trials to Complete 1st Set	−0.67**	36
TOH Total Score	0.45**	34
K-BIT2 Matrices	0.41	36
FAS Food	0.41	35
M-SVLT List A	0.45**	35
M-SVLT Cued Recall	0.31	34
Finger Spelling Test	0.36	35
Finger Spelling Test: Real Words	0.40	35
TOSWRF	0.59**	35
TSA Percent Correct	0.57	17
TSA Relativization % Correct	0.50	17
Print Letter Backward Span	0.42	26
Corsi Blocks Computer Forward	0.38	35
Corsi Blocks Computer Backward	0.48**	35
Corsi Blocks Manual Backward	0.39	35
ASL Letter Forward Span	0.36	35
ASL Digit Forward Span	0.40	35
ASL Digit Backward Span	0.38	35

**Significance at $p<0.01$, all others significant at $p<0.05$

Towers of Hanoi

The TOH is a measure of EF that requires both logical and abstract reasoning skills (Lezak et al. 2004), as well as the cognitive flexibility/shifting (Bull et al. 2004). It is also believed to measure implicit memory, strategy development, and high-order cognition (Davis et al. 1994). The TOH can be used in clinical practice to assess the EF areas of planning, inhibition, working memory, and visuospatial reasoning. Although the stimuli are visual and no verbal response is required, the participant must be able to understand and follow the directions and, as with other EF reasoning and problem-solving tasks, verbal mediation can be used to support performance.

For this study, the TOH was presented via computer using the Colorado Neuropsychology Tests, Tests (Davis et al. 1994) on a Twinhead Activecolor 486E Laptop running Windows 3.1. The participant is presented with a graphic representing a rectangular pegboard with three pegs. In the version used in the current study, five round disks are stacked on one peg with the largest disk at the base and each subsequent disk of diminishing size so that the smallest disk is at the top. The object is to move the disks from the initial stack on the right peg to an identical configuration on the far left peg. Only one disk may be moved at a time, and a larger disk cannot be placed on a smaller disk. This process requires planning as disks must be stacked in intermediary steps for a successful outcome. A trial can be completed in 31 moves, and is stopped if it is not successfully completed within 120 moves. The participant is presented with five trials of the task. Thus, when a successful strategy is developed, if the participant is able to retain and reproduce the strategy, future trials can be completed more efficiently. The minimum number of moves over the five trials is 155. Data are collected on the number of excess moves, number of Total Moves, and task time, and a total score is reported reflecting the number of trials successfully completed within 120 moves. In the current study, the computer administration from the Colorado Neuropsychological Battery was used.

Towers of Hanoi results. Over the five trials presented on the TOH, the performance of the participants in this study ranged from a minimal number of excess moves to being unable to complete any trial within the maximum number of moves allowed. The range of scores again suggest that while the average performance was adequate, some of the participants excelled while others had extremely limited ability to perform the task. Table 3.8 presents the descriptive statistics for the TOH.

As can be seen from Table 3.9, the TOH displays a pattern similar to that of the WCST in its relationship with measures of reading, nonverbal reasoning, naming fluency, and linguistic and visual working memory span. In this case, the strongest relationships appear to be with measures of nonverbal reasoning and fluency, and visual working memory span tests. These data are consistent with previous research suggesting that processing speed, working memory, and response inhibition are involved in performance of this test, particularly on the more complex TOH tasks such as the one used in this study (Lezak et al. 2004). Consistent with previous research using hearing college students (Welsh et al. 1999) the TOH demonstrated a weak to moderate relationship with the TOL,

Table 3.8 Towers of Hanoi (TOH)—descriptive statistics

Test	Scale	Range	N	Mean (SD)
TOH	Total Score	0–5	44	3.66 (1.46)
	Total Moves Trials (1–5)	163–600	44	390.36 (112.10)
	Total Time (min)	3–30	n/a	13.98 (5.97)

Table 3.9 Towers of Hanoi (TOH) Total Score—significant correlations

Test	r	N
PIAT Reading	0.40**	44
WCST Total Score	0.41	34
WCST Total Errors	0.39	34
WCST Categories Completed	0.45**	34
K-BIT2 Matrices	0.43**	44
Tower of London	0.36	43
F-A-S Food	0.45**	43
5–1–U	0.37	42
Print Letter Backward Span	0.53**	34
Print Digit Forward Span	0.37	41
Corsi Blocks Computer Backwards Span	0.49**	42
Corsi Blocks Manual Backwards Span	0.39	43
ASL Digit Forward Span	0.35	43
ASL Digit Backward Span	0.30	43

**Significance at $p<0.01$, all others significant at $p<0.05$

which could be explained in part by the differences in task demands over trials and the nature of the tasks (e.g., the TOH is a complex, repeated task, while the TOL uses different stimuli with increasing task demands). These tasks, although similar, have previously shown to be dissociated from one another in their measurement properties (Bull et al. 2004).

Mousley and Kelly (1998) used the TOH to investigate mathematics problem-solving strategies in deaf college students. Although their research aim was to explore and confirm different strategies for mathematics problem-solving, their data suggested that reading ability, as measured by the California Reading Test (CRT) at the time of college admission, was not significantly related to overall performance on the TOH, although stronger readers were better able to articulate the strategies used in solving the tower problems. While the PIAT-R Reading Comprehension and CRT both measure reading achievement, the differing task demands may be responsible for the conflicting outcomes. Additionally, the lack of significant correlations between the TOH and other reading measures in the current study does suggest that the relationship seen in the current study may relate to the specific type of reading task presented on the PIAT-R.

Tower of London

The second EF measure used was the TOL. The version used for this study was the TOL, Drexel Version: 2nd Edition (TOL^{DX}; Culbertson and Zillmer 2005). This version of the test offers standard scores and more difficult items than the original version developed by Shallice (1982). As with the above measures, this task requires abstract reasoning, and has been found to be affected by the ability to both inhibit responses and shift cognitive sets (Bull et al. 2004). As with the TOH, the TOL can be used in clinical practice to assess planning, inhibition, working memory, and visual-motor reasoning abilities. It is perhaps best known for its use in the assessment of frontal lobe abnormalities, brain injuries/lesions, autism, learning disabilities, and ADHD (Lezak et al. 2004); however, the research related to the diagnostic applicability of the TOL^{DX} for ADHD has yielded conflicting data (Culbertson and Zillmer 1998; Riccio et al. 2004). Riccio and colleagues concluded that while the TOL^{DX} appears to measure unique aspects of functioning and may provide valuable information, performance on this task does not appear to have direct diagnostic applications at this time.

The TOL is superficially similar to the TOH in that it requires the participant to move items (in this case, different colored beads) on pegboards. The TOL involves two pegboards, each with three pegs of increasing height. One pegboard is used by the examiner to present the model for each trial and the other is used by the examinee for the response. For the test, three colored beads (red, blue, and green) are stacked on the examiner's pegboard to create a target, which the examinee must match from a starting configuration set by the examiner on the response board. The participant is told that, as on the TOH, only one bead may be moved at a time and it must be placed on a peg before another bead is removed. Participants are also instructed that the shortest peg can only have one bead stacked on it at a time, the medium-height peg two, and the tallest peg three; the heights of the pegs enforce these constraints. One demonstration item is given, followed by two practice administrations and then ten problems are presented. This task is timed and takes approximately 10–15 min to complete. Starting and stopping the timer is not allowed due to potential interference with smooth administration and accurate time-recording (Culbertson and Zillmer 2005). Standard scores with a mean of 100 and SD of 15 are generated for the amount of time taken to start and complete each set and total test time, the number of moves per problem and total test moves, and number of time and rule violations, as well as the number of correct solutions attained in the minimum number of moves. This study focused on the Total Correct, Total Moves and number of Time Violation Scores.

Tower of London results. The participants in this study performed in an age appropriate manner on all TOL measures. However, as with the other EF measures, individual performances varied, with scores ranging from two SDs above the mean to nearly two SDs below the normative mean for the Total Correct to well below this level for the Total Moves and Time Violations. This suggests that even some students who were able to solve a number of the problems efficiently at times had difficulty with the task. Table 3.10 depicts the descriptive statistics for the TOL.

Table 3.10 Tower of London (TOL)—descriptive statistics for standard scores

Test	Scale	Range	N	Mean (SD)
Tower of London (TOL)	Total Correct Score	72–134	49	100.24 (15.91)
	Total Moves	60–130	49	95.90 (17.18)
	Time Violations	60–112	48	98.88 (14.84)

Table 3.11 Towers of London (TOL) Total Correct Score—significant correlations

Test	r	N
MRT-Short Form A	0.45	25
M-SVLT List B Recall	0.30	49
Towers of Hanoi	0.36	43
Tower of London Total Moves	0.81**	49
Print Letter Forward Span	0.35	36
Print Letter Backward Span	0.45**	35
Print Digit Forward Span	0.42**	45
Corsi Blocks Manual Backward Span	0.39**	49
ASL Letter Forward Span	0.31	49
ASL Letter Backward Span	0.33	49

**Significance at $p<0.01$, all others significant at $p<0.05$

Table 3.11 presents the significant correlations between the Tower of London Total Score and the other toolkit measures. Previous research with adults aged 16–33 has suggested that most TOL^{DX} scores have minimal relationships with other EF measures, with the few correlations observed primarily reflecting associations between time and rule violations and working memory and processing speed (Riccio et al. 2004). While no significant correlations between TOL and WCST were observed, as previously noted, despite differences between the specific tasks used in the two studies, the moderate correlation between TOH and TOL is consistent with the results of Welsh et al. (1999).

While no significant relationships between the TOL and standard learning trials on the task were observed, a low to moderate relationship was observed with the interference list trial of the verbal learning (M-SLVT). This trial would be expected to require increased involvement of cognitive shifting and response inhibition relative to the other verbal learning trials. The lack of correlation with the TOH and this task may relate to the differences between the two tower tasks, including the fact that all trials of the TOH are identical, while each trial differs on the TOL, requiring increased involvement of cognitive flexibility on the latter task. Interestingly, despite the lack of a significant relationship with the TOH, a moderate correlation was observed between the TOL and a mental rotation task, possibly due to the demand for ongoing visuospatial problem-solving and visualization.

Again consistent with Welsh et al. (1999), as with the TOH, the primary relationships appear to relate to spatial and linguistic sequencing and working memory.

3 Measures of General Cognitive Functioning

Table 3.12 Towers of London (TOL) Total Moves Score—significant correlations

Test	r	N
MRT-Short Form A	0.43	25
Tower of London Total Correct	0.81**	49
TOL Time Violations	0.35	48
Print Letter Forward Span	0.35	306

**Significance at $p<0.01$, all others significant at $p<0.05$

Table 3.13 Towers of London (TOL) Time Violations Score—significant correlations

Test	r	N
Tower of London Total Moves	0.35	49
5-1-U Animals Raw Score	0.32	45
Koo Phonological Awareness	−0.38	45
Lipreading Percent Words Correct	0.55**	35
Lipreading Percent Sentences Correct	0.58**	45
Corsi Blocks Manual Forward Span	0.51**	49

**Significance at $p<0.01$, all others significant at $p<0.05$

Indeed, while Welsh and colleagues used only visual working memory tasks, in this study, both the TOL and TOH were shown to relate to visual and linguistic working memory span. As can be seen in Table 3.12, an even more limited number of associations were found between the TOL Total Moves and the other measures. This was again consistent with the results of Riccio et al. (2004), who found only a weak relationship with the WCST Failure to Maintain Set.

While relatively few significant correlations were observed between the TOL Time Violations and the neuropsychological measures, relatively large associations were observed between this score and lipreading measures for both words and sentences correct (Table 3.13). This may relate to the finding by Riccio et al. (2004) that the only significant correlation between the TOL Time Violations and other scores was with processing speed. Lipreading requires rapid visual analysis in addition to English knowledge.

Overall Remarks

The data from this research suggest that the deaf college students in this study performed in a manner similar to expectations based on standard norms and research with hearing populations despite having scores at the lower end of the range below expectations for college students. Relationships of the EF measures studied here were generally consistent with those seen in previous research both with other deaf participants and hearing populations. For example, the correlations between the

WCST and language tasks in the current study are consistent with previous findings of language impacts on EF in deaf individuals (Edwards et al. 2011; Figueras et al. 2008; Rhine Kalback 2004). Similarly, previous research with hearing participants found a weak–moderate relationship between the TOH and TOL similar to that seen in the current study (Bull et al. 2004; Welsh et al. 1999). Associations have also been reported between working memory, inhibition, and fluid intelligence with the TOH (Zook et al. 2004). Consistent with the limited correlations seen with the TOL in the current study, Zook and colleagues found that the associations with the TOL were explained by the impact of fluid intelligence.

With the exception of the TOL, EF measures in our sample consistently demonstrated relationships with tests of linguistic (digit and letter spans), and also the visual (Corsi Blocks) working memory tasks. Although the relationships were generally moderate in strength and there were inconsistencies among the specific tasks correlating with the various EF measures, an overall pattern emerged suggesting that these measures of complex EF processes involve some degree of working memory across tasks. These data are again consistent with the above noted studies with both deaf and hearing populations. Thus, this association appears to reflect a more general relationship between these cognitive processes rather than characteristics unique to deaf populations.

References

Bavelier, D., Dye, M. W., & Hauser, P. C. (2006). Do deaf individuals see better? *Trends in Cognitive Science, 10*(11), 512–518.

Bishop, D. V. M. (1983). Comprehension of English syntax by profoundly deaf children. *Journal of Child Psychology and Psychiatry, 24*(3), 415–434.

Blennerhassett, L., Strohmeier, S. J., & Hibbett, C. (1994). Criterion-related validity of Raven's Progressive Matrices with deaf residential school students. *American Annals of the Deaf, 139*(2), 104–110.

Bond, T. G., & Fox, C. M. (2007). *Applying the Rasch model: Fundamental measurement in the human sciences*. Mahwah, NJ: Lawrence Erlbaum and Associates.

Bull, R., Espy, K. A., & Senn, T. E. (2004). A comparison of performance on the Towers of London and Hanoi in young children. *Journal of Child Psychology and Psychiatry, 45*(4), 743–754.

Corina, D., & Singleton, J. (2009). Developmental social cognitive neuroscience: Insights from deafness. *Child Development, 80*(4), 952–967.

Culbertson, W. C., & Zillmer, E. A. (1998). The Tower of London[DX]: A standardized approach to assessing executive functioning in children. *Archives of Clinical Neuropsychology, 13*, 285–301.

Culbertson, W. C., & Zillmer, E. A. (2005). *Tower of London Drexel University* (2nd ed.). New York: Multi-Health Systems.

Davis, H. P., Bajszar, G. M., & Squire, L. R. (1994). *Colorado neuropsychology tests: Explicit memory, implicit memory and problem solving (Version 2.0) [Computer program and test manual]*. Los Angles, CA: Western Psychological Services.

De Luca, C., & Leventer, R. (2008). Developmental trajectories of executive functions across the lifespan. In V. Anderson, R. Jacobs, & P. J. Anderson (Eds.), *Executive functions and the frontal lobes: A lifespan perspective* (pp. 23–56). New York: Taylor and Francis.

Delis, D. C., Kaplan, E., & Kramer, J. H. (2001). *Delis–Kaplan executive function system (D-KEFS)*. London: The Psychological Corporation.

Denckla, M. (2007). Executive function: Binding together the definitions of attention-deficit/hyperactivity disorder and learning disabilities. In L. Meltzer (Ed.), *Executive function in education: From theory to practice* (pp. 5–18). New York: The Guilford Press.

Edwards, L., Figueras, B., Mellanby, J., & Langdon, D. (2011). Verbal and spatial analogical reasoning in deaf and hearing children: The role of grammar and vocabulary. *Journal of Deaf Studies and Deaf Education, 16*(2), 189–197. doi:10.1093/deafed/enq051.

Emmorey, K., McCollough, S., Petrich, J., & Weisberg, J. (2011). Mapping word reading circuitry for skilled deaf readers.

Emmorey, K., & Petrich, J. (2012). Processing orthographic structure: Associations between print and fingerspelling. *Journal of Deaf Studies and Deaf Education, 17*, 194–204.

Figueras, B., Edwards, L., & Langdon, D. (2008). Executive function and language in deaf children. *Journal of Deaf Studies and Deaf Education, 13*(3), 362–377.

Fischer, K. W., & Daley, S. G. (2007). Connecting cognitive science and neuroscience: Potentials and pitfalls in inferring executive processes. In L. Meltzer (Ed.), *Executive function in education: From theory to practice* (pp. 5–18). New York: The Guilford Press.

Gioia, G., Isquith, P., Guy, S., & Kenworthy, L. (2000). *Behavior Rating Inventory of executive function (BRIEF)*. Lutz, FL: Psychological Assessment Resources, Inc.

Goetzinger, M. R., & Houchins, R. R. (1969). The 1947 colored Raven's progressive matrices with deaf and hearing subjects. *American Annals of the Deaf, 114*(2), 95–101.

Goetzinger, C. P., Wills, R. C., & Dekker, L. C. (1967). Non-language I.Q. tests used with deaf pupils. *Volta Review, 69*, 500–506.

Greve, K. W. (2001). The WCST-64: A standardized short-form of the Wisconsin Card Sorting Test. *The Clinical Neuropsychologist, 15*(2), 228–234.

Hauser, P. C., Lukomski, J., & Hillman, T. (2008). Development of deaf and hard-of-hearing students' executive function. In M. Marschark & P. C. Hauser (Eds.), *Deaf cognition* (pp. 268–308). Oxford: Oxford University Press.

Kaufman, A. S., & Kaufman, N. L. (2004). *Kaufman Brief Intelligence Test* (2nd ed.). Minneapolis, MN: Pearson, Inc.

Kongs, S., Thompson, L., Iverson, G., & Heaton, R. (2000). *Wisconsin Card Sorting Test-64 Card version: Professional manual*. Lutz, FL: Psychological Assessment Resources.

Lezak, M., Howieson, D., & Loring, D. (2004). *Neuropsychological assessment* (4th ed.). New York: Oxford University Press.

Linacre, J. M. (1994a). *Many facet Rasch measurement*. Chicago: MESA Press.

Linacre, J. M. (1994b). Sample size and item calibration stability. *Rasch Measurement Transactions, 7*(4), 328.

Linacre, J. M. (2006). *WINSTEPS Rasch measurement computer program*. Chicago. http://winsteps.com.

Maddox, W. T., Filoteo, V. J., Glass, B. D., & Markman, A. B. (2010). Regulatory match effects on a modified Wisconsin Card Sort Task. *Journal of International Neuropsychological Society, 16*, 352–359. doi:10.1017/S1355617709991408.

Mauk, G., & Mauk, P. (1992). Somewhere, out there: Preschool children with hearing impairment and learning disabilities. *Topics in Early Childhood Special Education: Hearing-impaired Preschoolers, 12*, 174–195.

Mauk, G., & Mauk, P. (1998). Considerations, conceptualizations, and challenges in the study of concomitant learning disabilities among children and adolescents who are deaf or hard of hearing. *Journal of Deaf Studies and Deaf Education, 3*, 15–34.

Meltzer, L., & Krishnan, K. (2007). Executive function difficulties and learning disabilities: Understandings and misunderstandings. In L. Meltzer (Ed.), *Executive function in education: From theory to practice* (pp. 77–105). New York: The Guilford Press.

Mousley, K., & Kelly, R. (1998). Problem-solving strategies for teaching mathematics to deaf students. *American Annals of the Deaf, 143*, 325–336.

Oberg, E., & Lukomski, J. (2011). Executive functioning and the impact of a hearing loss: Performance-based measures and the Behavior Rating Inventory of Executive Function (BRIEF). *Child Neuropsychology, 17*(6), 521–545.

Powell, K. B., & Voeller, K. K. S. (2004). Prefrontal executive function syndromes in children. *Journal of Child Neurology, 19*(1), 785–797.

Raven, J. C. (1960). *Guide to using the standard progressive matrices*. London: H.K. Lewis.

Rehkemper, G. M. (1996). *Executive functioning and psychosocial adjustment in deaf subjects with non-hereditary and hereditary etiologies*. Unpublished doctoral dissertation, Gallaudet University, Washington, District of Columbia.

Rhine, S. (2002). *Assessment of executive functioning in deaf and hard of hearing children*. Unpublished predissertation, Gallaudet University, Washington, District of Columbia.

Rhine Kalback, S. (2004). *The Assessment of developmental language differences, executive functioning, and social skills in deaf children*. Doctoral dissertation. Available from ProQuest Dissertations and Theses database (UMI Number: 3181454; AAT 3181454).

Riccio, C. A., Wolfe, M. E., Romine, C., Davis, B., & Sullivan, J. R. (2004). The Tower of London and neuropsychological assessment of ADHD in adults. *Archives of Clinical Neuropsychology, 19*, 661–671.

Samar, V., Parasnis, I., & Berent, G. (1998). Learning disabilities, attention deficit disorders, and deafness. In M. Marschark & M. Clark (Eds.), *Psychological perspectives on deafness* (Vol. 2, pp. 199–242). Mahwah, NJ: Lawrence Erlbaum Associates.

Schorr, E. A., Roth, F. P., & Fox, N. A. (2008). A comparison of the speech and language skills of children with cochlear implants and children with normal hearing. *Communication Disorders Quarterly, 29*(4), 195–210.

Schorr, E. A., Roth, F. P., & Fox, N. A. (2009). Quality of life for children with cochlear implants: Perceived benefits and problems and the perception of single words and emotional sounds. *Journal of Speech, Language, and Hearing Research, 52*(1), 141–152.

Shallice, T. (1982). Specific impairments of planning. *Philosophical Transcripts of the Royal Society of London, 298*, 199–209.

Sherer, M., Nick, T. G., Millis, S. R., & Novack, T. A. (2003). Use of the WCST and the WCST-64 in the assessment of traumatic brain injury. *Journal of Clinical and Experimental Neuropsychology, 25*(4), 512–520.

Somerville, J., Tremont, G., & Stern, R. (2000). The Boston Qualitative Scoring System as a measure of executive functioning in Rey–Osterrieth complex figure performance. *Journal of Clinical and Experimental Neuropsychology, 22*(5), 613–621.

Spreen, O., Risser, A., & Edgell, D. (1995). *Developmental neuropsychology*. New York, NY: Oxford University.

Strauss, E., Sherman, E., & Spreen, O. (2006). *A compendium of neuropsychological tests: Administration, norms, and commentary* (3rd ed.). New York: Oxford University Press.

Su, C. Y., Lin, Y. H., Kwan, A. L., & Guo, N. W. (2008). Construct validity of the Wisconsin Card Sorting Test-64 in patients with stroke. *Clinical Neuropsychology, 22*(2), 273–287.

Vernon, M., & Andrews, J. (1990). *The psychology of deafness: Understanding deaf and hard-of-hearing people*. New York, NY: Longman.

Welsh, M. C., Satterlee-Cartmell, T., & Stine, M. (1999). Towers of Hanoi and London: Contributions of working memory and inhibition to performance. *Brain and Cognition, 41*, 231–242.

Zook, N. A., Davalos, D. B., DeLosh, E. L., & Davis, H. P. (2004). Working memory, inhibition, and fluid intelligence as predictors of performance on Tower of Hanoi and London Tasks. *Brain and Cognition, 56*(3), 286–292.

Chapter 4
Measures of Visuospatial Ability

Donna A. Morere, Wyatte C. Hall, and Thomas Allen

Visuospatial functioning, while important for interaction with the world in general, is critical for deaf and hard of hearing individuals as it is the primary means of accessing language for this population. Whether the person uses American Sign Language (ASL), another signing or visual cuing system, or oral communication, visual access is the key to accurate language reception. Due to its spatial nature, full and accurate reception of ASL also depends on well-developed spatial processing (Bosworth et al. 2003). Indeed, an increasing body of research indicates that deaf individuals who have had early and ongoing exposure to and use of ASL process visuospatial information somewhat differently than their hearing peers and have enhancements in certain aspects of visuospatial processing (e.g., Bavelier et al. 2001, 2006; Bosworth and Dobkins 1999, 2002a, b; Hauser et al. 2007).

Clearly, visuospatial processing is important for the processing of ASL. While the relationship is not clear (Musselman 2000), and some have found little relationship between ASL skills and reading competence (Moores and Sweet 1990), recent research has supported ASL competence as a critical factor in the development of literacy for deaf signers based on the need for a strong first language (Chamberlain and Mayberry 2008; DeLana et al. 2007; Perfetti and Sandak 2000; Strong and Prinz 1997; Wilbur 2000). These relationships suggest that in addition to the visual capacity required to perceive print, visuospatial functioning may have unique associations with literacy and academic success in deaf students, particularly those for whom ASL is the primary mode of communication.

D.A. Morere (✉) • W.C. Hall
Department of Psychology, Gallaudet University,
800 Florida Avenue, NE, Washington, DC 20002, USA
e-mail: Donna.Morere@Gallaudet.edu; Wyatte.Hall@Gallaudet.edu

T. Allen
Science of Learning Center on Visual Language and Visual Learning,
Gallaudet University, SLCC 1223, 800 Florida Avenue, NE,
Washington, DC 20002, USA
e-mail: thomas.allen@gallaudet.edu

Despite its critical nature, due to time constraints only two measures of visuospatial functioning were selected for the VL2 Psychometric Toolkit. One represents visuospatial analysis and memory, while the other measures skills in mental rotation. As discussed below, each of these areas is significant in the ability to communicate effectively via ASL.

Visuospatial Memory

Visuospatial memory reflects the person's ability to retain and retrieve information about both the content and location of objects in space. In practice, this is typically a three-dimensional process, such as remembering both what book one has misplaced as well as where it was placed in the environment. Since ASL is a visuospatial language, the ability to retain and retrieve information related to both the content (handshapes, etc.) and spatial location relative to the general environment as well as to the signer is critical for effective reception and comprehension of ASL. Most visual memory research has focused on working memory (WM), and that is investigated in the chapter on memory; however, as memory in the visual modality is so critical for ASL, a measure of simple retention and retrieval was included as well. While ASL is three dimensional, few measures of three-dimensional memory are available, so a two-dimensional task was used which has the advantage of being brief and having a delayed recall trial. This latter is important, as it would have implications for learning in the visual modality.

The Brief Visuospatial Memory Test-Revised

Test Characteristics

The Brief Visuospatial Memory Test-Revised (BVMT-R: Benedict 1997) is a measure of visuospatial memory. It is used in both research and clinical practice, investigating a range of conditions, including brain injury, multiple sclerosis, sleep apnea, and cardiovascular disease (Allen and Gfeller 2011; Beglinger et al. 2009; Cohen et al. 2009; Lim et al. 2007). The task involves presentation of six geometric figures presented in two rows of three designs. On each of three learning trials, the participant is allowed to see the design array for 10 s and is then asked to draw the items from memory, placing them in the correct locations on the page. Each drawing is scored for both location and accuracy, with two points awarded for an item drawn accurately in the correct location, one point if either the location or design was inaccurate, and zero if both were inadequate. The test has three learning trials on the immediate recall task, a delayed recall task following a 25-min delay, and a recognition trial on which the test items must be selected from among a set of 12

4 Measures of Visuospatial Ability

Table 4.1 BVMT-R—descriptive statistic

Test	Scale	Range	N	Mean (SD)
BVMT-R T-Scores	Total Recall	20–66	48	36.75 (13.33)
	Delayed Recall	20–63	48	35.56 (14.16)
	Discrimination Index (Index Score)	−1 to 6	46	5.53 (1.47)

designs. Performance on this task is affected by visual perception, visual memory (for both content and location), the graphomotor skills required for drawing, and, to a lesser extent, the organization of visuospatial information. Despite its graphomotor demands, this measure correlates more highly with visual memory tasks (with or without a drawing component) than with visual construction tasks without a memory component (Beglinger et al. 2009; Benedict 1997).

With the exception of the Discrimination Index, the scores are reflected in age-normed T-scores, with a mean of 50 and standard deviation of 10. The Discrimination Index reflects the difference between the number of correctly recognized items and the number of incorrectly identified foils. The highest and lowest possible scores are 6 and −6, respectively. The manual reports inter-rater reliability coefficients in the 0.90's and test–retest reliability coefficients between 0.60 and 0.84 for the free recall trials (Benedict et al. 1996).

Results

As can be seen in Table 4.1, which presents the descriptive statistics for the BVMT-R, contrary to expectations that deaf individuals would perform well on measures of visual memory, the group mean on the BVMT-R was more than one standard deviation below the normative mean on the learning trials and delayed recall trials. Nonetheless, the mean performance on the recognition task approached the maximum possible score, suggesting adequate encoding of the stimuli in memory despite the inadequate retrieval and production of the designs. Future research using these data could investigate the nature of the limitations on the recall tasks. Relevant questions include whether the low T-scores are related to errors in location or content, or whether the productions were poorly executed and therefore not given full credit despite adequate recall. The latter could relate to either poor motor control or limitations in executive functioning (EF) resulting in hurried drawings or drawings produced with inadequate care.

Table 4.2 presents the significant correlations between the BVMT-R Total Recall and the other Toolkit measures. Overall, the BVMT-R Total Recall correlated significantly with the measure of nonverbal intelligence as well as a number of WM, EF, and academic and linguistic measures, including the measures of linguistic memory. The fact that the BVMT-R Total Correct correlates with the Tower of London, WCST Total Correct, and WCST Categories Completed as well as the

Table 4.2 BVMT-R Total Recall—significant correlations

Test	R	N
BVMT Delayed Recall	0.78**	48
BVMT Discrimination Score	0.44**	48
Mental Rotation Test	0.41*	25
WJ-III: Reading Fluency	0.38**	47
WJ-III: Writing Fluency	0.42**	47
WJ-III: Academic Knowledge	0.38**	47
WJ-III: Passage Comprehension	0.35*	45
PIAT: Reading Comprehension	0.43**	48
WCST Total Correct	0.37*	36
WCST Categories Completed	0.38*	36
K-BIT2 Matrices	0.39**	48
Tower of London	0.37*	47
F-A-S: Food	0.31*	47
5-1-U	0.38**	48
5-1-U: Food	0.35*	46
M-SVLT List A Total Recall	0.46**	47
M-SVLT List B Total Recall	0.32*	47
M-SVLT Cued Recall	0.33*	46
M-SVLT Delayed List A Free Recall	0.37*	46
M-SVLT Delayed Cued Recall	0.34*	45
Finger Spelling Test: Total	0.34*	47
Finger Spelling Test: Real Word	0.37**	47
Corsi Blocks Computer Backward Span	0.34*	46
Corsi Blocks Manual Backward Span	0.38**	47
ASL Letter Forward Span	0.33*	47
ASL Letter Backward Span	0.38**	47

**Significance at $p<0.01$, *significance at $p<0.05$

MRT suggests that the lower than expected mean performance may be at least partially related to the proposed impacts of EF, rather than visual memory limitations, at least within a subset of the participants. On the other hand, consistent with previous research using the BVMT-R and English list-learning tasks with hearing participants, correlations between the BVMT-R and the M-SVLT, a sign-based list learning task, suggest that memory may indeed be involved.

The moderate significant correlations between the BVMT-R and a range of academic tasks contrast with the results of the BVMT-R normative study, which found nonsignificant to weak, but significant, (largest $r=0.17$) correlations between education and BVMT-R scores using a nonclinical sample (Benedict et al. 1996). Allen and Gfeller (2011) evaluated college undergraduates and found that the BVMT-R loaded with the Hopkins Verbal Learning Test-Revised (HVLT-R), an English list learning task similar to the SVLT on a principal component analysis. Benedict and colleagues also administered the BVMT-R as part of a battery of neuropsychological measures, this time to a clinical sample, and found correlations with the HVLT, as well as other measures of memory and learning. These data are consistent with

Table 4.3 BVMT-R Delayed Recall—significant correlations

Test	R	N
BVMT Total Recall	0.78**	48
BVMT Discrimination Score	0.37*	48
Mental Rotation Test	0.41*	25
WJ-III: Writing Fluency	0.30*	47
WCST Total Correct	0.40*	36
WCST Categories Completed	0.33‡	36
M-SVLT List A Total Recall	0.46**	47
M-SVLT Delayed List A Free Recall	0.29‡	46
Corsi Blocks Computer Backward Span	0.29‡	46
Corsi Blocks Manual Backward Span	0.31*	47

**Significance at $p<0.01$, *$p<0.05$, ‡$p=0.05$

the current outcomes despite the differences in the populations. Interestingly, they found minimal correlations between the BVMT-R scores and the FAS. Thus, the relationships seen with verbal learning measures in previous studies with hearing participants appear to reflect the impact of memory-based relationships, since more purely linguistic measures were not reported to produce significant correlations with this task.

This contrasts somewhat with the current data; however, while there was no significant correlation between the BVMT-R Total Correct and the F-A-S in the current sample, the sign-based task, 5–1–U did correlate significantly with this task. Furthermore, both the sign- and English-primed Food fluency tasks produced significant correlations, suggesting some relationship between visual language fluency and this visual learning task. Based on these data, it appears that the greater relationships between linguistic measures and the BVMT-R observed in the deaf signers in this study may relate to the visual nature of the primary language of this population.

Interestingly, as seen in Table 4.3, BVMT-R Delayed Recall correlated with a smaller subset of these tests associated with the BVMT-R Total Correct, primarily those related to visuospatial skills or memory. This suggests that the relationship of the initial learning trials, reflected in the Total Correct score, with the academic skills and larger set of linguistic tasks is important primarily during the learning phase, and that the retention of the designs over time relates more strongly to visuospatial processing, EF, and memory and learning, including language-based learning.

Despite the more limited relationships associated with retrieval and reproduction of these designs following a delay, many of the same associations seen with the initial learning trials were again observed with the recognition task, as revealed in the correlations with the Discrimination Index, presented in Table 4.4. Thus, there appears to be some ongoing relationship between language, both signed and English-based, in the ability of the participant to discriminate between the designs that had been learned and similar foils. This may relate to the "self-talk" involved in the

Table 4.4 BVMT-R Discrimination Index—significant correlations

Test	R	N
BVMT Total Correct	0.44**	48
BVMT Delayed Recall	0.37*	48
WJ-III: Passage Comprehension	0.34*	43
WJ-III: Math Fluency	−0.31*	45
PIAT: Reading Comprehension	0.45**	46
WCST Total Correct	0.36*	34
WCST Categories Completed	0.50**	34
Towers of Hanoi	0.36*	43
F-A-S: Food	0.36*	45
5–1–U: Food	0.34*	44
M-SVLT Delayed Cued Recall	0.30‡	43
ASL-SRT Total Correct	0.45*	30
TOSWRF SS	0.33*	45
Test of Syntactic Ability Percent Correct	0.70**	20
TSA Relativization Percent Correct	0.60**	20
Corsi Blocks Manual Backward Span	0.50**	44
ASL Letter Forward Span	0.34*	45

**Significance at $p<0.01$, *$p<0.05$, ‡$p=0.05$

decision-making process when selecting recognized designs from among the larger set. Interestingly, the strongest relationship with this score involves the participant's understanding of syntax as reflected in the correlations with the TSA scores. It is unclear if this reflects the impact of English skills on the discrimination task or whether there is an underlying factor affecting both skills. There is also a continued involvement of EF, which is consistent with the need to carefully review the stimuli and reason through the decision-making process.

Overall, the relationships between the BVMT-R and other Toolkit measures reveal significant relationships between this task and other measures of visuospatial processing and memory. Executive control appears to be associated with performance at all levels of this task, while language, both English and ASL, appears to be most significant during the learning phase of the task and later discrimination between the test items and similar design foils. While previous research has found associations between the BVMT-R and English-based list learning tasks, the visual nature of ASL may contribute to the other associations between language and visual memory observed in this study. The significant relationships between reading skills and two aspects of this test despite a lack of relationships with educational level in hearing populations (Benedict et al. 1996) suggest that English language competence, as reflected in reading skills as well as other language measures, may be a significant contributor to performance on the learning and discrimination aspects of visual memory. This relationship may be further elucidated by the relationships between mental rotation and other Toolkit measures, discussed below.

Mental Rotation

Mental rotation ability is considered important for success in a variety of areas, particularly the academic and vocational fields involving mathematics and science (Moè and Pazzaglia 2010). Mental rotation is the ability to perceive and cognitively manipulate two- and three-dimensional objects from different spatial perspectives. This process is used in a variety of everyday tasks; for instance, simple navigation relies on mental rotation to establish direction within the physical environment. The cognitive process of mental rotation was first recognized by Shepard and Metzler (1971) who, when presenting two similar objects at different perspectives, found a linear progression between time requirement and the difference in angles between the objects. Essentially, during Shepard and Metzler's task, the more an object was rotated, the more time was needed to determine that the two objects were similar. This was significant for cognitive psychology as a field as it was the first experiment to conclusively demonstrate that objects exist as cognitive representations.

The speed of mental rotation has been found to increase with age and familiarity (Kail and Park 1990; Kail et al. 1980). This suggests that processing of mental rotation can become increasingly automatic with experience; however, there does appear to be a limit to the benefit of the aging effect as participants older than 55 responded both more slowly and less accurately than younger participants (Dror and Kosslyn 1994). Research has also indicated that both training (Feng et al. 2007) and increased level of effort expended (Moè and Pazzaglia 2010) can improve performance on mental rotation tasks.

As previously noted, mental rotation has been historically tied to math, particularly math reasoning skills (Lubinski and Benbow 2006; Prescott et al. 2010; Shea et al. 2001). Within this relationship, males typically outperform females on both standardized math testing and mental rotation tasks (Ariniello 2000) and this difference in gender performance has remained stable over time (Masters and Sanders 1993). However, this gender difference reportedly disappears when mental rotation is tested through three-dimensional stimuli (Neubauer et al. 2010). Although mental rotation is commonly considered to contribute to math ability (Casey et al. 1995), research in a sample of deaf signers suggests that this is not the case for deaf individuals who use ASL (Halper 2009).

Deaf individuals have shown enhanced performance on mental rotation tasks compared to hearing peers (Emmorey 2002; Emmorey et al. 1998; Marschark 2003). However, despite the previously discussed relationship between mental rotation and math skills in the general population, this enhanced mental rotation ability has not resulted in corresponding gains in math performance among deaf students, many of whom graduate from high school having a sixth- to seventh-grade math level (Kelly 2008; Nunes and Moreno 2002; Qi and Mitchell 2012). Instead, research has suggested that mental rotation may correlate with English skills for deaf students who report their primary mode of communication to be ASL (Halper 2009). This relationship is thought to be secondary to the effects of sign language fluency, not deafness itself, as the previously noted mental rotation advantage is seen in both hearing and deaf ASL users, but not oral deaf individuals (Emmorey 2002; Marschark 2003; Parasnis et al. 1996). Indeed, both deaf and hearing signers appear to have enhanced mental rotation skills even when acquisition of ASL skills did not occur until early adulthood (Martin 2010, September). ASL is a spatial language that incorporates mental rotation and spatial relationships into its linguistic structure (Bosworth et al. 2003), and measurement of this ability is critical to the understanding of the complex role that mental rotation plays in learning and in language for deaf individuals.

The Mental Rotation Test

Test Characteristics

The MRT is an adapted form of the Vandenberg Mental Rotation Test (MRT: Vandenburg and Kuse 1978) that reflects both spatial organization and the ability to mentally visualize and rotate three-dimensional shapes. Shortened versions of Forms A and C of the redrawn Vandenberg Mental Rotation Test (Peters et al. 1995) were used in the present research as part of the counter-balanced battery administered within the VL2 Toolkit project. The current discussion will focus on Form A, which represented the bulk of the data.

The full version of this test is administered in two 12-item sections, each of which has a 3-min time limit. The version used in the present research consisted of one 3-min administration of the test with a total of 12 questions. On each item, participants are asked to indicate which two (out of four) shapes are the same as a target shape. Items in which both of the correct responses were indicated were scored as correct, other responses were scored as incorrect. Split half reliability on the full version of the Vandenberg Mental Rotation Test given to a comparable deaf adult sample showed a high degree of correspondence between performance on the first and second halves of the test, and patterns such as gender differences in performance and relative performance on Forms A and C were consistent with outcomes on the full test (Halper et al. 2011, June). These indicators support the use of the MRT short version as a valid representation of the abilities measured by the test.

Results

Overall, the current data on the short form of the MRT are consistent with the outcomes for the full (24 item) version of the MRT Form A as reported by Peters and colleagues, on which a sample of college students achieved a mean of 10.82 (SD 4.98). This indicates that the current sample of deaf college students is performing in a manner consistent with previous studies of hearing peers. Table 4.5 presents the descriptive statistics for the MRT.

Table 4.5 MRT, Short Form A—descriptive statistics

Test	Subtest	Range	N	Mean (SD)
Mental Rotation	Form A—short form	1–12	25	5.16 (2.97)

Table 4.6 MRT, Short Form A—significant correlations

Test	R	N
WJ-III: Reading Fluency	0.58**	24
PIAT-R: Reading Comprehension	0.42*	25
Tower of London Total Score	0.45*	25
Tower of London Total Moves	0.43*	25
Tower of London: Time Violations	0.45*	24
ASL-SRT	0.60*	15
ASL Letter Backwards Span	0.46*	25

**Significance at $p < 0.01$, *significance at $p < 0.05$

Table 4.6 presents the significant correlations between the MRT and the other Toolkit measures. Although significant relationships were observed with a relatively limited number of the Toolkit measures, as anticipated, moderate to large correlations between mental rotation and reading skills were obtained. This relationship is not typically found in hearing samples, although it is consistent with the above noted outcomes with deaf college students. Additionally, consistent with Halper (2009), the typical association with math skills was not observed with this deaf sample. In addition to the relationships with reading measures, again as expected, a strong relationship was observed with the measure of ASL skill, and moderate correlations were obtained between the MRT and one of the EF measures as well as an ASL-based measure of WM.

Of the correlations found with MRT, the strongest relationship was with the WJ-III Reading Fluency, a measure of fast, accurate reading of simple sentences. While this is consistent with Halper's (2009) research indicating a relationship between mental rotation and English skills for deaf students, it is also possible that multiple cognitive processes are common between these two tasks. For example, they may employ visualization of the items during the comprehension and decision-making process, allowing more rapid analysis of the item. As this is a timed task, this may result in an improved score. Additionally, as discussed elsewhere in this volume, having mastery of ASL as a first language may be able to support the acquisition of English print (Freel et al. 2011). Given the relationship between ASL fluency and mental rotation, it is possible that a high score on the Reading Fluency subtest could be indicative of underlying ASL fluency rather than a direct relationship between mental rotation and reading fluency.

A similar argument could be made concerning the significant relationship between the MRT and the PIAT-R Reading Comprehension subtest. While untimed, this reading comprehension task involves increased visual involvement in the task itself, as the participant must select a picture (out of four) which best represents a sentence which has been read. Thus, the processing speed demands are diminished, but there are increased demands on short-term memory. As Kelly (2003a, b) noted,

Table 4.7 Rasch Analysis Person and Item Statistics: Mental Rotation Test

	Persons	Items
Mean raw scores	4.9 (out of 12)	10.2 (out of 25)
SD of raw scores	2.7	4.6
Mean Rasch measures	−0.61	0
SE of means (for measures)	0.28	0.38
Measure range	−2.88 to 2.10	−1.45 to 2.58
# with MSq out-fit >2.0	2	1
Reliability (KR-20)	0.73	–

stronger language skills can decrease the cognitive load on WM during reading, leaving more resources for comprehension. Thus, if the MRT is reflective of ASL skills, this may partially explain the correlation seen between the MRT and this untimed reading measure.

The TOL test, as a problem-solving task, is commonly given to assess EF skills. Participants must solve visual problems in a limited amount of time, making few errors in the process in order to achieve higher scores. Phillips et al. (1999) found that mental rotation, as a component of spatial memory, plays a role in TOL success.

The ASL-SRT is a research measure of receptive ASL skills which requires a complex mixture of visual–spatial abilities, short-term memory, and motor skills to properly reproduce the sentence. Given the close relationship between ASL and mental rotation reported in previous research, it is not surprising to see a strong correlation between mental rotation and the ASL-SRT. The intervening impact of ASL skills on the ASL Letter Span task, which requires the participant to view a sequence of signed letters and repeat them in reverse order, may partially explain the correlation with this task.

Rasch Analysis

(Note: a brief explanation of the Rasch analysis procedures used in this book is provided in Chap. 3, as an introduction to the discussion of the Rasch analysis conducted on the item data for the K-BIT2.)

Table 4.7 presents the Rasch statistics for the MRT, and Fig. 4.1 presents the map of person ability and item difficulty logit scores. Figure 4.1 shows that there is considerable overlap between person abilities and item difficulties and that the range of item difficulties has a spread from −1.45 to 2.58 logits. The total range of just over four logits is considered narrow for most tests developed for Rasch analysis (Wright and Stone 1979). Table 4.7 shows that the mean ability level of participants was −.61, indicating that the MRT was a difficult test for many of the study participants. The range of ability levels for participants was from −2.88 to 2.10, and Fig. 4.1 shows that five participants had logit scores that fell below the item difficulty logit score for the easiest item on the test.

4 Measures of Visuospatial Ability

Fig. 4.1 Rasch person ability by item difficulty map: Mental Rotation Test

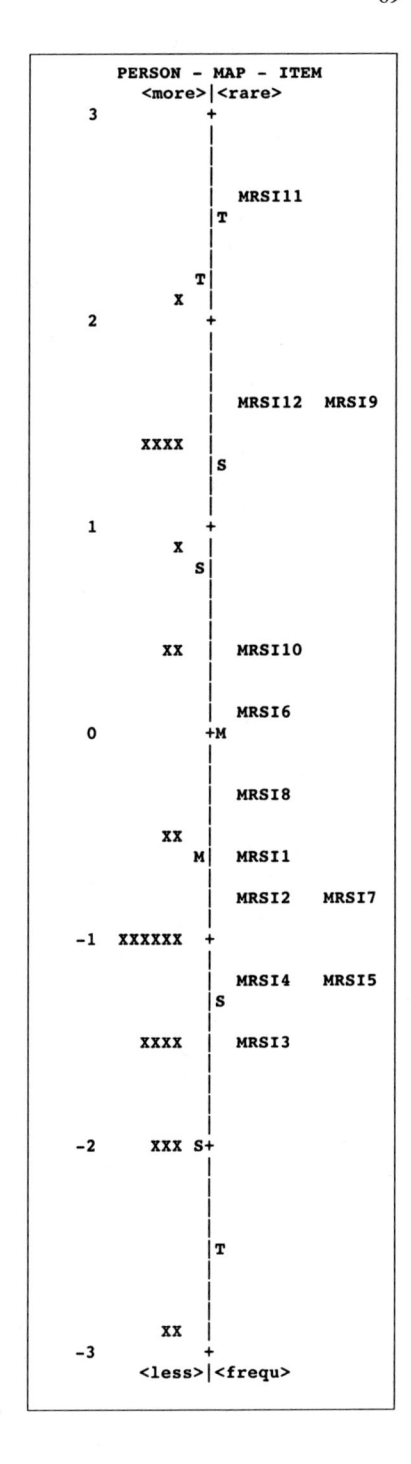

```
            PERSON - MAP - ITEM
              <more>|<rare>
         3         +
                   |
                   |
                   |
                   |  MRSI11
                   |T
                   |
                 T |
               X   |
         2         +
                   |
                   |
                   |
                   |  MRSI12   MRSI9
                   |
            XXXX   |
                   |S
                   |
         1         +
               X   |
                 S |
                   |
                   |
              XX   |  MRSI10
                   |
                   |  MRSI6
         0        +M
                   |
                   |  MRSI8
                   |
              XX   |
                 M |  MRSI1
                   |
                   |  MRSI2    MRSI7
        -1  XXXXXX +
                   |
                   |  MRSI4    MRSI5
                   |S
                   |
            XXXX   |  MRSI3
                   |
                   |
                   |
        -2   XXX  S+
                   |
                   |
                   |
                   |T
                   |
                   |
              XX   |
        -3         +
              <less>|<frequ>
```

The standard error for the Rasch person measure is 0.28 logits. This translates to a 95% confidence interval of ±0.55 logits, which is acceptable for an exploratory study (Linacre 1994). The standard error for the item difficulty measures is 0.38 logits, which is also acceptable. Table 4.7 shows that only 2 (out of 25) examinees had significant noise (Fit statistics >2) in their response patterns, as did only 1 of the 12 test items. This indicates a good "fit" of persons and items in this sample.

Finally, the KR20 reliability coefficient for this test (for these participants) is 0.73, a minimally acceptable level of internal test item consistency. In sum, this analysis reveals that the MRT was a difficult test with a narrow range of abilities measured. The standard errors for both persons and items were acceptable for an exploratory study. There was a good degree of fit between persons and items, and the internal consistency reliability was acceptable. Due to the small number of items, and the low number of participants taking this test, further research with larger samples, and, perhaps, a greater number of items covering a wider range of abilities would help to increase the test reliability and provide more stable estimates of examinee ability.

Conclusions

Overall, the data suggest that visuospatial functioning is significantly associated with literacy, ASL skills, and EF in this population. While visuospatial memory appears to have broader associations with academic functioning and linguistic memory, both English- and ASL based, the relationships with mental rotation were more restricted, focused on conceptually based reading comprehension (rather than that requiring a specific word to complete the task) and ASL skills. This suggests that while learning of this sample depends heavily on visual memory for both academic and language development (ASL and English), mental rotation has a more targeted impact on ASL skills. It is possible that the associations between mental rotation and the reading measures are mediated by ASL skills. This bears further investigation. Regardless, the associations between these visual measures and academic and linguistic functioning highlight the unique relationships among cognitive factors seen in this sample.

References

Allen, B. J., & Gfeller, J. D. (2011). The immediate post-concussion assessment and cognitive testing battery and traditional neuropsychological measures: A construct and concurrent validity study. *Brain Injury, 25*(2), 179–191.

Ariniello, L. (2000). *Gender and the brain*. Retrieved March 10, 2006, from web.sfn.org: web.sfn.org/content/Publications/BrainBrieffings/brain_lang_reading.htm.

Bavelier, D., Brozinsky, C., Tomann, A., Mitchell, T., & Liu, G. (2001). Impact of early deafness and early exposure to sign language on the cerebral organization for motion processing. *The Journal of Neuroscience, 21*(22), 8931–8942.

Bavelier, D., Dye, M. W. G., & Hauser, P. C. (2006). Do deaf individuals see better? *Trends in Cognitive Science, 10*, 512–518.
Beglinger, L. J., Duff, K., Moser, D. J., Cross, S. A., & Kareken, D. A. (2009). The Indiana Faces in Places Test: Preliminary findings on a new visuospatial memory test in patients with mild cognitive impairment. *Archives of Clinical Neuropsychology, 24*, 607–618.
Benedict, R. H. B. (1997). *Brief Visuospatial Memory Test-Revised (BVMT-R)*. Odessa, FL: The Psychological Corporation.
Benedict, R. H. B., Schretlen, D., Groninger, L., Dobraski, M., & Shpritz, B. (1996). Revision of the Brief Visuospatial Memory Test: Studies of normal performance, reliability, and validity. *Psychological Assessment, 8*, 145–153.
Bosworth, R. G., & Dobkins, K. R. (1999). Left hemisphere dominance for motion processing in deaf signers. *Psychological Science, 10*(3), 256–262.
Bosworth, R. G., & Dobkins, K. R. (2002a). Visual field asymmetries for motion processing in deaf and hearing signers. *Brain and Cognition, 49*(1), 152–169.
Bosworth, R. G., & Dobkins, K. R. (2002b). The effects of spatial selective attention on motion processing in deaf and hearing subjects. *Brain and Cognition, 49*(1), 170–181.
Bosworth, R. G., Wright, C. E., Bartlett, M. S., Corina, D. P., & Dobkins, K. R. (2003). Characterization of the visual properties of signs in ASL. In A. E. Baker, B. van den Bogaerde, & O. Crasborn (Eds.), *Cross-linguistic perspectives in sign language research*. Hamburg: Signum Press.
Casey, M. B., Nuttall, R., Pezaris, E., & Benbow, C. P. (1995). The influence of spatial ability on gender differences in mathematical college entrance test scores across diverse samples. *Developmental Psychology, 31*(4), 697–705.
Chamberlain, C., & Mayberry, R. I. (2008). ASL syntactic and narrative comprehension in skilled and less skilled adult readers: Bilingual-bimodal evidence for the linguistic basis of reading. *Applied PsychoLinguistics, 29*, 368–388.
Cohen, R. A., Poppas, A., Forman, D. E., Hoth, K. F., Haley, A. P., Gunstad, J., et al. (2009). Vascular and cognitive functions associated with cardiovascular disease in the elderly. *Journal of Clinical and Experimental Neuropsychology, 31*(1), 96–110. doi:10.1080/13803390802014594.
DeLana, M., Gentry, M., & Andrews, J. (2007). The efficacy of ASL/English bilingual education: Investigating public schools. *American Annals of the Deaf, 152*(1), 73–87.
Dror, I., & Kosslyn, S. (1994). Mental imagery and aging. *Psychology and Aging, 9*(1), 90–102.
Emmorey, K. (2002). The impact of sign language use on visuospatial cognition. In K. Emmorey (Ed.), *Language, cognition and the brain: Insights from sign language research*. Mahwah, NJ: Lawrence Erlbaum Associates.
Emmorey, K., Klima, E., & Hickok, G. (1998). Mental rotation within linguistic and non-linguistic domains in users of American Sign Language. *Cognition, 68*(3), 221–246.
Feng, J., Spence, I., & Pratt, J. (2007). Playing an action video game reduces gender differences in spatial cognition. *Psychological Science, 18*(10), 850–855.
Freel, B., Clark, D., Anderson, M., Gilbert, G., Musyoka, M., & Hauser, P. (2011). Deaf individuals' bilingual abilities: American sign language proficiency, reading skills, and family characteristics. *Psychology, 2*(1), 18–23.
Halper, E. B. (2009). *The nature of relationships between mental rotation, math, and English in deaf signers*. Doctoral dissertation. Available from Dissertations and Theses database. (UMI Number: 3388611).
Halper, E., Hall, W. C., & Morere, D. A. (2011, June). Short form of the mental rotation test with deaf participants. Poster presented at the American Academy of Clinical Neuropsychology (AACN) 9th annual conference, Washington, DC. Abstract in *The Clinical Neuropsychologist, 25*(4), 516–607.
Hauser, P. C., Cohen, J., Dye, M. W. G., & Bavelier, D. (2007). Visual constructive and visual-motor skills in deaf native signers. *Journal of Deaf Studies and Deaf Education, 12*, 148–157.
Kail, R., & Park, Y. (1990). Impact of practice on speed of mental rotation. *Journal of Experimental Child Psychology, 49*(2), 227–244.
Kail, R., Pellegrino, J., & Carter, P. (1980). Developmental changes in mental rotation. *Journal of Experimental Child Psychology, 29*, 102–116.

Kelly, L. (2003a). Considerations for designing practice for deaf readers. *Journal of Deaf Studies and Deaf Education, 8*(2), 171–186.

Kelly, L. (2003b). The importance of processing automaticity and temporary storage capacity to the differences in comprehension between skilled and less skilled college-age deaf readers. *Journal of Deaf Studies and Deaf Education, 8*(3), 230–249.

Kelly, R. (2008). Deaf learners and mathematical problem solving. In *Deaf Cognition* (pp. 226–249). New York: Oxford University Press.

Lim, W., Bardwell, W. A., Loredo, J. S., Kim, E., Ancoli-Israel, S., Morgan, E. E., et al. (2007). Neuropsychological effects of 2-week continuous positive airway pressure treatment and supplemental oxygen in patients with obstructive sleep apnea: A randomized placebo-controlled study. *Journal of Clinical Sleep Medicine, 3*(4), 380–386.

Linacre, J. M. (1994). Sample size and item calibration stability. *Rasch Measurement Transactions, 7*(4), 328.

Lubinski, D., & Benbow, C. P. (2006). Study of mathematically precocious youth after 35 years: Uncovering antecedents for the development of math-science expertise. *Perspectives on Psychological Science, 1*, 316–345.

Marschark, M. (2003). Cognitive functioning in deaf adults and children. In M. Marschark & P. Spencer (Eds.), *Oxford handbook of deaf studies, language, and education* (pp. 464–477). New York: Oxford University Press.

Martin, A. J. (2010, September). *Age of acquisition effects of American Sign Language on mental rotation*. Poster presented at the Theoretical Issues in Sign Language Research 2010 conference, West Lafayette, IN. Poster retrieved from http://www.purdue.edu/tislr10/pdfs/Martin%20AJ.pdf.

Masters, M., & Sanders, B. (1993). Is the gender difference in mental rotation disappearing? *Behavior Genetics, 23*(4), 337–341.

Moè, A., & Pazzaglia, F. (2010). Beyond genetics in mental rotation test performance: The power of effort attribution. *Learning and Individual Differences, 20*, 464–468.

Moores, D., & Sweet, C. (1990). Relationships of English grammar and communicative fluency to reading in deaf adolescents. *Exceptionality, 1*(2), 97–106.

Musselman, C. (2000). How do children who can't hear learn to read an alphabetic script? A review of the literature on reading and deafness. *Journal of Deaf Studies and Deaf Education, 5*(1), 9–31.

Neubauer, A., Bergner, S., & Schatz, M. (2010). Two- vs. three-dimensional presentation of mental rotation tasks: Sex differences and effects of training on performance and brain activation. *Intelligence, 38*(5), 529–539.

Nunes, T., & Moreno, C. (2002). An intervention program for promoting deaf pupils' achievement in mathematics. *Journal of Deaf Studies and Deaf Education, 7*(2), 120–133.

Parasnis, I., Samar, V., Bettger, J., & Sathe, K. (1996). Does deafness lead to enhancement of visual spatial cognition in children? Negative evidence from deaf nonsigners. *Journal of Deaf Studies and Deaf Education, 1*(2), 145–152.

Perfetti, C., & Sandak, R. (2000). Reading optimally builds on spoken language: Implications for deaf readers. *Journal of Deaf Studies and Deaf Education, 5*(1), 32–50.

Peters, M., Laeng, B., Latham, K., Jackson, M., Zaiyouna, R., & Richardson, C. (1995). A redrawn Vandenburg & Kuse mental rotations test: Different versions and factors that affect performance. *Brain and Cognition, 28*, 39–58.

Phillips, L., Wynn, V., Gilhooly, K., Salla, S., & Logie, R. (1999). The role of memory in the tower of london task. *Memory, 7*(2), 209–231.

Prescott, J., Gavrilescu, M., Cunnington, R., O'Boyle, M. W., & Egan, G. F. (2010). Enhanced brain connectivity in math-gifted adolescents: An fMRI study using mental rotation. *Cognitive Neuroscience, 1*(4), 277–288. doi:10.1080/17588928.2010.506951.

Qi, S., & Mitchell, R. E. (2012). Large-scale academic achievement testing of deaf and hard-of-hearing students: Past, present, and future. *Journal of Deaf Studies and Deaf Education, 17*(1), 1–18. doi:10.1093/deafed/enr028.

Shea, D., Lubinski, D., & Benbow, C. (2001). Importance of assessing spatial ability in intellectually talented young adolescents: A 20-year longitudinal study. *Journal of Educational Psychology, 93*(3), 604–614.

Shepard, R. N., & Metzler, J. (1971). Mental rotation of three-dimensional objects. *Science, 171*(3972), 701–703.

Strong, M., & Prinz, P. M. (1997). A study of the relationship between American Sign Language and English literacy. *Journal of Deaf Studies and Deaf Education, 2*(1), 37–46.

Vandenburg, S., & Kuse, A. (1978). Mental rotations, a group test of three-dimensional spatial visualization. *Perceptual and Motor Skills, 47*(2), 599–604.

Wilbur, R. P. (2000). The use of ASL to support the development of English and literacy. *Journal of Deaf Studies and Deaf Education, 5*(1), 81–104.

Wright, B. D., & Stone, M. H. (1979). *Best test design.* Chicago: MESA Press.

Chapter 5
Measures of Memory and Learning

Donna A. Morere

Learning and memory are critical components of functioning. They are required for all aspects of an individuals' interaction with the world: academic, vocational, and social. Measurement of visual memory and learning based on design reproduction is discussed in the chapter on visuospatial ability. The current chapter will focus on short-term sequential/working memory, both linguistic and visuospatial, and a sign-based list learning task.

Working/Short-Term Sequential Memory

The primary focuses of memory research in deaf populations have been short-term verbal sequential memory and working memory (WM), and more specifically linguistic sequential memory. This has largely focused on digit and letter span tasks. Research has, for the most part, demonstrated that deaf individuals as a whole perform poorly on verbal sequential recall tasks compared to data from the general population regardless of the format (signed, spoken, and print) of the stimuli and the response mode (Bellugi et al. 1975; Belmont and Karchmer 1978; Coryell 2001; Greenberg and Kusche 1987; Hanson 1982; Krakow and Hanson 1985; Liben and Drury 1977; Pintner and Paterson 1917; Tomlinson-Keasey and Smith-Winberry 1990; Waters and Doehring 1990; Wilson and Emmorey 1998). In contrast, performance of deaf subjects has been comparable to that of hearing subjects on linguistic memory tasks in which the order of recall was unimportant (Hanson 1982), and research with deaf children and adults has consistently demonstrated

---

D.A. Morere (✉)
Department of Psychology, Gallaudet University,
800 Florida Avenue, NE, Washington, DC 20002, USA
e-mail: Donna.Morere@Gallaudet.edu

sequential recall of nonlinguistic stimuli comparable to or exceeding that of hearing subjects, including sequential recall of nonlinguistic manual sequences (Tomlinson-Keasey et al. 1981; Ulissi et al. 1989), motoric reproduction of a sequence of lights (Tomlinson-Keasey and Smith-Winberry 1990), and visual–spatial memory span tasks (Geraci et al. 2008; Logan et al. 1996; Morere 1989; Wilson et al. 1997).

If deaf individuals do indeed have limited linguistic sequential or WM, this has a range of implications. For example, Hamilton (2011) in his review of memory and deaf learners suggested that this may limit the deaf individual's ability to understand syntactic order, limiting language development, and comprehension of signed or written material. Similarly, Marschark and Harris (1996) suggested that the limitations in syntactic knowledge in deaf children may relate to structures that must be held in verbal short-term memory (STM) while additional components of the message, which clarify the meaning, are received. While not definitive, a significant body of research has suggested that linguistic sequencing and WM are important for successful reading for hearing individuals (Baddeley 1986; Ellis 1990; Hansen and Bowey 1994; Levy and Carr 1990; Mann and Liberman 1984; Stanovich 1982; Torgesen et al. 1987; Wagner and Torgesen 1987). However, this is not a simple relationship as it is believed that there is a reciprocal interaction between verbal sequential processing and reading, as reading experience itself appears to promote certain cognitive functions including verbal sequential memory development (Ellis 1990; Share 1995).

There has been much controversy in the literature over the cause of the decreased linguistic spans seen in deaf signers (see Brownfeld 2010 for a recent comprehensive review). Wilson and Emmorey (1998) have proposed that a "sign length effect" similar to the word length effect seen for various spoken languages (Chincotta and Underwood 1997; Ellis and Hennelly 1980; Olazaran et al. 1996) may be occurring based on the impact of sign production time, since production of individual signs is generally more time consuming than production of individual words. However, as Gozzi et al. (2011) noted, this has not been supported by recent research. Indeed, while Wilson and Emmorey (1997) did find that sign production time affected recall for short versus long signs, when the impacts of rehearsal were controlled, the limitations in serial recall for signs did not appear to be secondary to this effect.

Other researchers have suggested that the capacities of auditory and visual WM differ, with auditory WM having a greater capacity (Boutla et al. 2004). Indeed, they found longer spoken English spans compared to American Sign Language (ASL) spans for hearing native ASL/English bilinguals, suggesting that it was the use of a visual language (ASL) rather than deafness itself which produced the shorter ASL spans. This is supported by the results of Coryell (2001), who found that deaf users of Cued Speech (CS) had linguistic spans more consistent with hearing participants on series of visually presented digits and words. Although the stimuli in the latter study were visually presented, it is assumed that the CS and hearing participants used English-based coding and rehearsal of the stimuli.

A third proposed explanation is that words or signs that are phonologically similar are harder to recall than those which are dissimilar, and since signed digits are more similar than spoken digits, this might explain the differences seen in digit spans

(Caplan and Waters 1994). Boutla and colleagues (2004) attempted to account for this by using signed letters for deaf participants compared to spoken numbers for the hearing participants, since a similar phonological similarity issue can impact letter recall for spoken letters. They suggested that neither phonological similarity nor a word length effect explained the differences and supported the modality-specific impact. However, Wilson and Emmorey (2006a) disputed this conclusion, stating that the use of digits for the hearing participants was inappropriate as recent research suggests that digits hold a unique position in STM and therefore produce higher scores despite comparable overall STM capacity. They compared printed and spoken digit and letter spans of hearing participants and spoken and signed letter spans of hearing and deaf participants, using letters which are relatively phonologically discrete for both signs and speech. Though the sample was small, they found higher digit spans for both spoken and print tasks, but comparable letter spans for speech and sign. Bavelier et al. (2006) contested these findings, suggesting that when phonological similarity of the spoken letters was reduced and speech and sign articulation rate equalized, sign spans for letters continued to be lower than those for spoken letter spans. Wilson and Emmorey (2006b) contested these results, and the controversy continued with Bavelier et al. (2008) continuing to report differential spoken and signed spans.

While the controversy continues, the preponderance of the evidence appears to support limits in sign spans compared to spoken spans, although the source of this difference continues to be unclear. In order to investigate the STM and WM (based on reverse spans), the current study used digit and letter spans, both signed and print-based. Although most previous research (with the exception of Bavelier et al. 2008) used only forward spans, both forward and reverse span tasks were used for all span tasks in this study. Similarly, while previous studies have compared tasks with spoken stimuli to those with signed or print-based stimuli, few have investigated two different visual linguistic formats (sign versus print) within a deaf signing population. This study provides the range of data that can allow for further analyses. Although forward span tasks may be considered short-term serial memory rather than WM tasks, as historically they have been combined with WM measures, for convenience these measures will be referred to as WM tasks within this chapter.

Measures of Working Memory

All of the measures of working and STM used span tasks, with the score being the number of items in the longest correctly replicated series. Thus, regardless of whether the stimuli were print-based, signed, or visuospatial, if a series of seven items were correctly reproduced, the score would be 7. The responses were recorded for later investigation, but the current analyses are restricted to the forward and reverse spans. It should be noted that while the digit and letter tasks are typically referred to as verbal memory tasks, as ASL is not a spoken language, these tasks will generally be labeled linguistic memory tasks.

Working Memory Measures: Linguistic Spans

Linguistic (verbal) immediate recall and WM are commonly measured using the ability to recall a string of numbers; either in the order given or in reversed order. Historically the forward span, or longest string of digits recalled in the correct order for the forward recall task, is seven plus or minus two (7 ± 2) for spoken English, and recent research suggests that this is also the case for phonologically discrete letters (Bavelier et al. 2006). However, Bavalier and colleagues' meta-analysis of signed letter spans in multiple studies in their lab using deaf native signers has indicated a span of approximately five, plus or minus one (5 ± 1). Previous research suggests that hearing individuals between the ages of 20 and 30 have a letter span consistent with their digit span, with a mean of 6.7 (Lezak et al. 2004) to 6.8 (Bavelier et al. 2006) for phonologically dissimilar letters.

To evaluate this area the digit and letter span tasks were administered using printed English and video-based ASL stimuli. The sign and print forms of the task were presented on separate days, with an average of approximately 1 week between the sessions. Administration of the digit and print versions of the tasks within a session was separated by at least one other task. The forward recall trial of each task was immediately followed by the backward recall trial of the task.

Print digit span forward and backward. The print digit span tasks, forward and backwards, were administered using the digit span task of the California Neuropsychology Tests (CNT; Davis et al. 1994) on a Twinhead Activecolor 486E Laptop running Windows 3.1. The digits were presented in a yellow square on a gray background. The numbers were presented, one per second, as white text within the square in the center of the screen which turns dark gray during the presentation. The numbers one through nine are then displayed in black print on yellow squares; the participants can respond either by using the mouse to click on the numbers in sequence or by typing the numbers in the appropriate sequence on the keyboard. The examiner also recorded the participant's response on a response sheet to ensure preservation of the response sequence. The participant initiates the presentation of each series by pressing the space bar. Sets of two trials of each string length were presented, the shortest of which was two digits long, increasing one digit per setup to a maximum of nine digits. No digits were repeated within a string, and no more than two consecutive numbers (e.g., 7–8) were presented within a string. The task was discontinued if the individual made an error on both trials within a set. On the forward task the participant was asked to repeat the sequence exactly as presented, while on the backward task they were instructed to reverse the sequence for the reproduction.

Print letter span forward and backward. The print letter span tasks, forward and backwards, were administered using letter lists created in the recall task of the CNT (Davis et al. 1994) on a Twinhead Activecolor 486E Laptop running Windows 3.1. The letters B, C, D, F, G, K, L, N, and S, which have low sign-based phonological similarity (Bavelier et al. 2008), were used. The letters were presented, one per second, in black print on a gray background within a blue frame in the center of the screen. The participant responded by typing the letters in the appropriate sequence on the keyboard. The examiner also recorded the participant's response on a response sheet to ensure preservation of the response sequence. Sets of two trials of each string length were presented, the shortest of which was two digits long, up to a maximum of nine letters. The task was discontinued if the individual made an error on both trials of the same length. On the forward task the participant was asked to repeat the sequence exactly as presented, while on the backward task they were instructed to reverse the sequence for the reproduction.

ASL letter and digit spans forward and backward. The ASL tasks were presented via video clips using an iMac with Mac OS X 10.4.11 software. AppleScript was used for the ASL condition of the forward and backward digit and letter span tasks. Each stimulus string was filmed as a separate video, which was presented in full screen mode using QuickTime. This approach allowed for standardized presentation of the signed stimuli. The movies showed the face and upper body of the signer who presented the digits or letters at 1-s intervals. The stimuli were signed without accompanying mouth movements to ensure that the participants based their responses on the signed stimuli rather than speechreading. The lists were signed by a Caucasian female native signer wearing a black shirt to provide contrast. The signer began and ended each letter or digit string with her arms at her sides. Digital editing software (iMovie HD) was used to crop each list to begin and end after 1.5 s. The participants responded by signing the strings in forward or reverse order, as required, with the responses recorded via videotape using a Sony Handycam Mini DV camera. The tasks were otherwise consistent with the printed forms.

Working Memory Measures: Visual/Spatial Spans

Visual (or spatial) span has been used as a visual equivalent of digit span tests (Kessels et al. 2000; Lezak et al. 2004; Vandierendonck et al. 2004). However, it should be noted that Wilde et al. (2004) determined that visual and digit span tasks have significant differences in task demands and outcomes, and may not yield analogous results. One difference they reported was the finding that although it is typical for forward spans to be longer on both tasks, longer reverse spans are more common in the normative sample for the visual task than the digit task. Even so, Park et al. (2002) determined that the two tasks are processed by separate, but closely related, visual and verbal STM stores. To evaluate spatial span, the modification of the original Corsi block task (Corsi 1972) reported by Kessels et al. (2000) was used. This is also the format used on the Wechsler Memory Scale, Third Edition (Wechsler 1997) and in previous research with deaf participants (Koo et al. 2008; Wilson et al. 1997). On this task, the individual is asked to repeat a sequence of locations indicated on an asymmetric array of blocks or locations on a computer screen. The current assessment was administered on identical spatial arrays on the manual and computer versions.

Corsi blocks manual version, forward and backward. The stimulus for the manual Corsi blocks is a square with an array of nine raised cubes. For the forward span task, the examiner touches the blocks in a sequence, one block per second.

The participant is then asked to replicate the sequence. For the backward span task, the participant is asked to repeat the sequence in reverse order. The task has a series of sets of patterns of increasing length, starting with a two item set up to a maximum series of nine blocks. No block is indicated twice in the same series. Each set has two trials, and the task continues until the participant makes an error on both trials in a set or until all of the sets are completed.

Corsi blocks computer version, forward and backward. The computer version of the spatial span task replicates this procedure using the visual span task of the CNT (Davis et al. 1994). The task presents the same array as yellow squares on a gray background. The sequence is initiated by the participant's pressing the space bar and is presented by the squares briefly turning dark gray in the order to be repeated. The sequence is repeated by the participant using a mouse to click on the squares, which briefly turn dark gray to verify their selection. As with the manual task, increasingly long pairs of sequences are presented until either all sets are presented or the participant misses both sequences in a set.

Results of Working Memory Tasks

Linguistic Spans: Print and ASL Digit/Letter Spans

Lezak et al. (2004) note that hearing individuals typically recall strings one to two digits longer in the forward sequence than when they are required to report the sequence in reverse order. Clinical observation has suggested more consistency between forward and reverse spans in deaf signers, and Wilson et al. (1997) reported comparable forward and reverse spans in deaf children. However, Brownfeld (2010) reported slight (less than one digit of mean span), but statistically significant, differences in forward and reverse spans in his study, with the forward spans being marginally longer. The current data also trend in this direction, with the forward spans averaging approximately half a digit longer than the reverse spans for all of the linguistic WM tasks.

The means for the current data, presented in Table 5.1, appear generally consistent with previous studies of deaf signers, with a mean span of 5–5.5 and standard deviations of about 1–1.5, although the forward digit span mean is marginally closer to 6 for both the print and signed administrations. Performances on the forward letter span tasks were similar to those on the digit spans.

Tables 5.2–5.9 present the significant correlations (at the $p<0.05$ or $p<0.01$ level) between the linguistic span tasks and the other VL2 Psychometric Toolkit tasks. Not surprisingly, the tasks are highly inter-correlated. Most of the linguistic span tasks have associations with some reading or other linguistic tasks and executive functioning (EF) measures. Some, but not all, of the tasks are correlated with other academic achievement tasks and the sign-based measure of learning and memory. Relationships of the specific tasks will be discussed below.

Table 5.1 Print and ASL Digit & Letters Spans—descriptive statistics

Test	Subtest	Range	N	Mean (SD)
English print	Digits Forward	3–9	45	5.71 (1.31)
	Digits Backward	0–9	45	5.07 (1.57)
	Letters Forward	3–8	36	5.58 (1.25)
	Letters Backward	3–7	35	4.97 (1.18)
ASL	Digits Forward	3–9	49	5.67 (1.25)
	Digits Backward	3–8	49	4.84 (1.21)
	Letters Forward	3–9	49	5.20 (1.22)
	Letters Backward	3–9	49	4.71 (1.49)

Table 5.2 Print Digit Forward—significant correlations

Test	r	N
WJ-III Academic Knowledge	0.31*	43
WJ-III Passage Comprehension	0.32*	43
Towers of Hanoi	0.37*	41
K-BIT2 Matrices	0.32*	45
Tower of London Total Correct	0.42**	45
Koo Phoneme Detection Test	0.33*	44
Print Letter Forward Span	0.36*	34
Print Letter Backward Span	0.48**	34
Print Digit Backward Span	0.36*	45
Corsi Blocks Computer Forward Span	0.48**	44
ASL Letter Forward Span	0.35*	45
ASL Letter Backward Span	0.35*	45
ASL Digit Forward Span	0.52**	45
ASL Digit Backward Span	0.43**	45

**Significance at $p<0.01$, *significance at $p<0.05$

Print Digits Forward. The Print Digit Forward task correlated at moderate levels with all of the other linguistic WM. Not surprisingly, the highest correlation was with the ASL Digit Span Forward. This suggests that despite the different stimulus languages, these tasks tap significantly overlapping cognitive processes. Interestingly, over the different span tasks, the correlations with the backward span tasks were generally comparable to those with the forward span tasks. As this range of WM tasks has not been studied in a single population, the implications of this lack of differential association between the forward and reverse span tasks are unclear. In addition to the correlations with the linguistic span tasks, the Print Digits Forward correlated at a moderate to high level with the forward task of the computer administered visual span task, consistent with the suggestion of Park et al. (2002), that the visual and linguistic short-term stores involve closely related cognitive processes.

Table 5.3 Print Digit Backward Span—significant correlations

Test	r	N
WJ-III Reading Fluency	0.46**	44
WJ-III Writing Fluency	0.33*	44
WJ-III Passage Comprehension	0.48**	43
PIAT-Reading	0.44**	45
WCST Total Correct	0.48**	33
WCST Total Errors	0.40*	33
WCST Perseverative Errors	0.39*	33
WCST Trials to Complete 1st set	−0.39*	33
F-A-S Animals	0.31*	45
F-A-S Food	0.31*	45
M-SVLT Delayed Cued Recall	0.34*	43
Finger Spelling Test	0.31*	45
Finger Spelling Test Fake Word	0.32*	45
TSA Percent Correct	0.48**	22
TSA Relativization	0.45*	22
Print Letter Forward Span	0.39*	34
Print Letter Backward	0.43*	34
Print Digit Forward Span	0.36*	45
ASL Letter Forward Span	0.50**	45
ASL Letter Backward Span	0.42**	45
ASL Digit Backward Span	0.47**	45

**Significance at $p \leq 0.01$, *significance at $p < 0.05$

Table 5.4 Print Letters Forward—significant correlations

Test	r	N
W-III Reading Fluency	0.53**	36
WJ-III Writing Fluency	0.50**	36
WJ-III Academic Knowledge	0.54**	35
WJ-III Passage Comprehension	0.39*	35
WJ-III Math Fluency	0.34*	36
Tower of London Total Correct	0.35*	36
Tower of London Total Moves	0.35*	36
F-A-S	0.58**	36
F-A-S Animals	0.38*	36
F-A-S Food	0.39*	36
5–1–U	0.40*	36
5–1–U Animals	0.34*	35
5–1–U Food	0.36	35
M-SVLT List A Total	0.35*	36
M-SVLT Cued Recall	0.40*	36
M-SVLT Delayed Cued Recall	0.35*	35
M-SVLT Recognition Number Correct	0.37*	35
ASL-SRT	0.45*	24
Finger Spelling Test Total Correct	0.46**	36

(continued)

Table 5.4 (continued)

Test	r	N
Finger Spelling Test Real Word	0.46**	36
Finger Spelling Test Fake Word	0.44**	36
Print Digit Forward Span	0.36*	34
Print Digit Backward Span	0.39*	34
ASL Letter Forward Span	0.64**	36
ASL Letter Backward Span	0.43**	36
ASL Digit Forward Span	0.50**	38
ASL Digit Backward Span	0.61**	36

**Significance at $p < 0.01$, *significance at $p < .05$

Table 5.5 Print Letters Backwards—significant correlations

Test	r	N
WJ-III Passage Comprehension	0.39	33
WCST Total Correct	0.51**	26
WCST Total Errors	0.58**	26
WCST Perseverative Errors	0.46	26
WCST Categories Completed	0.42	26
Towers of Hanoi	0.53**	34
K-BIT2 Matrices	0.34	35
Tower of London Total Correct	0.45	35
Tower of London Total Moves	0.35	36
M-SVLT List A Total	0.57**	35
M-SVLT List B Total	0.39	35
M-SVLT Cued Recall	0.38	35
Print Digit Forward Span	0.48**	34
Print Digit Backward Span	0.43**	34
Corsi Blocks Computer Backwards Span	0.36	35
Corsi Blocks Manual Backwards Span	0.34	35
ASL Letter Backwards Span	0.48**	35
ASL Digit Forwards Span	0.36	35

**Significance at $p < 0.01$, all others significant at $p < 0.05$

Table 5.6 ASL Digits Forward Span—significant correlations

Test	r	N
WJ-III Academic Knowledge	0.39**	46
PIAT-Reading	0.31	47
WCST Categories Completed	0.40	35
Towers of Hanoi	0.35	43
Koo Phoneme Detection Test	0.52**	46
Print Letter Forward Span	0.50**	36
Print Letter Backward Span	0.36	35
Print Digit Forward Span	0.52**	45
ASL Letter Forward Span	0.41**	49
ASL Digit Backward Span	0.40**	49

**Significance at $p < 0.01$, all others significant at $p < 0.05$

Table 5.7 ASL Digits Backward Span—significant correlations

Test	r	N
WJ-III Reading Fluency	0.29*	46
WJ-III Math Fluency	0.42**	49
PIAT-Reading	0.30*	47
WCST Total Correct	0.44**	35
WCST Categories Completed	0.38*	35
WCST Trials to Complete 1st set	−0.34*	35
Towers of Hanoi	0.30*	43
K-BIT2 Matrices	0.29*	47
F-A-S	0.37*	49
F-A-S Food	0.34*	49
ASL-SRT	0.35*	33
Finger Spelling Test Real Word	0.29*	49
TSA Percent Correct	0.44**	23
TSA Relativization Percent	0.51*	23
Print Letter Forward Span	0.61**	36
Print Digit Forward Span	0.43**	45
Print Digit Backward Span	0.47**	45
ASL Letter Forward Span	0.75**	49
ASL Letter Backward Span	0.55**	49
ASL Digit Forward Span	0.40**	49

**Significance at $p < 0.01$, *significance at $p < 0.05$

Performance on this task was also moderately associated with performance on two WJ-III tasks which involve English reading comprehension, vocabulary, and academic knowledge as well as a measure of knowledge of English phonology. While sequential recall has typically been associated with reading success in hearing populations (Baddeley 1986; Ellis 1990; Hansen and Bowey 1994; Levy and Carr 1990; Wagner and Torgesen 1987), research with deaf participants have had more mixed outcomes. In contrast to the current significant low to moderate correlation found in the current sample, Coryell (2001) did not find significant correlations between performance on verbal sequential recall tasks and the WJ Reading Comprehension subtest for a sample of signing deaf college students, although she did for deaf users of CS. On the other hand, consistent with the current data, Koo et al. (2008) found statistically significant moderate correlations between verbal sequential processing tasks and WJ Passage Comprehension for a group of deaf participants. Additionally, again consistent with the current data, they did not obtain a significant correlation between these tasks and the Test of Silent Word Reading Fluency (TOSWRF), a measure of rapid word identification. These inconsistencies suggest that while there appears to be some relationship between verbal sequential processing and reading skills in deaf college students, this relationship needs additional study in order to clarify the factors that may mediate the presence or absence of the associations seen in this population.

The Print Digit Forward task also correlated moderately with the measure of cognitive abilities and two measures of EF. While this may reflect the impact of higher order control on these measures, it should be noted that attention is also a factor in the performance of all four of these tasks. Thus, this may simply reflect the individual's management of attention and concentration rather than higher order executive control.

Print Digits Backward. Not unexpectedly, the correlations between the Print Digits Backward and other Toolkit measures, presented in Table 5.3, overlap significantly with those of the forward span of this task. It correlates significantly at moderate levels with most of the other linguistic WM tasks. In addition to the moderate relationships with reading tasks, moderate correlations were observed with measures of reading and writing fluency, rapid English-primed categorical word retrieval, knowledge of English syntax, and reception of fingerspelled words. It is not clear if this is specific to automaticity with English language structures or general linguistic fluency (regardless of the language), but higher performance on all of these measures is associated with well-developed language skills allowing for fluent word and sentence recognition, retrieval, and use.

A moderate relationship was found with a categorically cued delayed recall trial of the sign-based list recall task, possibly reflecting the influence of categorical fluency intersecting with the memory aspects of both tasks. While the backward span task also produced moderate correlations with EF tasks, in this case, all correlations were with the Wisconsin Card Sorting Test (WCST) scores, which have a greater emphasis on cognitive flexibility and inhibiting responses. This may relate to the demand of backwards span tasks that the participant inhibit the tendency to repeat the sequence in the order administered (particularly since they just completed a task on which that response was required) and hold the numbers in memory while repeating them in the reverse order. Overall, this task appears to relate to a similar set of Toolkit measures to those of the related forward span task, but adds relationships with cognitive processes specifically required for the more demanding reverse span task.

Print Letters Forward. The Print Letter Forward task correlates a broader array of measures than the Print Digit Forward task, as seen in Table 5.4. While there is significant overlap with the measures discussed above, there was a greater relationship with the signed list learning task. Additionally, this measure correlated moderately with the ASL-SRT, a task developed to measure receptive ASL skills. This suggests that for the letter-based serial recall task, both English and ASL skills provide a foundation for linguistic serial recall. Interestingly, a broader array of linguistic fluency tasks was significantly associated with this task than with the previous measure. All of the categorical fluency tasks and both the letter- and handshape-based tasks were significantly associated with this measure, with a strong correlation being observed between this task and the letter-based fluency task. The strongest relationship was with the ASL Letter Span Forward, the analogous task presented through the manual alphabet; however, while the large correlation suggests that the two tasks are closely related, the presentation in different modalities does appear to produce some differences in the task.

Table 5.8 ASL Letters Forward Span—significant correlations

Test	r	N
WJ-III Reading Fluency	0.50**	46
WJ-III Writing Fluency	0.46**	46
WJ-III Passage Comprehension	0.38**	47
WJ-III Math Fluency	0.38**	49
PIAT-Reading	0.39**	47
WCST Total Correct	0.37*	35
WCST Total Errors	0.40*	35
WCST Categories Completed	0.36*	35
Tower of London Total Correct	0.31*	49
F-A-S	0.39**	49
F-A-S Food	0.35*	49
5-1-U Food	0.33*	46
M-SVLT Delayed Cued Recall	0.42**	47
ASL-SRT	0.43*	33
Finger Spelling Test Total Correct	0.44**	49
Finger Spelling Test Real Words	0.47**	49
Finger Spelling Test Fake Words	0.36*	49
TOSWRF	0.36*	46
TSA	0.59**	23
TSA Relativization	0.58**	23
Print Letter Forward Span	0.64**	36
Print Digit Forward Span	0.35*	45
Print Digit Backward Span	0.50**	45
ASL Letter Backward Span	0.62**	49
ASL Digit Forward Span	0.41**	49
ASL Digit Backward Span	0.75**	49

**Significance at $p<0.01$, *significance at $p<0.05$

The Print Letter Forward task correlates with a wider range of linguistic tasks, both memory and non-memory, than the related digit task. This may relate to the associations between reading and related linguistic tasks and alphabetic automaticity, which would be expected to support letter recall. As with the forward print digits task, while it correlates with EF measures, this did not include the WCST. This suggests that while some degree of executive control is involved, likely associated with attention management, the key aspects of the WCST, cognitive flexibility and response inhibition, are not primary factors on this task.

Print Letters Backward. Table 5.5 presents the significant correlations between the Print Letter Forward task and the other Toolkit measures. Moderate correlations were again observed with most other WM measures, including both reverse visual span tasks. Moderate to strong associations were also found between this task and the sign-based list learning task as well as a wide range of EF measures, suggesting that this task requires significant involvement of executive control systems, including those associated with response inhibition. Interestingly, the only non-memory language measure with which this task was significantly associated was the WJ-III

5 Measures of Memory and Learning

Table 5.9 ASL Letter Backward Span—significant correlations

Test	r	N
MRT Short Form A	0.46*	25
WJ-III Reading Fluency	0.56**	46
WJ-III Writing Fluency	0.43**	46
WJ-III Academic Knowledge	0.44**	46
WJ-III Passage Comprehension	0.57**	47
PIAT-Reading	0.50**	47
WCST Total Correct	0.34*	35
K-BIT2 Matrices	0.29*	47
Tower of London Total Correct	0.33*	49
F-A-S	0.41**	49
F-A-S Food	0.39**	49
5-1-U Animals	0.39**	46
5-1-U Food	0.51**	46
M-SVLT List A Total Recall	0.40**	49
M-SVLT Cued Recall	0.31*	48
M-SVLT Delayed List A Total Recall	0.29*	48
M-SVLT Delayed Cued Recall	0.42**	47
M-SVLT Recognition Number Correct	0.35*	47
ASL-SRT	0.45**	33
Finger Spelling Test Total	0.45**	49
Finger Spelling Test Real Word	0.48**	49
Finger Spelling Test Fake Word	0.35*	49
TOSWRF	0.36*	46
TSA Percent Correct	0.49*	23
TSA Relativization Percent	0.57**	23
Print Letter Forward Span	0.43**	36
Print Letter Backward Span	0.48**	35
Print Digit Forward Span	0.35*	45
Print Digit Backward Span	0.42**	45
Corsi Blocks Manual Backward Span	0.34*	49
ASL Letter Forward Span	0.62**	49
ASL Digit Backward Span	0.55*	49

**Significance at $p<0.01$, *significance at $p<0.05$

Passage Comprehension. It is possible that since this task involves reading of paragraphs, this association may reflect some involvement of WM in the WJ-III task.

ASL Digits Forward. As the students involved in this study are expected to be bilingual in ASL and English (at least in print form), similar relationships might be expected between the other Toolkit measures and both the print- and ASL-based WM tasks. While some differences were noted, in general this appeared to be the case. This task correlates highly with both of the forward print span tasks and moderately with most of the other linguistic WM tasks. Interestingly, although this task was presented using signed numbers, as with the Print Digits Forward, it correlated significantly with the Koo Phoneme Detection Test, which measures awareness of English phonology. Measures of phonological awareness are commonly associated with digit recall in hearing populations (Hansen and Bowey 1994; Mann and Liberman 1984), and this has been associated with processing of verbal sequential information in a phonological loop (Baddeley 2000, 2003). However, this has not consistently been the case with deaf participants (Koo et al. 2008), and alternative processes related to the visual nature of the stimuli, such as sign-based encoding and rehearsal systems have been proposed (Wilson and Emmorey 1997). Thus, the processes underlying linguistic WM in deaf individuals represent a continued area of controversy (Rudner and Ronnberg 2008). In his review of studies of memory processes in deaf individuals, Hamilton (2011) concluded that while deaf individuals are less likely than their hearing peers to use phonological encoding, "When employed, phonological or articulatorily based encoding has been shown to facilitate sequential recall by deaf [individuals]" (p. 407). The correlations seen between the English phonology and WM in this study may reflect subsets of individuals within this participant population who utilize speech-based encoding to varying degrees. Further analysis of the current data may yield information about the associations between demographic factors and the outcomes of these measures. Certainly the current data provide fuel for the continued controversy in this area.

ASL Digits Backward. As with print-based reverse digit span task, the sign-based reverse digit task correlated with a wider range of Toolkit measures, including a wider array of language and reading tasks. Again consistent with its print-based form, moderate to large associations were noted with most linguistic WM tasks as were moderate correlations with the WCST scores and some verbal fluency tasks, suggesting similar associations to those previously discussed with the print-based form.

One notable difference between the outcomes of the print- and sign-based reverse digit task was the presence of both a weak, but significant association between the current task and the nonverbal intelligence measure and a moderate correlation with the ASL-SRT, which would be expected to reflect both receptive sign skills and visuospatial memory. These correlations suggest that while the print and signed forms of this task represent largely overlapping processes, the sign-based task also engages more ASL and visuospatial processing than the print-based task.

ASL Letters Forward. Interestingly, as seen in Table 5.8, the sign-based forward letter span task again mirrors the print-based equivalent in the majority of its associations. Both have significant associations with academic achievement and English language and reading tasks as well as the other linguistic WM tasks. Both also produced similar correlations with the receptive fingerspelling tasks, which require similar reception of signed letters. While both produced moderate correlations with verbal fluency and sign-based list learning tasks, fewer such correlations were observed with the current letter span task than with the print-based version. Similarly, while both versions of the forward letter span task correlated moderately with EF tasks, as on the digit span tasks, only on the signed form was the WCST represented. As with the signed reverse digit task, a moderate correlation was observed between the ASL Letters Backwards and the ASL-SRT. Thus, as with the signed digit tasks, while the sign-based letter span task appears to represent a similar set of cognitive processes to the print-based task, the signed nature of the task is reflected in its association with the measure of sign skills.

ASL Letters Backward. Consistent with the above noted similarities in Toolkit relationships between the print- and sign-based linguistic span tasks, the ASL Letter Backward Span task shares many correlational relationships with its print-based equivalent; however, this form of the task produced a much broader range of correlations. While the print-based version correlated significantly with only one measure of reading, the ASL-based form produced significant moderate to large correlations with all of the reading measure as well as other measures of English knowledge. Although both reverse letter span tasks produced significant correlations with the other WM tasks and the signed list learning task, in contrast to the print version, the signed letters backwards also correlated significantly with most measures of word/sign fluency. More notably, as with the ASL Letters Forward, this task correlated significantly with both the ASL-SRT and the receptive fingerspelling task. Furthermore, this task produced a significant correlation with the mental rotation test. These data again suggest overlapping processes measured by the print and signed forms of these tasks, but greater impact of visuospatial and sign-based reception for the sign-based measures.

Visual/Spatial Spans: Corsi Blocks Manual and Computer Version

Research has typically reflected a one to two unit lower recall for visual span tasks compared to digit spans (Lezak et al. 2004); however, clinical experience has suggested that deaf individuals may have spatial spans more consistent with their linguistic spans. In their normative study, Kessels et al. (2000) reported a mean forward span of 6.2 with a standard deviation of 1.3 compared to the commonly cited English digit span of 7 with a standard deviation of 2 originally reported by Miller (1956). As previously noted, while these types of tasks are similar to linguistic span tasks, they utilize both overlapping and unique sets of cognitive processes in the general population (Park et al. 2002; Wilde et al. 2004). Wilson et al. (1997) reported statistically significant differences in spatial spans for the deaf and hearing children in their study (5.56 and 5.00, respectively), while Koo et al. (2008) found no significant differences in the spatial spans of the deaf and hearing adult groups in their study.

As can be seen in Table 5.10, in contrast to the typical expectation in the general population, despite similar standard deviations, the mean spatial span appears to be about one unit longer than the linguistic spans for the current sample, with a mean of over six for the forward spans, and reverse spans about half a point lower for each version of the task. These data are consistent with the forward spans reported by Kessels et al. (2000) for his normative sample.

Corsi Blocks Manual Forward. As can be seen in Table 5.11, the Manual version of the Corsi blocks forward produced a single significant correlation with the Tower of London Total Correct. This is surprising, as Park et al. (2002) used the manual Corsi blocks test and found moderate to strong correlations with a wide range of tasks, including visual memory, list recall, and digit span tasks in a sample of hearing adults. While a number of the linguistic WM tasks also correlated with the Tower of London, consistent with the Park et al. study, the other tasks also produced significant correlations with other measures. It is unclear why this task yielded this

Table 5.10 Corsi Blocks Manual and Computer Version Forward and Backward Spans—descriptive statistics

Test	Subtest	Range	N	Mean (SD)
Corsi Blocks—manual	Forward	4–8	49	6.33 (1.11)
	Backward	3–9	49	5.80 (1.12)
Corsi Blocks—computer	Forward	4–8	47	6.74 (1.17)
	Backward	0–8	46	5.24 (1.52)

Table 5.11 Corsi Blocks Manual Version Forward Span—significant correlations

Test	r	N
Tower of London Total Correct	0.51**	48

**Significance at $p<0.01$

single correlation; however, as can be seen in Table 5.13, the computer version of this task yielded a larger, but still relatively small set of significant relationships. The most surprising aspect of this outcome is the lack of correlations with other WM tasks. This outcome deserves further investigation.

Corsi Blocks Manual Backward. In contrast to the limited relationships found with the forward span task, the computer administered reverse span task produced a similar set of correlations to those seen with the linguistic reverse span tasks (Table 5.12). Not unexpectedly, it produced a moderate correlation with the computer administered version of the same task. It also correlated moderately with both the print and signed reverse letter span tasks. As with the linguistic WM tasks, it correlated moderately with the EF measures, and, as with the other reverse span tasks, it produced moderate to large correlations with the WCST. Despite the lack of verbal stimuli, this task produced moderate correlations with the reading comprehension tasks as well as writing fluency and the sign-based fluency task and the associated categorical fluency tasks. It also produced weak to moderate correlations with the receptive fingerspelling tasks and the cued recall trial of the signed list learning task. Overall, despite being a visuospatial task, this measure produced a similar set of correlations to those of the linguistic WM tasks.

Corsi Blocks Computer Forward. As previously noted, while it produced more significant correlations than the computer administered forward spatial span task, relatively few correlations were obtained (Table 5.13). Not unexpectedly, it correlated with the computer administered reverse span task. Also, as with the manual reverse span task, this measure correlated moderately with both reading comprehension measures. Finally, consistent with the ASL letter and digit span forward tasks, it produced a moderate correlation with the WCST Categories Completed. As this relationship was not seen with the forward print digit and letter tasks, this may represent some aspect of visual WM.

Table 5.12 Corsi Blocks Manual Version Backward Span—significant correlations

Test	r	N
WJ-III Writing Fluency	0.32*	46
WJ-III Passage Comprehension	0.29*	47
PIAT-Reading	0.36*	47
WCST Total Correct	0.51**	35
WCST Categories Completed Raw Score	0.39*	35
WCST Trials to Complete 1st Set	−0.34*	35
Towers of Hanoi	0.39*	43
K-BIT2 Matrices	0.41**	47
Tower of London Total Correct	0.39**	49
5-1-U	0.43**	47
5-1-U Animals	0.31*	46
5-1-U Food	0.41**	46
M-SVLT Cued Recall	0.32*	48
Finger Spelling Test Total	0.29*	49
Finger Spelling Test Real Words	0.29*	49
Print Letter Backward Span	0.34*	35
Corsi Blocks Comp. Backward Span	0.42**	46
ASL Letter Backward Span	0.34*	49

**Significance at $p<0.01$, *significance at $p<0.05$

Table 5.13 Corsi Blocks Computer Version Forward—significant correlations

Test	r	N
WJ-III Passage Comprehension	0.35*	45
PIAT-Reading	0.43**	47
WCST Categories Completed	0.39*	35
Corsi Blocks Computer Backward Span	0.31*	46

**Significance at $p<0.01$, *significance at $p<0.05$

Corsi Blocks Computer Backward. The computer administered form of the visual reverse span task produced correlations with a subset of the tasks with which the equivalent manual task correlated (Table 5.14). The correlations with the reading comprehension tasks and the measure of knowledge of English syntax were again seen, as were the relationships with the EF measures, including all of the WCST scores. Not surprisingly, the other spatial span tasks except the manually administered forward span task were correlated with it, as well as two of the print-based WM tasks. Overall, despite its visual nature, this task was significantly associated with reading comprehension. This is consistent with the conclusion of Park et al., that the linguistic and visual WM processes are closely related despite their differences, and the similarities and relationships may be enhanced in deaf users of ASL.

Table 5.14 Corsi Blocks Computer Version Backward Span—significant correlations

Test	r	N
WJ-III Passage Comprehension	0.30	44
PIAT-Reading	0.36	46
WCST Total Correct	0.49**	35
WCST Total Errors	0.37	35
WCST Categories Completed	0.49**	35
WCST Trials to Complete 1stSet	0.46**	34
Towers of Hanoi	0.49**	42
K-BIT2 Matrices	0.31	46
TSA Total Percent Correct	0.59**	22
TSA Pronominalization Percent	0.44	22
Print Letter Backward Span	0.36	35
Print Digit Forward Span	0.48**	44
Corsi Blocks Computer Forward Span	0.31	46
Corsi Blocks Manual Backward Span	0.42**	46

**Significance at $p<0.01$, all others significant at $p<0.05$

Linguistic Learning and Memory

Linguistic, or verbal, memory is critical for both academic skill development and functioning on a day-to-day basis. Historically, assessment of linguistic memory in deaf individuals has depended on the use of English-based memory tasks and clinical judgment. One measure of paired recall has been published (Pollard et al. 2005), but this provides only a limited picture of the deaf person's memory. A story recall task has also been developed using ASL (Pollard et al. 2007); however, this task does not have published norms and has been studied only with individuals fluent in linguistically correct ASL and may not be appropriate to individuals who use more flexible or English-like signing. English-based measures are often not readily signed, and when stimuli must be fingerspelled due to the lack of an appropriate sign, the task is significantly altered. Additionally, while word lists are typically selected with factors such as phonological similarity controlled, the relevant signs may have formational similarities which alter the difficulty of the task. The measure selected for this study was developed specifically for signing deaf individuals and takes advantage of current technology to allow for standardized administration.

Morere Signed Verbal Learning Test

The Morere Signed Verbal Learning Test (M-SVLT) is a revision of the Signed Verbal Learning Test (SVLT) originally developed using a videotaped administration

(Morere et al. 1992). It is a list learning task similar to the California Verbal Learning Test (CVLT; Delis et al. 1987). The M-SVLT was developed to evaluate linguistic list memory in deaf users of ASL, and includes five learning trials, an interference list, and short- and long-delay free and cued recall trials followed by a recognition trial. The stimuli were selected to take into consideration not only English-based phonological and orthographic similarities, but also sign-based similarities.

Instrument Design and Administration

The SVLT was administered through video clips presented on an iMac with Mac OS X 10.4.11 software. The items were signed by a native deaf user of ASL who was videotaped presenting each list and the instructions separately. The signs were presented at 1-s intervals, with the signer's hands returning to her sides at the end of each sign. The task was administered in full screen mode using QuickTime. The participant then signed the responses, which were recorded using videotape. The examiner recorded the responses at the time, when possible, but all responses were reviewed using the videotape to ensure accurate scoring.

The instrument presents the examinee with a list of 16 items to be packed for a move (List A). The items represent four categories, with four items each from the kitchen, study/office, bedroom, and garage. The items are intermingled, and the categories are not mentioned during the learning trials. List A is presented five times, with instructions that these are the items to be packed during the week, and the participant should remember as many signs as possible in any order and repeat them following each presentation. After they finished their response, before the next trial was presented, the participant was asked if they were ready for the next movie. Following the fifth trial, the participants were presented with an interference list of 16 items which a friend would help them pack on the weekend (List B), containing 4 items each from 2 categories shared with List A, and 4 items each from 2 unshared categories. Care was taken in limiting the number of signs which were visually similar, both within and between lists. Most items on the sign lists varied by at least two parameters (e.g., handshape, location, and movement of the sign) from all other items on the list.

Following interference list (List B) recall, subjects were asked to recall List A (the things packed during the week). They were then presented with the categories of the List A rooms and asked to recall as many List A items as possible related to each category. A 20–30 min delay followed the cued recall trial during which unrelated visual activities were performed. Afterward, free recall of List A was again requested, followed by cued recall based on the room categories, and then a recognition trial, on which the participant was asked to identify items from the learning list within a set of 40 signs representing the target signs from list A. The foils represented six potential error types: (1) items from the interference list that shared categories with List A; (2) interference list items from unshared categories; (3) novel items sharing a List A category, but not formationally similar (sharing at least two parameters) to List A items; (4) novel items which shared a List A category and at least two formational parameters with one of the List A items; (5) novel items not sharing a List A category, but formationally similar to a List A sign; (6) novel items neither categorically nor formationally similar to the stimulus list.

M-SVLT Descriptive Data

Due to task and linguistic differences, a direct comparison between the results of the M-SVLT and the CVLT would not be appropriate. However, a general estimate of current participants' performance relative to the general population may be made by comparing the results obtained to the performance of young adults on the CVLT. The normative data on the original CVLT were updated in 2000 (Norman et al. 2000). The CVLT included a group of participants ages 17–40, who averaged more than 1 year of college education. This represents a sample comparable to the current participants.

On the M-SVLT, the total words recalled from the five trials for the current sample was nearly identical to the normative mean of 56.13 and standard deviation of 9.45 from the CVLT study (Table 5.15). Similarly, the current sample performed in a manner consistent with the List B recall on the CVLT on which the mean was 7.76 and standard deviation 2.16. Cued recall data were not provided for the CVLT in the updated norms, but the short-delay free recall (mean 11.69, standard deviation 2.69) and long-delay free recall (mean 12.05, standard deviation 2.78) were consistent with the outcomes on the SVLT. This suggests that given linguistic access, the deaf participants in the current study perform in a comparable manner to hearing peers on list learning tasks and retain the information learned in a manner similar to their hearing counterparts. This comparability with hearing performance on free recall tasks is consistent with previous research suggesting that while ordered linguistic recall was lower for deaf groups, recall of linguistic information not requiring retention of the sequence was comparable for deaf and hearing groups (Boutla et al. 2004; Hanson 1982). Hamilton (2011) suggests that the relative strength in the area of free recall may be valuable in learning academic information, such as learning of sets of related information in subject areas such as geography and biology.

M-SVLT Correlations

Overall, the SVLT scores correlated at moderate to high levels with each other. All of the recall trials produced significant correlations with all other recall trials, while the recognition trial correlated significantly with all four of the target list recall trials which trained the items to be recognized. All of the scores also produced significant correlations with at least one reading measure, with most producing multiple significant correlations with reading measures. Other relationships, which varied somewhat among the various SVLT subtests, include language, fluency, EF, and WM measures. These will be discussed below.

5 Measures of Memory and Learning 95

Table 5.15 Morere Signed Verbal Learning Test (M-SVLT)—descriptive statistics

Test	Subtest	Range	N	Mean (SD)
SVLT (raw scores)	List A Total (trials 1–5)	33–75	49	54.80 (9.55)
	List B Recall	2–12	49	6.65 (2.43)
	List A Short Delay Free Recall	0–16	49	10.88 (4.14)
	List A Short Delay Cued Recall	3–16	48	11.06 (2.78)
	Long Delay List A Free Recall	0–16	48	10.71 (3.87)
	Long Delay List A Cued Recall	5–16	47	11.53 (2.55)
	Recognition Total Correct	22–40	47	34.38 (4.12)

Table 5.16 M-SVLT List A Total Recall—significant correlations

Test	r	N
WJ-III Reading Fluency	0.35*	46
WJ-III Academic Knowledge	0.48**	46
WJ-III Passage Comprehension	0.40**	47
PIAT Reading	0.40**	47
WCST Total Correct	0.59**	35
WCST Categories Completed	0.45**	35
WCST Trials to Complete 1st Set	−0.35*	35
M-SVLT List B Recall	0.49**	49
M-SVLT List A Free Recall	0.48**	49
M-SVLT Cued Recall	0.62**	48
M-SVLT Delayed List A Free Recall	0.62**	48
M-SVLT Delayed Cued Recall	0.65**	47
M-SVLT Recognition Number Correct	0.52**	47
Finger Spelling Test Total Correct	0.29*	49
Finger Spelling Test Real Word	0.29*	49
Finger Spelling Test Fake Word	0.28*	49
TOSWRF	0.41**	46
Print Letter Forward Span	0.35*	36
Print Letter Backward Span	0.57**	35
ASL Letter Backward Span	0.40**	49

**Significance at $p<0.01$, *significance at $p<0.05$

List A Total Recall Correlations. Table 5.16 presents the significant correlations between the M-SVLT List A Total Recall and the other Toolkit measures. This represents the combined number of correctly recalled items over the five learning trials. Not surprisingly, the total score over the initial learning trials was correlated with the other scores on the SVLT. The strongest relationships were with the delayed recall trials, suggesting that efficiency of initial learning was associated with better later recall of the items. The strong relationships with both cued recall trials suggest that categorical organization of the items may be associated with enhanced learning of the lists.

The moderate to strong associations with the WCST may represent the memory demands involved in that EF task, or it could be associated with the need for attention and organization demands of both tasks. The associations with the linguistic WM tasks likely reflect the shared requirements for attention and short-term linguistic memory. These attention and linguistic memory demands in conjunction with the need for receptive language are also likely responsible for the weak, but significant correlations with the receptive fingerspelling tasks. Finally, consistent with research involving hearing children (Cornwall 1992), list learning was significantly correlated with all of the reading tasks. While, as previously discussed, verbal sequential memory has been implicated in reading success, this has been less studied with unordered recall, and since performance on this type of task is consistent between hearing and deaf populations, this may have implications for reading assessment and intervention in this population. Similarly, consistent with Hamilton's (2011) suggestion, this task correlated significantly with the WJ-III Academic Knowledge subtest, which is heavily influenced by vocabulary in academic subject areas including biology and social studies.

List B Recall Correlations. As the interference list, List B represents the only trial requiring the participants to remember and reproduce a different set of words. This requires the participant to suppress the list learned over the initial five trials while repeating this new list, which included some items from categories shared with List A. Interestingly, while it did correlate with one EF measure, this was not the WCST, which requires this type of response suppression and cognitive flexibility (Table 5.17). While the Towers of London do require altering strategies on each trial, the core process which these two tasks share is unclear. On the other hand, the moderate correlation with the reverse Print Letters task does suggest the WM component of analyzing information cognitively while making a decision.

Although they involved learning separate lists, the correlations between this task and the other SVLT learning and recall trials are to be expected. The other interesting relationships were the moderate correlations between this task and two fluency tasks, the WJ-III Reading Fluency and the sign-primed categorical fluency task involving foods. While language fluency is at the core of all of these tasks, it is possible that other latent relationships may underlie these associations.

List A Short-Delay Free Recall Correlations. Not unexpectedly, fewer measures correlated with the free recall of List A following the interference list than with the initial learning trials (Table 5.18). This is likely due to the fact that this trial did not require either the language reception process or the initial learning of the items, but simply the recall of the items initially learned. Thus, it is not surprising that it correlated significantly with the other List A tasks. Also, since the participant had to "deselect" the items from List B, which had been learned immediately prior to this task and which included items which shared categories with the target list, it is not surprising that a moderate correlation was obtained between these two tasks.

5 Measures of Memory and Learning

Table 5.17 M-SVLT List B—significant correlations

Test	r	N
WJ-III Reading Fluency	0.32*	46
Tower of London Total Correct	0.30*	49
5–1–U Food	0.31*	46
M-SVLT List A Total Recall	0.49**	49
M-SVLT List A Free Recall	0.36*	49
M-SVLT Cued Recall	0.39**	48
M-SVLT Delayed List A Free Recall	0.42**	48
M-SVLT Delayed Cued Recall	0.38*	47
Print Letter Backward Span	0.39*	35

**Significance at $p<0.01$, *significance at $p<0.05$

Table 5.18 M-SVLT List A Free Recall—significant correlations

Test	r	N
WJ-III Academic Knowledge	0.32	46
WJ-III Passage Comprehension	0.38**	47
PIAT-Reading	0.32	47
M-SVLT List A Total	0.48**	49
M-SVLT List B Recall	0.36	49
M-SVLT Cued Recall	0.69**	48
M-SVLT Delayed List A Free Recall	0.77**	48
M-SVLT Delayed Cued Recall	0.51**	47
Koo Phoneme Detection Test	0.31	46
Lip Reading Percent Words Correct	0.41	24

**Significance at $p<0.01$, all others significant at $p<0.05$

Interestingly, both reading comprehension tasks as well as the previously discussed WJ-III Academic Knowledge subtest also produced moderate correlations, again supporting the involvement of linguistic memory in these tasks even when the memory and learning task is sign based and the academic tasks are English based. The most interesting correlations were the moderate correlations between the English-based measures of phoneme detection and speech reading. It is unclear if these relationships represent an underlying linguistic process, attention, or some other underlying process affecting these tasks. As with many of the tasks discussed in this volume, further analyses of the current data as well as additional data collection would allow for further insight into these relationships.

List A Short-Delay Cued Recall Correlations. Interestingly, a larger set of tasks correlated significantly with the cued recall trial presented immediately following the Short-Delay Free Recall trail (Table 5.19). It correlated at moderate to high levels with all of the other SVLT subtests. Consistent with the outcomes on other

Table 5.19 M-SVLT List A Cued Recall—significant correlations

Test	r	N
WJ-III Reading Fluency	0.41**	46
WJ-III Writing Fluency	0.42**	45
WJ-III Academic Knowledge	0.42**	45
WJ-III Passage Comprehension	0.47**	46
PIAT-Reading	0.46**	46
WCST Trials to Complete 1st Task	−0.37	34
5–1–U Total	0.32	46
5–1–U Animals	0.33	45
5–1–U Food	0.46**	45
M-SLVT List A Total Recall	0.62**	48
M-SVLT List B Recall	0.38**	48
M-SVLT List A Free Recall	0.69**	48
M-SVLT Delayed List A Free Recall	0.65**	47
M-SVLT Delayed Cued Recall	0.70**	46
M-SVLT Recognition Number Correct	0.40**	46
ASL-SRT	0.44	33
Finger Spelling Test Total Correct	0.29	48
Finger Spelling Test Real Words	0.29	48
TOSWRF	0.38**	45
Print Letter Forward	0.40**	36
Print Letter Backward	0.38**	35
Corsi Blocks Manual Backward Span	0.32	48
ASL Letter Backward Span	0.31	48

**Significance at $p<0.01$, all others significant at $p<0.05$

memory measures, academic and reading tasks produced moderate correlations with this subtest. Despite the task demands, only one EF measure produced a significant correlation; however, moderate correlations were observed with one visuospatial as well as three linguistic WM tasks. The linguistic tasks all involved letters; however, despite the signed nature of the current task, two of the three linguistic WM tasks were print based. It is less surprising that significant, but weak, correlations were observed between this task and the receptive fingerspelling tasks. Perhaps the most interesting correlations were the moderate relationships seen with the sign-based verbal fluency tasks. It is possible that this relationship is related to the use of sign- and category-based search and retrieval strategies which would be important for both tasks. Previous research with hearing populations has produced moderate correlations between verbal memory tasks and measures of verbal fluency (Duff et al. 2005) using spoken English tasks, suggesting a relationship between linguistic memory and fluency independent of the specific language or modality involved.

List A Long-Delay Free Recall Correlations. A similar set of relationships to those seen with the List A Short-Delay Free Recall task were observed following a 20–30 min delay (Table 5.20). Moderate to large correlations were obtained for all

5 Measures of Memory and Learning

Table 5.20 M-SVLT Delayed List A Free Recall—significant correlations

Test	r	N
WJ-III Reading Fluency	0.42**	45
WJ-III Writing Fluency	0.37	45
WJ-III Academic Knowledge	0.43**	45
WJ-III Passage Comprehension	0.40**	46
PIAT-Reading	0.47**	46
5–1–U Food	0.41**	45
M-SVLT List A Recall	0.62**	48
M-SVLT List B Recall	0.42**	48
M-SVLT List A Free Recall	0.77**	48
M-SVLT Cued Recall	0.65**	47
M-SVLT Delayed Cued Recall	0.61**	47
M-SVLT Recognition Number Correct	0.57**	46
TSA Pronominalization Percent Correct	0.53**	23
TSA Relativization Percent Correct	0.46	23
Lip Reading Percent Words Correct	0.46	24
ASL Letter Backward Span	0.29	48

**Significance at $p<0.01$, all others significant at $p<0.05$

other SVLT scores. As with the short-delay task, significant correlations were observed with the sign-based categorical fluency task related to food as well as to measures of reading and other aspects of English knowledge and skill. While there was overlap in the measures with which the two trials correlated, there were differences. The delayed recall task correlated with a larger set of reading measures, and while both free recall tasks correlated with a measure of speechreading, the current measure correlated with a measure of English syntax while the short-delay task correlated with a measure of English phonological awareness.

List A Long-Delay Cued Recall correlations. As with the Short-Delay Cued Recall Task, this score correlated with a broad range of tasks, including all other SVLT measures and all of the reading, writing, and academic knowledge (Table 5.21). Both cued recall tasks also correlated significantly with measures of receptive fingerspelling and linguistic WM. Both also correlated with one WCST measure. Where the two diverged, is a lack of correlation with the sign-based linguistic fluency and receptive ASL tasks on the delayed trial. While receptive language may be less critical for the delayed task, language is clearly critical, the broad relationships with academic skills suggest categorically organized memory may be important for academic skill development.

Number of Recognition Correct Responses Correlations. The final SVLT task represents the ability of the participant to discriminate between the items from List A and foils represented by the above described potential errors. As with the other delayed recall tasks, it correlated significantly with reading and other language-related academic tasks (Table 5.22). It correlated significantly with all of the List A SVLT tasks, but not with the List B task. Consistent with the benefit of categorical organization for long-term memory, it correlated moderately with the two sign-primed categorical

Table 5.21 M-SVLT Delayed List A Cued Recall—significant correlations

Test	r	N
WJ-III Reading Fluency	0.40	44
WJ-III Writing Fluency	0.37	45
WJ-III Academic Knowledge	0.46**	44
WJ-III Passage Comprehension	0.35	45
PIAT-Reading	0.43**	45
WCST Total Correct	0.33	35
M-SVLT List A Total Recall	0.65**	47
M-SVLT List B Recall	0.36	47
M-SVLT List A Free Recall	0.51**	47
M-SVLT Cued Recall	0.70**	46
M-SVLT Delayed List A Free Recall	0.61**	47
M-SVLT Recognition Number Correct	0.39**	46
Finger Spelling Test Total Correct	0.31	47
Finger Spelling Test Real Words	0.30	47
Finger Spelling Test Fake Words	0.31	47
TOSWRF	0.38	44
Print Letter Forward Span	0.35	35
Print Digit Backward Span	0.34	43
ASL Letter Forward Span	0.42**	47
ASL Letter Backward Span	0.42**	47

**Significance at $p<0.01$, all others significant at $p<0.05$

Table 5.22 M-SVLT Number of Recognition Correct—significant correlations

Test	r	N
WJ-III Reading Fluency	0.42**	44
WJ-III Academic Knowledge	0.41**	44
WJ-III Passage Comprehension	0.40**	45
PIAT-Reading	0.35	45
5–1–U Animals	0.30	44
5–1–U Food	0.47**	44
M-SVLT List A Total Recall	0.52**	47
M-SVLT Cued Recall	0.40**	46
M-SVLT Delayed List A Free Recall	0.57**	46
M-SVLT Delayed Cued Recall	0.39**	46
Print Letter Forward Span	0.37	35
Corsi Blocks Computer Backward Span	0.30	44
ASL Letter Backward Span	0.35	47

**Significance at $p<0.01$, all others significant at $p<0.05$

fluency tasks. Correlations were also observed with three WM tasks, one each visual, print, and ASL. As with the other SVLT tasks, this measure appears to reflect a significant relationship between linguistic long-term memory and academic success. This occurred despite the fact that the memory task is sign based, with neither English stimuli nor responses, while the academic tasks were primarily English based.

Conclusions

Overall, these data indicate that all aspects of WM are important for academic skill development. Furthermore, linguistic learning and memory, even when ASL based, is significantly associated with a broad range of academic skills, including reading and writing as well as subject area content. While further research is certainly required, these data suggest that ASL skills may provide a route for academic skill success.

References

Baddeley, A. D. (1986). *Working memory*. New York: Clarendon.
Baddeley, A. (2000). The episodic buffer: A new component of working memory? *Trends in Cognitive Sciences, 4*, 417–423.
Baddeley, A. (2003). Working memory: Looking back and looking forward. *Nature Reviews Neuroscience, 4*, 829–839.
Bavelier, D., Newport, E. L., Hall, M. L., Supalla, T., & Boutla, M. (2006). Persistent difference in short-term memory span between sign and speech: Implications for cross-linguistic comparisons. *Psychological Science, 17*, 1090–1092.
Bavelier, D., Newport, E. L., Hall, M. L., Supalla, T., & Boutla, M. (2008). Ordered short-term memory differs in signers and speakers: Implications for models of short-term memory. *Cognition, 10*, 433–459.
Bellugi, U., Klima, E., & Siple, P. (1975). Remembering in sign. *Cognition, 3*, 93–125.
Belmont, J. M., & Karchmer, M. A. (1978). Deaf people's memory: There are problems testing special populations. In M. M. Gruneberg, P. E. Morris, & R. N. Sykes (Eds.), *Practical aspects of memory* (pp. 581–588). London: Academic.
Boutla, M., Supalla, T., Newport, E., & Bavelier, D. (2004). Short-term memory: Insights from sign language. *Nature Neuroscience, 7*, 997–1002.
Brownfeld, A. (2010). *Memory spans in the visual modality: A comparison between American Sign Language and print in deaf signers*. Doctoral dissertation. Available from ProQuest Dissertations and Theses database (UMI No. 3415574).
Caplan, D., & Waters, G. S. (1994). Articulatory length and phonological similarity in span tasks: A reply to Baddeley and Andrade. *Quarterly Journal of Experimental Psychology, 47A*, 1055–1062.
Chincotta, D., & Underwood, G. (1997). Digit span and articulatory suppression: A cross-linguistic comparison. *European Journal of Cognitive Psychology, 9*(1), 89–96.
Cornwall, A. (1992). The relationship of phonological awareness, rapid naming, and verbal memory to severe reading and spelling disability. *Journal of Learning Disabilities, 25*(8), 532–538. doi:10.1177/002221949202500808.
Corsi, P. M. (1972). *Human memory and the medial temporal region of the brain*. Doctoral dissertation. Available from ProQuest Dissertations and Theses database, AAT NK14430.
Coryell, H. R. (2001). Verbal sequential processing skills and reading ability in deaf individuals using cued speech and signed communication. *Dissertation Abstracts International, 62*(10), 4812B. UMI No. 3030003.

Davis, H. P., Bajszar, G. M., & Squire, L. R. (1994). *Colorado neuropsychology tests: Explicit memory, implicit memory and problem solving (Version 2.0) [Computer program]*. Los Angles, CA: Western Psychological Services.

Delis, D. C., Kramer, J. H., Kaplan, E., & Ober, B. A. (1987). *The California Verbal Learning Test*. San Antonio, TX: Psychological Corporation.

Duff, K., Schoenberg, M. R., Scott, J. G., & Adams, R. L. (2005). The relationship between executive functioning and verbal and visual learning and memory. *Archives of Clinical Neuropsychology, 20*, 111–122.

Ellis, N. (1990). Reading, phonological skills and short-term memory: Interactive tributaries of development. *Journal of Research in Reading, 13*(2), 107–122.

Ellis, N. C., & Hennelly, R. A. (1980). A bilingual word-length effect: Implications for intelligence testing and the relative ease of mental calculation in Welsh and English. *British Journal of Psychology, 71*, 43–51.

Geraci, C., Gozzi, M., Papagno, C., & Cecchetto, C. (2008). In R. M. de Quadros (Ed.), *Sign Languages: Spinning and unraveling the past, present and future*. Petrópolis/RJ, Brazil: Editora Arara Azul. http://www.editora-arara-azul.com.br/EstudosSurdos.php. downloaded 3/19/08.

Gozzi, M., Geraci, C., Cecchetto, C., Perugini, M., & Papagno, C. (2011). Looking for an explanation for the low sign span. Is order involved? *Journal of Deaf Studies and Deaf Education, 16*(1), 101–107.

Greenberg, M. T., & Kusche, C. A. (1987). Cognitive, personal and social development of deaf children and adolescents. In M. C. Wang, M. C. Reynolds, & H. J. Walberg (Eds.), *Handbook of special education: Research and practice* (Low incidence conditions, Vol. 3, pp. 95–129). New York: Pergamon Press.

Hamilton, H. (2011). Memory skills of deaf learners: Implications and applications. *American Annals of the Deaf, 156*(4), 402–423.

Hansen, J., & Bowey, J. A. (1994). Phonological analysis skills, verbal working memory, and reading ability in second-grade children. *Child Development, 65*(3), 938–950.

Hanson, V. L. (1982). Short-term recall by deaf signers of American Sign Language: Implications of encoding strategy for order recall. *Journal of Experimental Psychology: Learning, Memory, and Cognition, 8*(6), 572–583.

Kessels, R. P. C., van Zandvoort, M. J. E., Postma, A., Kappelle, L. J., & de Haan, E. H. F. (2000). The Corsi Block-Tapping Task: Standardization and normative data. *Applied Neuropsychology, 7*(4), 252–258.

Koo, D. S., Crain, K., LaSasso, C., & Eden, G. F. (2008). Phonological awareness and short-term memory in hearing and deaf individuals of different communication backgrounds. *Annals of the New York Academy of Sciences, 1145*, 83–99. doi:10.1196/annals.1416.025.

Krakow, A., & Hanson, V. L. (1985). Deaf signers and serial recall in the visual modality: Memory for signs, fingerspelling, and print. *Memory and Cognition, 13*, 265–272.

Levy, B. A., & Carr, T. H. (1990). Component process analysis: Conclusions and challenges. In T. H. Carr & B. A. Levy (Eds.), *Reading and its development: Component skills approaches* (pp. 423–437). San Diego: Academic Press, Inc.

Lezak, M. D., Howieson, D. B., & Loring, D. W. (2004). *Neuropsychological assessment* (4th ed.). NY: Oxford University Press.

Liben, L. S., & Drury, A. M. (1977). Short-term memory in deaf and hearing children in relation to stimulus characteristics. *Journal of Experimental Child Psychology, 24*, 60–73.

Logan, K., Maybery, M., & Fletcher, J. (1996). The short-term memory of profoundly deaf people for words, signs, and abstract spatial stimuli. *Applied Cognitive Psychology, 10*(2), 105–119.

Mann, V. A., & Liberman, I. Y. (1984). Phonological awareness and verbal short-term memory: Can they presage early reading problems? *Journal of Learning Disabilities, 17*, 592–599.

Marschark, M., & Harris, M. (1996). Success and failure in learning to read: The special case (?) of deaf children. In C. Cornoldi & J. Oakhill (Eds.), *Reading comprehension difficulties: Processes and intervention* (pp. 279–300). Mahwah, NJ: Lawrence Erlbaum Associates.

Miller, G. A. (1956). The magical number seven, plus or minus two: Some limits on our capacity for processing information. *Psychological Review, 63*, 81–97.

Morere, D. A. (1989). *Serial and simultaneous processing in deaf versus hearing adolescence.* Doctoral dissertation. Available from ProQuest Dissertations and Theses database. AAT 9009506.

Morere, D. A., Fruge', J. G., & Rehkemper, G. M. (1992, August). *Signed Verbal Learning Test: Assessing verbal memory of deaf signers.* Poster presented at the 100th Annual Convention of the American Psychological Association, Washington, DC.

Norman, M. A., Evans, J. D., Miller, W. S., & Heaton, R. K. (2000). Demographically corrected norms for the California Verbal Learning Test. *Journal of Clinical and Experimental Neuropsychology, 22*(1), 80–94.

Olazaran, J., Jacobs, D. M., & Stern, Y. (1996). Comparative study of visual and verbal short-term memory in English and Spanish speakers: Testing a linguistic hypothesis. *Journal of the International Neuropsychological Society, 2*(2), 105–110.

Park, D. C., Hedden, T., Davidson, N. S., Smith, P. K., Lautenschlager, G., & Smith, A. D. (2002). Models of visuospatial and verbal memory across the adult life span. *Psychology and Aging, 17*(2), 299–320. doi:10.1037//0882-7974.17.2.299.

Pintner, R., & Paterson, D. (1917). A comparison of deaf and hearing children in visual memory for digits. *Journal of Experimental Psychology, 2*, 76–88.

Pollard, R. Q., Jr., Rediess, S., & DeMatteo, A. (2005). Development and validation of the Signed Paired Associates Test. *Rehabilitation Psychology, 50*(3), 258–265. doi:10.1037/0090-5550.50.3.258.

Pollard, R. Q., Jr., Rediess, S., DeMatteo, A., & Lentz, E. (2007). A prose recall test using stories in American Sign Language. *Rehabilitation Psychology, 52*(1), 11–24. doi:10.1037/0090-5550.52.1.11.

Rudner, M., & Ronnberg, J. (2008). Explicit processing demands reveal language modality-specific organization of working memory. *Journal of Deaf Studies and Deaf Education, 13*(4), 466–484. doi:10.1093/deafed/enn005.

Share, D. L. (1995). Phonological recoding and self-teaching: *sine qua non* of reading acquisition. *Cognition, 55*, 151–218.

Stanovich, K. E. (1982). Individual differences in the cognitive processes of reading: I. Word decoding. *Journal of Learning Disabilities, 15*, 485–493.

Tomlinson-Keasey, C., Smith, C., & Hale, S. (1981). *Can deaf individuals process sequential material?* Paper submitted to the Ninth Annual International Neuropsychological Society, Atlanta, GA.

Tomlinson-Keasey, C., & Smith-Winberry, C. (1990). Cognitive consequence of congenital deafness. *Journal of Genetic Psychology, 151*(1), 103–115.

Torgesen, J. K., Rashotte, C. A., Greenstein, J., Houck, G., & Portes, P. (1987). Academic difficulties of learning disabled children who perform poorly on memory tasks. In H. I. Swanson (Ed.), *Memory and learning disabilities: Advances in learning and behavioral disabilities* (pp. 305–333). Greenwich, CT: JIA Press.

Ulissi, S. M., Brice, P. S., & Gibbins, S. (1989). Use of the Kaufman-assessment battery for children with the hearing impaired. *American Annuals of the Deaf, 134*, 283–286.

Vandierendonck, A., Kemps, E., Fastame, M. C., & Szmalec, A. (2004). Working memory components of the Corsi blocks task. *British Journal of Psychology, 95*, 57–79.

Wagner, R. K., & Torgesen, J. (1987). The nature of phonological processing and its causal role in the acquisition of reading skills. *Psychological Bulletin, 101*, 192–212.

Waters, G. S., & Doehring, D. G. (1990). Reading acquisition in congenitally deaf children who communicate orally: Insights from an analysis of component reading, language, and memory skills. In T. H. Carr & B. A. Levy (Eds.), *Reading and its development*. San Diego, CA: Academic.

Wechsler, D. (1997). *Wechsler Memory Scale—Third Edition: Administration and scoring manual.* San Antonio, TX: The Psychological Corporation.

Wilde, N. J., Strauss, E., & Tulsky, D. S. (2004). Memory span on the Wechsler scales. *Journal of Clinical and Experimental Neuropsychology, 26*(4), 539–549.

Wilson, M., Bettger, J. G., Niculae, I., & Klima, E. S. (1997). Modality of language shapes working memory: Evidence from digit span and spatial span in ASL signers. *Journal of Deaf Studies and Deaf Education, 2*(3), 150–160.

Wilson, M., & Emmorey, K. (1997). Working memory for sign language: A window into the architecture of the working memory system. *Journal of Deaf Studies and Deaf Education, 2*(3), 121–130.

Wilson, M., & Emmorey, K. (1998). A "word length effect" for sign language: Further evidence for the role of language in structuring working memory. *Memory and Cognition, 26*, 584–590.

Wilson, M., & Emmorey, K. (2006a). Comparing sign language and speech reveals a universal limit on short-term memory capacity. *Psychological Science, 17*(8), 682–683.

Wilson, M., & Emmorey, K. (2006b). No difference in short-term memory span between sign and speech. *Psychological Science, 17*(8), 1093–1094.

Part III
Academic Achievement

Historically, reading and academic achievement of deaf and hard of hearing (D/HOH) individuals has been limited compared to that of hearing individuals. While the range of reading skills is comparable to that of their hearing peers, D/HOH adults' average reading skills have been below expectations. The following chapters will discuss these delays and the data obtained using the VL2 Toolkit measures.

These data were collected in order to document current reading, writing, and math skills in a college age deaf sample and in order to investigate the relationships between academic achievement and parameters such as language, memory, and visuospatial functioning as well as demographic factors, which will be addressed in a later chapter. Standardized measures of academic achievement developed for the general population were used to measure academic skills. While all instructions were adapted for presentation in sign, all scoring of the tests within this section were scored in the standard manner.

Chapter 6
Measures of Reading Achievement

Donna A. Morere

Introduction

Limitations in reading skills have been a major issue in the education of deaf children for decades, with little change in the outcomes over the past half century (Allen 1994; Conrad 1970; Furth 1966; Karchmer and Mitchell 2003; Moores 2001; Moores 2009; Quigley and Kretschmer 1982). While some deaf students do excel at reading, the 1990 SAT-8 Reading Comprehension data for 18 year olds indicated that the median reading level of the profoundly deaf students yielded a grade equivalent of 3.8 and even those with a mild to moderate hearing loss averaged a grade equivalent of 5.4, and the Stanford Achievement Test, 9th Edition data are consistent with those outcomes (Holt 1993; Holt et al. 1997; Qi and Mitchell 2012). Furthermore, the majority of deaf elementary through high school aged students test at "Below Basic" levels (less than partial mastery) on reading, vocabulary, and language skills, and Basic (partial mastery) or below for math and spelling when compared to standard educational expectations (Traxler 2000). Traxler noted that a significant portion of hearing students have similar skill limitations; however, the deaf students as a whole lagged behind their hearing peers. Qi and Mitchell reviewed three decades of SAT data and found minimal change. This is consistent with previous research suggesting limited gains in reading and other academic skills over the past half century (Allen 1994; Karchmer and Mitchell 2003; Moores 2001). While Qi and Mitchell noted that there are issues with standardized testing for this population, the consistency of the data are indicative of a lack of progress in this area which needs to be better understood and addressed.

The source of this lack of reading achievement despite adequate cognitive potential has been a source of controversy. Indeed, recent papers published in journals

---

D.A. Morere (✉)
Department of Psychology, Gallaudet University,
800 Florida Avenue, NE, Washington, DC 20002, USA
e-mail: Donna.Morere@Gallaudet.edu

related to deaf education have argued for and against a range of approaches, including a focus on training in English phonology (Allen et al. 2009; Mayberry et al. 2011; Trezek et al. 2007; Wang et al. 2008); use of ASL to support literacy (Chamberlain and Mayberry 2008; Wilbur 2000); morphemic support of literacy through the use of manual English systems (Nielsen et al. 2011), and the use of fingerspelling as a bridge to reading (Haptonstall-Nykaza and Schick 2007).

Perhaps the most contentious discussion has been related to the need for training in phonological awareness. Among the proponents, Trezek et al. (2010) have presented theory, research, and curricula to support their contention, while Mayberry et al. (2011) and Allen et al. (2009) are among those who cite research suggesting that English phonology may not be a critical factor in reading skill development and propose that deaf readers may be accessing alternative pathways to reading. Additionally, it is also possible that even for those with skills in English phonology the development of phonological awareness occurs through the process of learning to read rather than as a means of basic reading skill development (Kyle and Harris 2011).

There is a significant body of research which indicates that regardless of whether phonological awareness is necessary for reading skill development, it is not *sufficient* for reading comprehension beyond the single word level (Kelly 2003a, b; Musselman 2000). Factors that affect reading comprehension include knowledge of syntax and grammar, depth and breadth of vocabulary, range of knowledge as well as topic specific knowledge, understanding of figurative language and idioms, working memory capacity, and a range of other cognitive processes (Kelly 1996, 2003a, b; Musselman 2000; Paul 2003; Schirmer and Williams 2003; Trezek et al. 2010). Imagine a reader who only knows the literal meaning of each word in the sentence attempting to understand text such as, "It was raining cats and dogs yesterday when I ran into Mary. She was sporting a killer dress with spaghetti straps in knock-your-eyes-out pink and green." Clearly word identification is inadequate for comprehension of such passages. Even something as simple and commonplace as "I threw up" could be perplexing for a reader depending on literal analysis of the words.

Research has suggested that factors which predict reading success include earlier vocabulary, speechreading, and letter-sound knowledge (Kyle and Harris 2011); speed and accuracy of word recognition (Brown and Brewer 1996; Waters and Doehring 1990); student communication skills and parental participation in education (Anita et al. 2009); processing automaticity and working memory capacity (Kelly 2003b); and early language skills in English (DesJardin et al. 2009) or ASL (Chamberlain and Mayberry 2008). The involvement of language skills in both English and ASL supports the contention of Perfetti and Sandak (2000) that a critical factor in reading achievement of deaf individuals is early access to and mastery of a first language. This is also consistent with the findings of Marschark et al. (2009) that a key factor in the academic success (or lack thereof) of college students is language skill and fluency and that the frequently discussed limitations in reading skills are actually secondary to a lack of facility with their primary language. They indicated that the deaf students may be able to access information best through reading rather than through-the-air communication, be it oral English or ASL. An interesting (and somewhat disconcerting) outcome of their study was the participants' belief that they understood more of a signed lecture than was apparent through direct measurement. A later study by Marschark et al. (2012) found that the amount of print exposure, as measured by accurate recognition of book and magazine titles (but not self-reports of time spent reading), predicted academic outcomes and English and reading skills at moderate to strong levels for deaf college students. This suggests that deaf students may depend more on reading to acquire information than their hearing peers despite difficulties they may have with reading. Additionally, these data indicate that the volume of reading affects skills in both reading and English: increased quantity of reading enhances both reading and English skills.

While a comprehensive review of the literature on reading skills of deaf individuals is not possible in this chapter, a brief summary was presented above in order to lay the groundwork for many of the factors investigated in the current study. While not all of the factors previously associated with reading skills in deaf students were investigated, it was possible to investigate the relationships of many of these factors, such as working memory, linguistic fluency, and language skills, with the following measures of reading skills.

Woodcock-Johnson III (WJ-III) Tests of Achievement

The majority of the measures of academic achievement are from the WJ-III Tests of Achievement (Woodcock et al. 2001). This is a standardized battery of educational tests, normed on a large US sample. The full achievement battery contains 22 tests that take anywhere from 3 to 12 min each to administer. In the VL2 Toolkit study, subtests from the WJ-III were used to evaluate academic skills in the areas of reading, math, writing, and general school-based knowledge. The subtests were selected to allow for appropriate administration to deaf individuals (i.e., spoken instructions, stimuli, or responses were able to be performed using ASL), with the aim of evaluating a broad spectrum of academic ability.

WJ-III Reading Fluency

Test Characteristics

The WJ-III Reading Fluency subtest measures basic reading comprehension at the sentence level. This subtest is timed and therefore reflects adequacy of both cognitive fluency and basic reading skills. The participant reads a series of brief sentences (e.g., "All cats have slimy fur.") and makes a determination of whether or not they are correct. They are told to complete as many items as possible within a 3-min period. The response is made simply by circling the correct letter to indicate a yes/no determination. Since the accuracy of the sentence depends on some world

Table 6.1 Woodcock-Johnson Tests of Achievement (WJ-III) Reading Fluency—descriptive statistics

Test	Subtest	Range	N	Mean SS (SD)
WJ-III Achievement	Reading Fluency	72–131	47	99.87 (16.45)

knowledge, the Reading Fluency subtest also evaluates the individual's general fund of information in addition to speed and accuracy of reading comprehension. As with all WJ-III measures, age-based norms were used to derive Standard Scores, which have a mean of 100 and a standard deviation of 15 using the WJ-III Normative Update Compuscore and Profiles Program (Version 3.0) (WJ-III NU Compuscore; Schrank and Woodcock 2007).

Results

As can be seen in Table 6.1, the participants' performance mean on the WJ-III Reading Fluency subtest was solidly average compared to the standard age-based norms. Although below expectations for college students, this suggests that when asked to use relatively restricted vocabulary and simple sentence structure, this sample of deaf individuals was able to read, comprehend, and make judgments about written information with the speed and accuracy expected of individuals of their age. However, based on the average performances obtained on the other toolkit reading measures, performance on more complex sentence comprehension may be weaker in the deaf population than expected of average hearing students. Individual performance ranged from nearly two standard deviations below the normative mean to two standard deviations above the mean. While the former suggests the inclusion of students who may struggle with college reading demands, the latter suggests the typical upward range of Reading Fluency expected of this population. Table 6.1 presents the descriptive statistics for the Reading Fluency subtest of the WJ-III.

As can be seen from Table 6.2, the WJ-III Reading Fluency correlated significantly with a wide range of other Toolkit measures. Consistent with the strong correlation between these two tests in the norming sample reported in the WJ-III Normative Update Technical Manual (McGrew et al. 2007), the strongest correlation (0.73) was with WJ-III Writing Fluency. These are both timed measures involving knowledge of written English, and this correlation is consistent with a strong relationship between fluency of receptive and expressive print skills. Not surprisingly, moderate correlations, in the mid- to upper-sixties, were also seen with the two untimed reading comprehension tasks. Interestingly, moderate to strong correlations were observed with the Fingerspelling Tests, with higher correlations seen with the real words compared to the pseudowords. Despite the differences in task administration, this is consistent with the correlations reported by McGrew et al. between Reading Fluency and the two spelling tests on which the Fingerspelling Test was based. This suggests that this test may tap similar constructs to those measured by the spelling tests, and the pattern of the stronger correlation with the Real Word score suggests

6 Measures of Reading Achievement

Table 6.2 Woodcock-Johnson Tests of Achievement (WJ-III) Reading Fluency—significant correlations

Test	R	N
BVMT Total Recall	0.38**	47
MRT Short Version Form A	0.58**	24
WJ-III: Writing Fluency	0.73**	46
WJ-III: Academic Knowledge	0.60**	46
WJ-III: Passage Comprehension	0.64**	44
PIAT: Reading Comprehension	0.68**	47
F-A-S	0.53**	46
F-A-S: Animals	0.55**	46
F-A-S: Food	0.55**	46
5–1–U: Animals	0.52**	45
5–1–U: Food	0.64**	45
M-SVLT List A Total Recall	0.35*	46
M-SVLT: List B Recall	0.32*	46
M-SVLT Cued Recall	0.41**	46
M-SVLT Delayed List A Recall	0.42**	45
M-SVLT Delayed Cued Recall	0.37**	44
M-SVLT Recognition # Correct	0.42**	44
ASL Sentence Reproduction Test	0.45**	32
Finger Spelling Test: Total	0.68**	46
Finger Spelling Test: Real Word	0.69**	46
Finger Spelling Test: Fake Word	0.61**	46
TOSWRF	0.44**	46
TSA Relativization Percent Correct	0.51*	22
Print Letter Forward Span	0.53**	36
Print Digit Backward Span	0.46**	44
ASL Letter Forward Span	0.50**	46
ASL Letter Backward Span	0.56**	46
ASL Digit Backward Span	0.29*	46

**Significance at $p<0.01$; *significance at $p<0.05$

that reception of the real words may be supported by reading skills and English word knowledge.

Again consistent with the correlation between Reading Fluency and a linguistic fluency task (Retrieval Fluency) on the WJ-III reported in the Technical Manual, moderate correlations were observed between Reading Fluency and the word fluency tasks, both letter based and categorical. However, significance was not achieved with the sign-based fluency task (5–1–U); again suggesting that English fluency and word retrieval support Reading Fluency. A weaker, but still moderate correlation was noted with the Test of Silent Word Reading Fluency (TOSWRF), a speeded task which requires only word recognition, not comprehension. A significant, but much weaker correlation was observed between Reading Fluency and the ASL Sentence Reproduction Test. This suggests that while knowledge of ASL can support Reading Fluency, tasks reflecting English knowledge are more strongly related to this task.

A moderate correlation was also observed with the Mental Rotation Task. This is consistent with, although slightly higher than, the correlation between Reading Fluency and the analogous task of WJ-III task of Block Rotation for the 20–39 age group reported in the manual to the WJ-III Diagnostic Supplement to the Tests of Cognitive Abilities (Schrank et al. 2003). Moderate correlations were also observed between Reading Fluency and both print and sign-based working memory tasks as well as for several scores from a sign-based list learning task (M-SVLT), suggesting that linguistic short-term/working memory and learning are both associated with Reading Fluency. A weak, but statistically significant, correlation was noted between Reading Fluency and a measure of visual memory. Interestingly, no significant correlations were observed between this task and measures of executive functioning in this sample. Overall, the correlations observed were consistent with previous research and expectations based on related research for the novel tasks examined in this study.

WJ-III Passage Comprehension

Test Characteristics

The Passage Comprehension subtest measures reading comprehension at the paragraph level by requiring the participant to produce a specific word to fill in a blank late in the paragraph. The test starts with simple, brief statements. As the test progresses, the sentence structure, vocabulary, and content become increasingly complex. Passage Comprehension relies on the integration of the words and syntax of the text combined with prior knowledge of the topic in order to derive the meaning of the paragraph and retrieve the appropriate response. The use of imagery-based strategies can enhance performance; however, both English knowledge and the participant's fund of information affect the ability to use the context of the paragraph to identify the required word. It should be noted that the participants signed their responses, and conceptually appropriate responses were scored as correct.

Results

The data presented in Table 6.3 indicate that the participants' mean performance on the WJ-III Passage Comprehension subtest was two-thirds of a standard deviation below the age-based normative mean. While this is still within the average range, it is at the lower end of that range and somewhat below expectations for typical college students. The range of the scores indicates that some students' skills are likely quite limited while others' skills are quite advanced. Thus, the outcomes of this measure suggest that the deaf students in this sample exhibit a wide range of reading comprehension skills.

Table 6.4 presents the significant correlations between the WJ-III Passage Comprehension and the other toolkit measures. In addition to the relatively high

Table 6.3 Woodcock-Johnson Tests of Academic Achievement (WJ-III) Passage Comprehension—descriptive statistics

Test	Subtest	Range	N	Mean SS (SD)
WJ-III Achievement	Passage Comprehension	69–120	47	90.32 (10.16)

Table 6.4 Woodcock-Johnson Tests of Achievement (WJ-III) Passage Comprehension—significant correlations

Test	R	N
WJ-III: Reading Fluency	0.64**	44
WJ-III: Writing Fluency	0.57**	44
WJ-III: Academic Knowledge	0.74**	44
PIAT- Reading Comprehension	0.75**	45
WCST Total Correct	0.40*	33
WCST Categories Completed	0.36*	33
F-A-S	0.44**	47
F-A-S Animals	0.51**	47
F-A-S Food	0.48**	47
5-1-U Food	0.48**	44
M-SVLT List A Total Recall	0.39**	47
M-SVLT List A Free Recall	0.38**	47
M-SVLT: Cued Recall	0.47**	46
M-SVLT Delayed List A Free Recall	0.40**	46
M-SVLT Delayed Cued Recall	0.35*	45
M-SVLT Recognition Number	0.40**	45
ASL-SRT	0.39*	33
Finger Spelling Test	0.55**	47
Finger Spelling Test: Real Word Correct	0.54**	47
Finger Spelling Test: Fake Word Correct	0.52**	47
TOSWRF	0.36*	44
TSA Percent Correct	0.45*	22
TSA Relativization Percent Correct	0.61**	22
Lip Reading Percent Words Correct	0.44*	22
Lip Reading Percent Sentences Correct	0.44*	22
Print Letter Forward Span	0.39*	35
Print Letter Backward Span	0.39*	33
Print Digit Forward Span	0.32*	43
Print Digit Backward Span	0.48**	43
Corsi Blocks Computer Forward Span	0.35*	45
Corsi Blocks Computer Backward Span	0.30*	44
Corsi Blocks Manual Backward Span	0.29*	47
ASL Letter Forward Span	0.38**	47
ASL Letter Backward Span	0.57**	47

**Significance at $p < 0.01$; *significance at $p < 0.05$

(0.64) correlation with Reading Fluency, Passage Comprehension produced strong correlations with WJ-III Academic Knowledge and the Peabody Individual Achievement Test-Revised (PIAT-R) Reading Comprehension subtests. As both are measures of reading comprehension, a strong relationship between the W-III Passage Comprehension and PIAT-R Reading Comprehension is expected. However, the strong (0.74) correlation with Academic Knowledge is higher than the reported correlations (0.55–0.58) for the comparable age groups in the WJ-III norming sample (McGrew et al. 2007). Since reading is not required for the Academic Knowledge task, it would appear that the impact of fund of information and vocabulary required for that task also has a significant impact on the performance on Passage Comprehension. This greater dependence on reading for the fund of information in the deaf sample compared to the hearing normative group is consistent with the results of the study by Marschark et al. (2009) which indicated that deaf college students depend more on print for information than their hearing peers.

A strong correlation was observed between Passage Comprehension and the Relativization score on the Test of Syntactic Ability (TSA), which reflects skills with accurate understanding of relative clauses, one of the weaker areas of the TSA for this sample. It is likely that the moderate correlation reflects the use of the more complex sentence structures only in the more advanced items on the Passage Comprehension test, reflecting the need for greater automaticity with complex sentence structures seen as critical for advanced reading comprehension by Kelly (2003b). Consistent with the normative data reported by McGrew et al. (2007), a moderate correlation was also found between Passage Comprehension and the WJ-III Writing Fluency subtest, which reflects expressive functioning in print while the Passage Comprehension reflects receptive print knowledge. Again consistent with the normative data, as with Reading Fluency, Passage Comprehension was moderately correlated with both measures of word fluency (but not sign fluency) and fingerspelling. This task produced moderate correlations with a much broader range of working memory tasks, both linguistic and visuospatial. This may again be reflective of the interaction between automaticity with reading skills and the working memory capacity which Kelly (2003b) found to be important for reading comprehension in deaf college students.

Moderate correlations were also observed with a range of scores on the signed memory and learning task as well as the measures of receptive ASL, which may reflect the participants' ability to benefit from signed input to enhance their fund of information, supporting top-down analysis of the text. Similarly, moderate correlations were observed with the scores on the measure of receptive speechreading, suggesting that the ability to use receptive oral English skills may provide similar access to incidental as well as direct learning of information. The influences of executive control, which manages the juggling of cognitive processes involved in reading cited by Kelly (2003a), were apparent in the moderate correlations with scores on the Wisconsin Card Sorting Test (WCST).

6 Measures of Reading Achievement

Table 6.5 Rasch Analysis Person and Item Statistics: Woodcock-Johnson Reading Passage Comprehension

	Persons	Items
Mean Raw Scores	33.2 (out of 47)	23.1 (out of 47)
SD of raw scores	5.0	14.1
Mean Rasch measures	0.51	0
SE of means (for measures)	0.30	0.60
Measure range	−5.53 to 5.01	−5.06 to 5.59
# with MSq out-fit >2.0	3	1
Reliability (KR-20)	0.88	–

Rasch Analysis

(Note: a brief explanation of the Rasch analysis procedures used in this book is provided in Chap. 3, as an introduction to the discussion of the Rasch analysis conducted on the item data for the K-BIT2.)

Table 6.5 presents the Rasch statistics for the Woodcock-Johnson Passage Comprehension test (WJPC), and Fig. 6.1 presents the map of person ability and item difficulty logit scores for the WJPC. Figure 6.1 shows that there are very wide ranges of both item difficulties and person abilities. As noted in Table 6.5, items range in difficulty from −5.06 to 5.59 logits (a 10.65 point spread). Person abilities range from −5.53 to 5.01 logits (an equally large 10.54 point spread), which is also an indication of considerable range in student performance. The mean Rasch measures for both persons and items are moderately close (0.51 for persons and 0 for items). The higher mean Rasch measure for persons (compared to items) is due to a clustering of very easy items at the bottom of the item logit scale.

The standard errors for the Rasch person and item measures are 0.30 and 0.60, respectively. These translate to 95% confidence intervals of ±0.59 logits and 1.18 logits, respectively. While the ±0.59 confidence interval for person ability estimates are acceptable for an exploratory study (Linacre 1994), the ±1.18 confidence interval for item parameters is reason for concern that the item difficulty parameters are highly unstable. (This could be anticipated with the high standard deviation among item scores = 14.1.) Regarding the fit to the Rasch model, Table 6.5 shows that only 3 (out of 47) participants and only 1 (out of 47) items show patterns of responses that are "noisy" (i.e., participants who either made lucky guesses to difficult items, careless responses to easy items, or who demonstrated idiosyncratic response patterns). These are excellent fit statistics for developing a Rasch-based test, but are hindered by high standard errors for the estimates of the item difficulty parameters. A study with an increased number of participants to produce more stable estimates would be warranted.

Finally, the KR20 reliability coefficient for this test (for these participants) is a very high 0.88 indicating an exceptionally high level of internal test item consistency. In sum, the WJPC test produced an acceptable array of Rasch statistics, both for persons and items, but large standard errors for the item measures caused by large performance variance and a small number of participants undermine some confidence in the results.

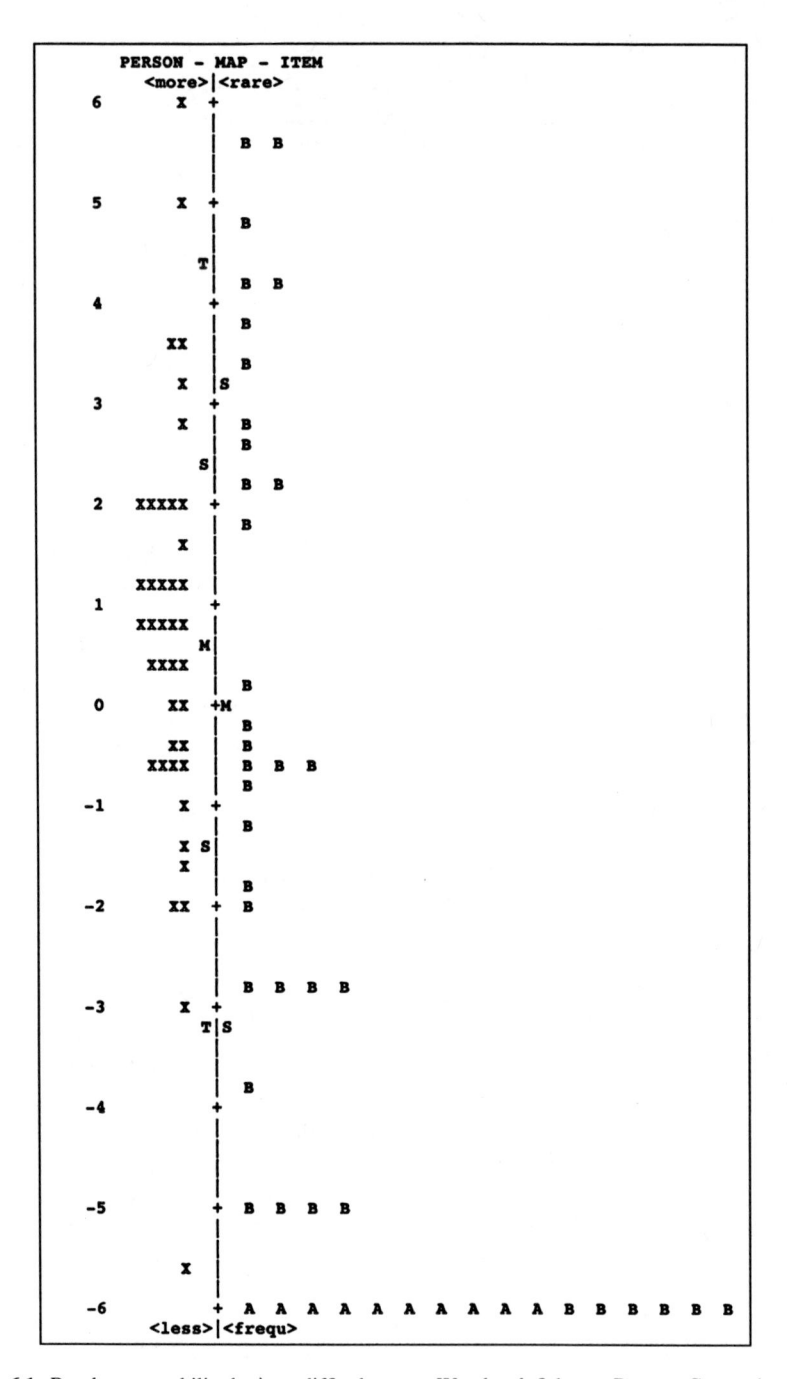

Fig. 6.1 Rasch person ability by item difficulty map: Woodcock-Johnson Passage Comprehension

Additional Reading Measures

Peabody Individual Achievement Test-Revised: Reading Comprehension

Test Characteristics

The PIAT-R (Markwardt 1998) is a measure assessing academic achievement across six broad domains that include general information, reading recognition, reading comprehension, mathematics, spelling, and written expression. Of these, only the Reading Comprehension subtest was utilized for the present research. This subtest evaluates reading comprehension at the sentence level via a nonverbal response method. Participants are required to indicate their answer by selecting one of the four pictures which best represents the meaning of the sentence they have read. This method of response avoids the impact of expressive limitations in English on the participant's ability to demonstrate understanding of English print. While the PIAT-R Reading Comprehension task is not timed, one is not allowed to look back at the sentence once the pictures are presented; thus the response must be made on their original understanding of the sentence. This task starts with simple sentences and increases in complexity as the test progresses. On the more advanced items, the sentences are designed so that erroneous interpretations are more likely based on expectations, and the foils are designed to reflect these expectations. For example, the accurate interpretation of a sentence might be that a feather is carrying a boy, and one of the foils would depict a boy carrying a feather. Errors are also designed to reflect inadequacies of vocabulary or incautious reading of a word. Thus, in the previous example another foil might be a father carrying a boy. The 1997 normative update provides grade-based norms for grades k through 12 and age-based norms for ages 5–22 years, 11 months old. For the purpose of this study, age-based norms were used, with those ages 23 and above scored based on the age 22–11 norms. As with the WJ-III, Standard Scores are used, with a mean of 100 and standard deviation of 15.

Results

The data in Table 6.6 indicate that the mean performance on the PIAT-R Reading Comprehension subtest was nearly two standard deviations below the normative mean. The scores ranged from three standard deviations below the normative mean to more than one standard deviation above. The scores obtained at the high end of this range indicate that at least a portion of the participants were able to read and understand both common sense and nonsensical items presented with complex sentence structures. However, the low end of the range indicates that a significant portion of the participants struggled with this task.

Those who struggled with this task may have made unintentional word substitutions or tried to make sense of the material based on expectations rather than accurately analyzing more complex sentence structures. This latter may be based on the tendency of deaf readers to depend on context more than their hearing counterparts (Marschark and Harris 1996), as the use of context would guide the reader to interpret sentences based on expectations when unfamiliar words are confronted and encourage the selection of foils intended to represent more likely interpretations than the nonsensical meanings of some later items.

As can be seen in Table 6.7 significant correlations were observed between the PIAT-R and large set of other Toolkit measures. Many of the correlations with other measures were closely aligned with those seen with the WJ-III Passage Comprehension, with which there was a strong correlation. For example, the correlation between the PIAT-R Reading Comprehension and the WJ-III Academic Knowledge was consistent with that between the latter measure and the WJ-III Passage Comprehension. Moderate correlations were again seen with the WJ-III Reading Fluency and Writing Fluency, Fingerspelling, particularly of real words, and TSA Relativization. Significant relationships were again observed with some working memory tasks, although in this case more sign based and visual working memory tasks were involved, perhaps reflecting the increased use of visualization and focus on general meaning of the sentence rather than the need to retrieve a specific word. The use of visualization may have also been responsible for the correlations between this test and two measures which did not correlate significantly with Passage Comprehension: the Mental Rotation Test and the K-BIT2 Matrices, both of which require visualization and visuospatial reasoning for effective performance. Additionally, a somewhat stronger relationship was observed between this test and the measure of receptive ASL, a language involving ongoing use of visualization.

However, as with the WJ-III Passage Comprehension, moderate correlations were obtained between Reading Comprehension and the sign-based list learning and speechreading scores, in addition to moderate to strong correlations with the linguistic fluency tasks. Indeed, despite the need to remember the meaning of the sentence in order to respond, the correlations with the memory tasks were generally similar to those with the WJ-III tasks. Interestingly, scores on this test correlated significantly with a broader range of scores on the WCST and an additional executive functioning task, the Towers of Hanoi. It is possible that this relates to the fact that the participant must understand the sentence and then apply it to the pictures without referring back to the text. Thus, the person must plan their anticipated response in advance of the presentation of the response options. Additionally, since some items reflect nonsensical sentences, the person cannot use general expectations and available context to guess the correct response and must inhibit the tendency to select responses that seem more likely rather than the one which accurately represents the nonsensical sentence. The impact of executive control on reading comprehension bears further investigation.

6 Measures of Reading Achievement

Table 6.6 Peabody Individual Achievement Test, Revised (PIAT-R) Reading Comprehension—descriptive statistics

Test	Subtest	Range	N	Mean SS (SD)
PIAT-R	Reading Comprehension	55–117	48	74.48 (14.59)

Table 6.7 Peabody Individual Achievement Test, Revised (PIAT-R) Reading Comprehension—significant correlations

Test	r	N
MRT Short Form A	0.42*	25
WJ-III Reading Fluency	0.68**	47
WJ-III Writing Fluency	0.61**	47
WJ-III Academic Knowledge	0.73**	47
WJ-III Passage Comprehension	0.75**	45
WCST Total Correct	0.44**	36
WCST Categories Completed	0.47**	36
WCST Trials to Complete 1st Task	−0.33*	36
Towers of Hanoi	0.40**	44
K-BIT2: Matrices	0.43**	48
F-A-S	0.36*	47
F-A-S Animals	0.48**	47
F-A-S Food	0.55**	47
5–1–U Animals	0.31*	46
5–1–U Food	0.50**	46
M-SVLT List A Total Recall	0.40**	47
M-SVLT List A Free Recall	0.32*	47
M-SVLT Cued Recall	0.45**	46
M-SVLT Delayed List A Free Recall	0.47**	46
M-SVLT Delayed Cued Recall	0.42**	45
M-SVLT Recognition Number Correct	0.35*	45
ASL Sentence Reproduction Test	0.53**	32
Finger Spelling Test Total Correct	0.61**	47
Finger Spelling Test Real Words Correct	0.61**	47
Finger Spelling Test Fake Words Correct	0.58**	47
TOSWRF	0.44**	47
TSA Percent Correct	0.55**	22
TSA Relativization Percent Correct	0.60**	22
Lip Reading Percent Words Correct	0.44*	24
Lip Reading Percent Sentences Correct	0.48*	24
Print Digit Backward Span	0.44**	45
Corsi Blocks Computer Forward Span	0.43**	47
Corsi Blocks Computer Backward Span	0.36*	46
Corsi Blocks Manual Backward Span	0.36*	47
ASL Letter Forward Span	0.39**	47
ASL Letter Backwards Span	0.50**	47
ASL Digit Forward Span	0.31*	47
ASL Digit Backward Span	0.30*	47

**Significance at $p<0.01$; *significance at $p<0.05$

Table 6.8 Rasch Analysis Person and Item Statistics: PIAT-Reading

	Persons	Items
Mean raw scores	55.6 (out of 82)	29.8 (out of 47)
SD of raw scores	14.3	13.4
Mean Rasch measures	1.37	0
SE of means (for measures)	0.31	0.31
Measure range	−2.57 to 5.90	−4.04 to 5.22
# with MSq out-fit >2.0	8	12
Reliability (KR-20)	0.96	–

Rasch Analysis

(Note: a brief explanation of the Rasch analysis procedures used in this book is provided in Chap. 3, as an introduction to the discussion of the Rasch analysis conducted on the item data for the K-BIT2.)

Table 6.8 presents the Rasch statistics for the Peabody Individual Achievement Test-Reading Comprehension (PIAT-R) and Fig. 6.2 presents the map of person ability and item difficulty logit scores for the PIAT-R. Figure 6.2 shows that there is a wide range of item difficulties, and a wide range of achievement levels among participants. As noted in Table 6.8 items range in difficulty from −4.04 to 5.22 logits, representing a large spread of over 9 logits. Person abilities range from −2.57 to 5.90 logits (a spread of 8.47 logits), which is also an indication of considerable range in ability on the PIAT-R test for this group of participants. The mean ability level for participants is 1.37 (quite a bit higher than the anchored mean of 0 for item difficulties), due to a group of easy items at the lower end of the scale, as can be seen in Fig. 6.2.

The standard errors for both the Rasch person measure and the item measure are 0.31 logits. These translate to 95% confidence intervals of ±0.61 logits, which, as with many of the other measures reported in this volume, are acceptable for an exploratory study (Linacre 1994). Regarding the fit to the Rasch model, Table 6.8 shows that 8 (out of 47) participants and 12 (out of 82) items show patterns of responses that are "noisy" (i.e., participants who either made lucky guesses to difficult items, careless responses to easy items, or who demonstrated idiosyncratic response patterns). It would certainly be worthwhile to scrutinize the characteristics of these individuals and items with poorly fitting patterns of responses.

Finally, the KR20 reliability coefficient for this test (for these participants) is 0.96, indicating an exceptionally high level of internal test item consistency. In sum, the PIAT-R provides very interesting results, given the wide variability in participant performance and in item difficulty, the large number of items, and the exceptionally high reliability, in spite of the cadres of both participants and items with poorly fitting patterns of responses. Perhaps, given the length of the test, some participants were beneficiaries of good guesses as they hastened through the more difficult items at the end of the test, or, perhaps the number of easy items on the test provoked carelessness among these items. A more provocative reason would be that there might be an

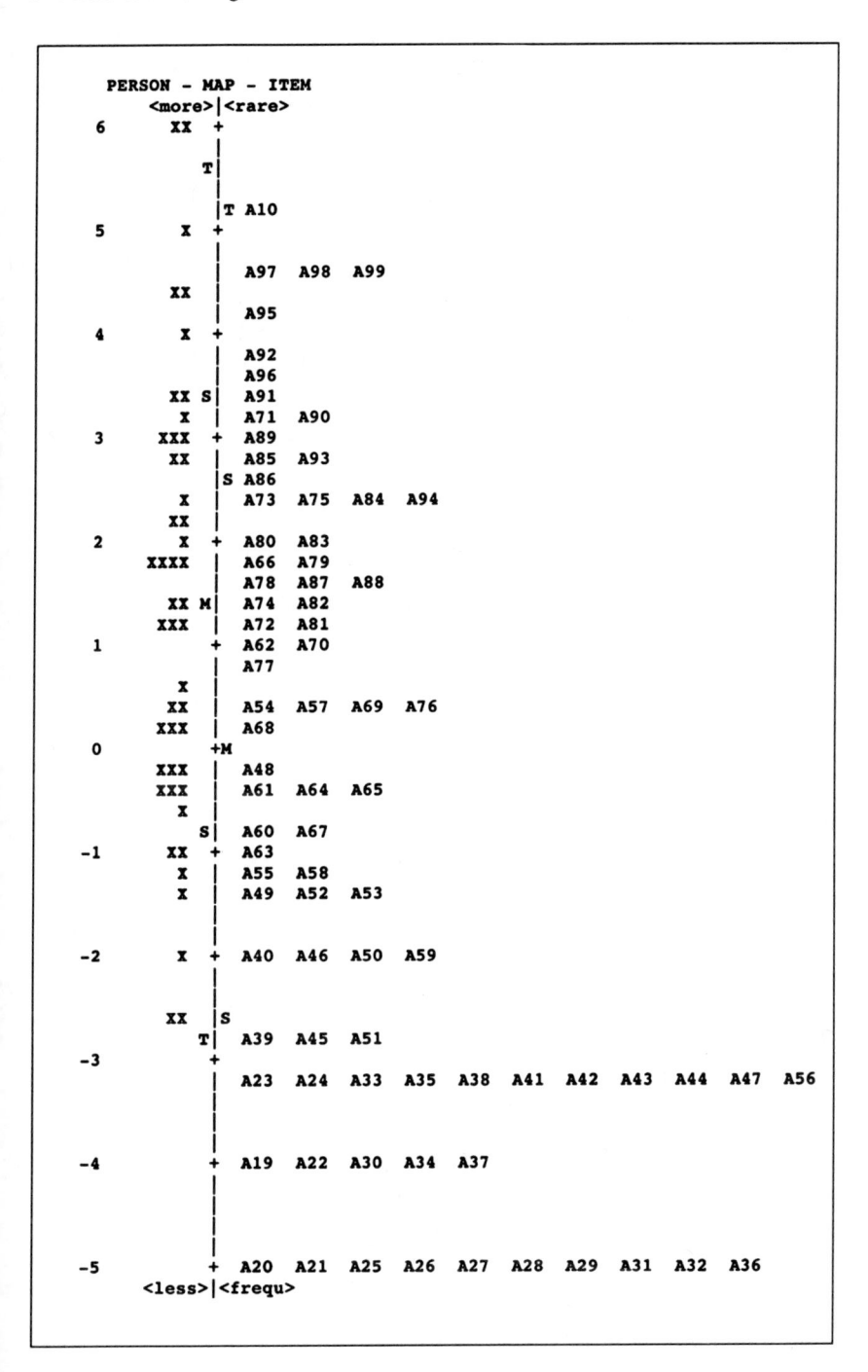

```
PERSON - MAP - ITEM
         <more>|<rare>
   6        XX  +
                |
                T|
                 |
                 |T A10
   5         X  +
                 |
                 |   A97  A98  A99
            XX   |
                 |   A95
   4         X  +
                 |   A92
                 |   A96
            XX  S|   A91
             X   |   A71  A90
   3       XXX  +   A89
            XX   |   A85  A93
                |S  A86
             X   |   A73  A75  A84  A94
            XX   |
   2         X  +   A80  A83
          XXXX   |   A66  A79
                 |   A78  A87  A88
            XX  M|   A74  A82
           XXX   |   A72  A81
   1            +   A62  A70
                 |   A77
             X   |
            XX   |   A54  A57  A69  A76
           XXX   |   A68
   0            +M
           XXX   |   A48
           XXX   |   A61  A64  A65
             X   |
                S|   A60  A67
  -1        XX  +   A63
             X   |   A55  A58
             X   |   A49  A52  A53
                 |
                 |
  -2         X  +   A40  A46  A50  A59
                 |
                 |
            XX  |S
                T|   A39  A45  A51
  -3            +
                 |   A23  A24  A33  A35  A38  A41  A42  A43  A44  A47  A56
                 |
                 |
                 |
  -4            +   A19  A22  A30  A34  A37
                 |
                 |
                 |
                 |
  -5            +   A20  A21  A25  A26  A27  A28  A29  A31  A32  A36
         <less>|<frequ>
```

Fig. 6.2 Rasch person ability by item difficulty map: PIAT-R

Table 6.9 Test of Silent Word Reading Fluency (TOSWRF)—descriptive statistics

Test	Scale	Range	N	Mean SS (SD)
TOSWRF	Total Score	70–132	47	102.51 (15.64)

element of multidimensionality to this test giving some participants either an advantage or a disadvantage to their performance due to their skills or deficits on a potential secondary dimension. Intriguingly, some of the correlational data presented in Chap. 4 on visuospatial skills suggest that this may be the case. In any event, further analysis of the Toolkit database and additional research on the use of the PIAT and its relationship to measures of other neurocognitive skills is warranted.

Test of Silent Word Reading Fluency

Test Characteristics

The TOSWRF (Mather et al. 2004) measures an individual's ability to recognize words quickly and accurately. This test presents a series of words as a string of letters without spaces to differentiate between words. The participant must identify individual words by drawing lines between the final letter of one word and initial letter of the next word in the sequence. Because the TOSWRF is a timed task, time spent on deliberation detracts from the score. The norms for this test range from ages 6 years, 6 months through 17 years, 11 months; thus, this measure was used and scored using the upper age range for students 17–0 to 17–11. Despite the potential concerns with out of age testing, this measure has been used effectively in previous research with deaf college students (e.g., Kearly 2008; Koo et al. 2008) and is considered appropriate due to its lack of oral demands and normative data through early adulthood. As with the above measures, Standard Scores with a mean of 100 and standard deviation of 15 are derived.

Results

In the present study, the participant's performance was on par with that of the normative data provided for 17-year-old students. It should be noted that because the normative group was younger than the average participant, the results might slightly overestimate the skills of the participants. Nonetheless, the outcomes presented in Table 6.9 suggest that deaf students have, at minimum, adequate recognition (as distinct from understanding of word meaning) of English words compared to typical high school seniors.

As with the other academic measures, participants' individual performances on this subtest ranged from two standard deviations below to two standard deviations above the normative mean. As with the reading measures from the WJ-III,

Table 6.10 Test of Silent Word Reading Fluency (TOSWRF)—significant correlations

Test	r	N
WJ-III Reading Fluency	0.44**	46
WJ-III Writing Fluency	0.31*	46
WJ-III Academic Knowledge	0.30*	46
WJ-III Passage Comprehension	0.36*	44
PIAT Reading	0.44**	47
WCST Total Correct	0.53**	35
WCST Total Errors	0.51**	35
WCST Categories Completed	0.59**	35
WCST Trials to Complete 1st Set	−0.36*	35
K-BIT2 Matrices	0.34*	47
F-A-S	0.29*	46
F-A-S Food	0.39**	46
5-1-U Animals	0.36*	45
5-1-U Food	0.43**	45
M-SVLT List A Total Recall	0.41**	46
M-SVLT Cued Recall	0.38**	45
M-SVLT Delayed Cued Recall	0.38*	44
ASL-SRT	0.41*	31
Finger Spelling Test Total Correct	0.53**	46
Finger Spelling Test Real Words	0.54**	46
Finger Spelling Test Fake Words	0.48**	46
TSA Percent Correct	0.46*	22
ASL Letter Forward Span	0.36*	46
ASL Letter Backward Span	0.36*	46

**Significance at $p<0.01$; *significance at $p<0.05$

this suggests that the participant population included both individuals who would likely struggle with college level reading demands, as well as those who would likely be able to perform such tasks with ease.

Table 6.10 presents the significant correlations between the TOSWRF and the other Toolkit measures. This task produced a more modest set of correlations than the previous reading measures. As both are WJ-III Reading Fluency and the TOSWRT are measures of reading with time constraints, a significant correlation between the two was expected. The fact that the WJ-III task requires comprehension and consideration of the accuracy of the sentences while the TOSWRF only requires word recognition in context may account for the moderate size of the relationship. This was also the case with the PIAT-R Reading Comprehension, although again the correlation was more modest than the strong correlation seen with a similar sample of deaf college students in the study by Kearly (2008). That study also produced moderate correlations between the TOSWRF and a rhyme-based measure of phonological awareness using pictorial stimuli, while the phonological awareness task used in the current study did not correlate with the TOSWRF. This would appear to reflect, at least to some degree, the differences in the tasks.

Consistent with the other reading measures, significant correlations were observed between this task and measures of linguistic fluency, fingerspelling, sign-based memory and learning, working memory, and receptive sign skills, although for many of these areas of functioning a smaller set of significant correlations were observed than with the other reading tasks. It should be reiterated that this task focuses on word recognition rather than comprehension, and this may be responsible for the smaller set of relationships observed. This is simply a cognitively less complex task. However, strong correlations were observed with several scores from the WCST, reflecting the executive control required to perform the visual search task, self-check prior to responding, and inhibit impulsive responses which would result in errors (e.g., marking after "in" in the string "interiordoor"). The strong relationships with the Fingerspelling Test scores may suggest that students supported their responses with fingerspelling, that alphabetic knowledge and word recognition are important for both tasks, or that both reflect an underlying facility with English.

Summary of Findings for Reading Measures

Reading in all of its forms (comprehension, word recognition, and fluency) is clearly associated with language skills, both English and ASL, in this population. Receptive language and linguistic memory as well as working memory are significant factors in reading skills. The fund of information reflected in Academic Knowledge was strongly associated with reading comprehension measures, suggesting that deaf students do indeed have an interactive relationship between reading and general knowledge. Executive functioning and linguistic fluency were also found to be important factors in reading for this sample. On the other hand, knowledge of English phonology did not appear to have a significant relationship with the reading measures in this study. This suggests that, at least for this sample of deaf college students who, for the most part, identify ASL as their primary mode of communication, the complex task of reading depends on a wide range of cognitive processes and skills, but does not appear to depend on English-based phonological awareness.

References

Allen, T. E. (1994). *Who are the deaf and hard-of-hearing students leaving high school and entering postsecondary education?* Paper submitted to Pelavin Research Institute as part of the project, *A comprehensive evaluation of postsecondary educational opportunities for students who are deaf or hard of hearing*. Available at http://research.gallaudet.edu/AnnualSurvey/whodeaf.php.

Allen, T. E., Clark, M. D., delGiudice, A., Koo, D., Lieberman, A., Mayberry, R., et al. (2009). Phonology and reading: A response to Wang, Trezek, Luckner, and Paul. *American Annals of the Deaf, 154*(4), 338–345.

Anita, S. D., Jones, P. B., Reed, S., & Kreimeyer, K. H. (2009). Academic status and progress of deaf and hard-of-hearing students in general education classrooms. *Journal of Deaf Studies and Deaf Education, 14*(3), 293–311.

Brown, P., & Brewer, L. (1996). Cognitive processes of deaf and hearing skilled and less skilled readers. *Journal of Deaf Studies and Deaf Education, 1*(4), 263–270.

Chamberlain, C., & Mayberry, R. I. (2008). ASL syntactic and narrative comprehension in skilled and less skilled adult readers: Bilingual-bimodal evidence for the linguistic basis of reading. *Applied PsychoLinguistics, 29*, 368–388.

Conrad, R. (1970). Short-term memory processes in the deaf. *British Journal of Psychology, 61*(2), 179–185.

DesJardin, J. L., Ambrose, S. E., & Eisenberg, L. S. (2009). Literacy skills in children with cochlear implants: The importance of early oral language and joint storybook reading. *Journal of Deaf Studies and Deaf Education, 14*(1), 22–43.

Furth, H. G. (1966). *Thinking without language*. New York: Free Press.

Haptonstall-Nykaza, T. S., & Schick, B. (2007). The transition from fingerspelling to English print: Facilitating English decoding. *Journal of Deaf Studies and Deaf Education, 12*, 172–183. doi:10.1093/deafed/enm003.

Holt, J. (1993). Stanford Achievement Test–8th Edition: Reading comprehension subgroup results. *American Annals of the Deaf, 138*(2), 172–175.

Holt, J. A., Traxler, C. B., & Allen, T. E. (1997). *Interpreting the scores: A user's guide to the 9th Edition Stanford Achievement Test for educators of deaf and hard-of-hearing students*. Washington, DC: Gallaudet Research Institute.

Karchmer, M. A., & Mitchell, R. E. (2003). Demographic and achievement characteristics of deaf and hard-of-hearing students. In M. Marschark & P. E. Spencer (Eds.), *Deaf studies, language, and education* (pp. 21–37). New York: Oxford University Press.

Kearly, D. J. (2008). *Eye movements of deaf readers*. Unpublished doctoral dissertation, Gallaudet University.

Kelly, L. (1996). The interaction of syntactic competence and vocabulary during reading by deaf students. *Journal of Deaf Studies and Deaf Education, 1*(1), 75–90.

Kelly, L. (2003a). Considerations for designing practice for deaf readers. *Journal of Deaf Studies and Deaf Education, 8*(2), 171–186.

Kelly, L. (2003b). The importance of processing automaticity and temporary storage capacity to the differences in comprehension between skilled and less skilled college-age deaf readers. *Journal of Deaf Studies and Deaf Education, 8*(3), 230–249.

Koo, D., Crain, K., LaSasso, C., & Eden, G. (2008). Phonological awareness and short-term memory in hearing and deaf individuals of different communication backgrounds. *Annals of the New York Academy of Sciences, 1145*, 83–99.

Kyle, F. E., & Harris, M. (2011). Longitudinal patterns of emerging literacy in beginning deaf and hearing readers. *Journal of Deaf Studies and Deaf Education, 16*(3), 289–304.

Linacre, J. M. (1994). Sample size and item calibration stability. *Rasch Measurement Transactions, 7*(4), 328.

Markwardt, F. C. (1998). *Peabody Individual Achievement Test—Revised normative update*. Minneapolis, MN: Pearson.

Marschark, M., & Harris, M. (1996). Success and failure in learning to read: The special case (?) of deaf children. In C. Cornoldi & J. Oakhill (Eds.), *Reading comprehension difficulties: Processes and intervention* (pp. 279–300). Mahwah, NJ: Lawrence Erlbaum Associates.

Marschark, M., Sapere, P., Convertino, C., Mayer, C., Wauters, L., & Sarchet, T. (2009). Are deaf students' reading challenges really about reading? *American Annals of the Deaf, 15*(4), 357–370. doi:10.1353/aad.0.0111.

Marschark, M., Sarchet, T., Convertino, C., Borgna, G., Morrison, C., & Remelt, S. (2012). Print exposure, reading habits, and reading achievement among deaf and hearing college students. *American Annals of the Deaf, 17*(1), 61–74. doi:10.1093/deafed/enr044.

Mather, N., Hammill, D. D., Allen, E. A., & Roberts, R. (2004). *Test of silent word reading fluency*. Austin, TX: PRO-ED.

Mayberry, R. I., del Giudice, A. A., & Lieberman, A. M. (2011). Reading achievement in relation to phonological coding and awareness in deaf readers: A meta-analysis. *Journal of Deaf Studies and Deaf Education, 16*(2), 164–188.

McGrew, K. S., Schrank, F. A., & Woodcock, R. W. (2007). *Technical manual, Woodcock-Johnson III normative update*. Rolling Meadows, IL: Riverside Publishing.

Moores, D. F. (2001). *Educating the deaf: Psychology, principles and practices* (5th ed.). Boston: Houghton Mifflin.

Moores, D. F. (2009). Cochlear failures. *American Annals of the Deaf, 53*(5), 423–424.

Musselman, C. (2000). How do children who can't hear learn to read an alphabetic script? A review of the literature on reading and deafness. *Journal of Deaf Studies and Deaf Education, 5*(1), 9–31.

Nielsen, D. C., Luetke, B., & Stryker, D. S. (2011). The importance of morphemic awareness to reading achievement and the potential of signing morphemes to supporting reading development. *Journal of Deaf Studies and Deaf Education, 16*(3), 275–288. doi:10.1093/deafed/enq063.

Paul, P. V. (2003). Processes and components of reading. In M. Marschark & P. E. Spencer (Eds.), *Deaf studies, language, and education* (pp. 97–109). New York: Oxford University Press.

Perfetti, C., & Sandak, R. (2000). Reading optimally builds on spoken language: Implications for deaf readers. *Journal of Deaf Studies and Deaf Education, 5*(1), 32–50.

Qi, S., & Mitchell, R. E. (2012). Large-scale academic achievement testing of deaf and hard-of-hearing students: Past, present, and future. *Journal of Deaf Studies and Deaf Education, 17*(1), 1–18. doi:10.1093/deafed/enr028.

Quigley, S., & Kretschmer, M. (1982). *The education of deaf children*. London: Edward Arnold Publishers.

Schirmer, B. R., & Williams, C. (2003). Approaches to teaching reading. In M. Marschark & P. E. Spencer (Eds.), *Deaf studies, language, and education* (pp. 110–122). New York: Oxford University Press.

Schrank, F. A., Mather, N., McGrew, K. S., & Woodcock, R. W. (2003). *Manual. Woodcock-Johnson III diagnostic supplement to the tests of cognitive abilities*. Itasca, IL: Riverside.

Schrank, F. A., & Woodcock, R. W. (2007). *WJ III normative update compuscore and profiles program (Version 3.0) [Computer software]. Woodcock-Johnson III*. Rolling Meadows, IL: Riverside.

Traxler, C. B. (2000). The Stanford Achievement Test, 9th Edition: National norming and performance standards for deaf and hard-of-hearing students. *Journal of Deaf Studies and Deaf Education, 5*, 337–348.

Trezek, B. J., Wang, Y., & Paul, P. V. (2010). *Reading and deafness: Theory, research and practice*. Clifton Park, NY: Cengage Delmar Learning.

Trezek, B. J., Wang, Y., Woods, D. G., Gampp, T. L., & Paul, P. V. (2007). Using Visual Phonics to supplement beginning reading instruction for students who are deaf/hard of hearing. *Journal of Deaf Studies and Deaf Education, 12*(3), 373–384.

Wang, Y., Trezek, B. J., Luckner, J. L., & Paul, P. V. (2008). The role of phonology and phonologically related skills in reading instruction for students who are deaf or hard of hearing. *American Annals of the Deaf, 153*(4), 396–407.

Waters, G. S., & Doehring, D. G. (1990). Reading acquisition in congenitally deaf children who communicate orally: Insights from an analysis of component reading, language, and memory skills. In T. H. Carr & B. A. Levy (Eds.), *Reading and its development*. San Diego, CA: Academic.

Wilbur, R. P. (2000). The use of ASL to support the development of English and literacy. *Journal of Deaf Studies and Deaf Education, 5*(1), 81–104.

Woodcock, R. W., McGrew, K. S., & Mather, N. (2001). *Examiner's manual. Woodcock-Johnson III Tests of Achievement*. Itasca, IL: Riverside Publishing.

Chapter 7
Measures of Writing, Math, and General Academic Knowledge

Donna A. Morere

Introduction

Despite the efforts of educators working with deaf students, academic achievement of deaf and hard of hearing individuals has been limited compared to that of hearing individuals. The majority of deaf elementary through high school aged students test at "Below Basic" levels (less than partial mastery) on reading, vocabulary, and language skills, and Basic (partial mastery) or below for math and spelling when compared to standard educational expectations (Traxler 2000). The data presented in this chapter were collected in order to document current writing and math skills and general academic knowledge in a college age deaf sample and in order to investigate the relationships between such achievement and parameters such as language, memory, and visuospatial functioning.

Standardized measures of academic achievement developed for the general population were used. While all instructions were adapted for presentation in sign, all scoring of the tests within this section were scored in the standard manner. The measures of academic achievement in this chapter are from the Woodcock-Johnson III (WJ-III) Tests of Achievement (WJ-III; Woodcock et al. 2001). This is a standardized battery of educational tests normed on a large US sample. The full achievement battery contains 22 tests that take anywhere from 3 to 12 min each to administer. In the VL2 Toolkit study, subtests from the WJ-III were used to evaluate academic skills in the areas of reading, math, writing, and general school-based knowledge. The subtests were selected to allow for appropriate administration to deaf individuals (i.e., spoken instructions, stimuli, or responses were able to be performed using ASL), with the aim of evaluating a broad spectrum of academic ability.

D.A. Morere (✉)
Department of Psychology, Gallaudet University,
800 Florida Avenue, NE, Washington, DC 20002, USA
e-mail: Donna.Morere@Gallaudet.edu

Writing

WJ-III Writing Fluency Subtest

The WJ-III Writing Fluency subtest measures the ability to quickly write a series of short, simple sentences, each of which uses a set of three words and describes a drawing. Minor errors, such as omission of articles, are allowed. This test measures both fluency and speed of writing and relies on fluid access to both the grammatical and semantic organization of words. Performance can be enhanced through practice. As with all WJ-III measures, age-based norms were used to derive Standard Scores, which have a mean of 100 and a standard deviation of 15 using the WJ-III Normative Update Compuscore and Profiles Program (Version 3.0) (WJ-III NU Compuscore; Schrank and Woodcock 2007).

Compared to the standard age-based norms, the participants' performance on WJ-III Writing Fluency subtest was in the average range. While this does not evaluate the participants' ability to produce more complex sentences or demonstrate complete accuracy in sentence construction, it does suggest that they are able to generate simple, complete sentences with the speed and general accuracy typical of individuals of their age.

As with Reading Fluency, individual performances on this subtest ranged from two standard deviations below the normative mean to more than two standard deviations above the mean. While the former suggests the inclusion of students who might expected to struggle with college writing demands, the latter suggests the typical upward range of Writing Fluency expected of college students. Table 7.1 presents the descriptive statistics for the Writing Fluency subtest of the WJ-III.

Table 7.2 presents the significant correlations between the WJ-III Writing Fluency and the other Toolkit measures. Moderate to strong correlations were observed between Writing Fluency and the WJ-III Reading Fluency, Reading Comprehension, and Academic Knowledge, as well as the PIAT-R Reading Comprehension, TSA, and TOSWRF, all of which represent English reading and vocabulary skills. The correlations with the other WJ-III tasks are consistent with, although slightly higher than, the relationships in the norming sample reported in the WJ-III Normative Update Technical Manual (McGrew et al. 2007). Generally moderate significant relationships were also obtained between this task and all of the verbal fluency measures, whether ASL or English based, again generally consistent with the relationships seen with a similar word fluency task on the WJ-III. Moderate to large significant relationships were also observed with measures of

Table 7.1 WJ-III Writing Fluency—descriptive statistics

Test	Subtest	Range	N	Mean SS (SD)
WJ-III Achievement	Writing Fluency	70–136	47	96.47 (15.90)

Table 7.2 WJ-III Writing Fluency—significant correlations

Test	r	N
WJ-III: Reading Fluency	0.73**	46
WJ-III Academic Knowledge	0.47**	46
WJ-III: Passage Comprehension	0.57**	44
PIAT-R	0.61**	47
F-A-S	0.38**	46
F-A-S: Animals	0.54**	46
F-A-S: Food	0.52**	46
5–1–U	0.29*	47
5–1–U Animals	0.32*	45
5–1–U Food	0.51**	45
M-SVLT: Cued Recall	0.42**	45
M-SVLT: Delayed List A Recall	0.37*	45
ASL Sentence Reproduction Test	0.60**	31
Finger Spelling Test: Total	0.60**	46
Finger Spelling Test: Real Word	0.60**	46
Finger Spelling Test: Fake Word	0.54**	46
TOSWRF	0.31*	46
TSA Percent Correct	0.47*	22
TSA Relativization Percent Correct	0.50*	22
Print Letter Forward Span	0.50**	36
Print Digit Backward Span	0.33*	44
Corsi Blocks Manual Backward Span	0.32*	46
ASL Letter Forward Span	0.46**	46
ASL Letter Backward Span	0.43**	46

**Significance at $p<0.01$; *significance at $p<0.05$

sign-based reception and memory tasks. These results suggest that language and linguistic fluency and memory are significantly associated with performance on this task in addition to academic skills. Finally, moderate relationships were observed with all of the measures of linguistic short term/working memory as well as visual working memory. These data support the multiple impacts of language (ASL and English), linguistic fluency and memory, and English vocabulary and literacy on the ability to perform the Writing Fluency task.

Math Skills

In addition to the issues associated with reading and writing, achievement in math has been below expectations compared to typical peers, particularly in the area of math problem solving (Kelly and Gaustad 2007; Mousley and Kelly 1998; Nunes and Moreno 2002; Traxler 2000). The source of this is unclear, but educational approaches have been implicated, in addition to potential impacts of language and differences in cognitive processing and experience (Kelly et al. 2003). These latter sources appear to

Table 7.3 WJ-III Math Fluency—descriptive statistics

Test	Subtest	Range	N	Mean SS (SD)
WJ-III Achievement	Math Fluency	69–130	49	94.45 (13.75)

be supported by the work of Kritzer (2009), who found that 4–6-year-old deaf children—even those with deaf parents and native sign skills—were behind the hearing norms on measures of early math skills. This suggests that the issues with academic achievement begin well before the students begin school, and that having deaf parents and early linguistic access alone is not enough to ensure success, at least for mathematical achievement.

WJ-III Math Fluency Subtest

The Math Fluency subtest of the WJ-III measures the ability of the participant to perform simple calculations quickly and accurately. This subtest is timed and therefore targets the speed and fluency with which one can comprehend symbolic material. Unlike higher order math, the Math Fluency subtest is designed to evaluate "Speeded (automatic) access to and application of digit-symbol arithmetic procedures" (Wendling et al. 2007, p. 2).

On the WJ-III Math Fluency subtest, the participant's performance was on par with the standard age-based norms. While this subtest does not measure calculation skill beyond single digit multiplication, it does indicate that the average participant was able to perform simple math calculations with the speed and accuracy typical of individuals of their age.

As with the other fluency tasks, individual performances on this subtest ranged from two standard deviations below the normative mean to two standard deviations above the mean. This again suggests the inclusion of students who might be expected to struggle with college level math skills as well as those who are in the typical upward range of Math Fluency expected of college students. Table 7.3 presents the descriptive statistics for the Math Fluency subtest.

Table 7.4 presents the significant correlations between the WJ-III Math Fluency and the other Toolkit measures. It is interesting that Math Fluency has relatively limited relationships with the other tests, and the associations observed appear to relate primarily to cognitive flexibility and linguistic short-term/working memory. This makes some practical sense, as Math Fluency requires the participant to quickly switch between performance of addition, subtraction, and—on later items—multiplication. Errors on this task often relate to use of the wrong math function, and individuals who struggle with cognitive flexibility may be slowed in their performance of this task even if they do not make errors. Similarly, as this requires mental math, the relation to short-term and working memory is reasonable.

Table 7.4 WJ-III Math Fluency—significant correlations

Test	r	N
WCST Perseverative Errors	0.37*	35
Print Letter Forward Span	0.33*	36
ASL Letter Forward Span	0.38**	49
ASL Digit Backward Span	0.42**	49

**Significance at $p<0.01$; *significance at $p<0.05$

General Academic Knowledge

WJ-III Academic Knowledge Subtest

The WJ-III Academic Knowledge subtest measures general academic knowledge as well as knowledge of subject specific information, including science, social studies, and geography. Participants are required to respond to each question with a word matching one of a limited set of words considered correct for each question. Thus, the nature of the response demand reflects categorical memory, subject-related vocabulary, and general knowledge of the topic. Performance on this subtest is enhanced in those who have access to language-rich and academically oriented environments (Wendling et al. 2007).

The participants' performance on the WJ-III Academic Knowledge subtest was one standard deviation below the age-based normative mean. Thus, the mean score on this test was within what is generally considered the low average range, and is well below expectations for typical college students. Despite this poor overall performance, some individual participants performed one standard deviation above the mean, suggesting both adequate knowledge and subject relevant vocabulary. However, the lower end of the range included students whose performance was approximately two and a half standard deviations below the normative mean. These participants would be expected to struggle significantly on college level content and their performance likely reflects limitations on both academic content and the relevant English vocabulary. Table 7.5 depicts the descriptive statistics for the Academic Knowledge subtest.

Table 7.6 presents the significant correlations between the WJ-III Academic Knowledge and the other Toolkit measures. This task produced significant correlations with a wide range of Toolkit measures. Strong correlations were obtained with all measures of reading comprehension and moderate correlations with most other tasks reflective of writing and English reception regardless of whether through reading, speechreading, or fingerspelling. English-based rapid word retrieval and phonological awareness were also moderately associated with this task. These data suggest that a strong background and skills in English are involved in success on this task.

The lack of a significant correlation with the ASL-SRT may relate to characteristics of that test in its current form rather than a limited impact of ASL skills, particularly in light of the broad associations found between this task and the sign-based memory and learning task, which suggest that linguistic memory is important, regardless of the language

Table 7.5 WJ-III Academic Knowledge—descriptive statistics

Test	Subtest	Range	N	Mean SS (SD)
WJ-III Achievement	Academic Knowledge	63–116	47	84.32 (11.62)

Table 7.6 WJ-III Academic Knowledge—significant correlations

Test	r	N
BVMT Total Recall	0.38**	47
WJ-III: Reading Fluency	0.60**	46
WJ-III: Writing Fluency	0.47**	46
WJ-III: Passage Comprehension	0.74**	44
PIAT- Reading Comprehension	0.73**	47
K-BIT2 Matrices	0.32*	47
F-A-S	0.41**	46
F-A-S Animals	0.44**	46
F-A-S Food	0.34*	46
M-SVLT List A Total	0.48**	46
M-SVLT List A Free Recall	0.32*	46
M-SVLT: Cued Recall	0.42**	45
M-SVLT: Delayed List A Free Recall	0.43**	45
M-SVLT: Delayed Cued Recall	0.46**	44
M-SVLT: Recognition # Correct	0.41**	44
Finger Spelling Test: Total	0.49**	46
Finger Spelling Test: Real Word	0.48*	46
Finger Spelling Test: Fake Word	0.47**	46
Koo Test of Phonological Awareness	0.44**	46
TOSWRF	0.30*	46
TSA Pronominalization Percent Correct	0.51*	22
TSA Relativization Percent Correct	0.44*	22
Lip Reading Percent Words Correct	0.43*	24
Lip Reading Percent Sentences Correct	0.42*	24
Print Letter Forward Span	0.54**	35
Print Digit Forward Span	0.31*	44
Print Digit Backward Span	0.36*	44
ASL Letter Backward Span	0.44**	46
ASL Digit Forward Span	0.39**	46

**Significance at $p<0.01$; *significance at $p<0.05$

involved. Similarly, moderate significant relationships were observed between this task and measures of linguistic immediate recall and working memory, both ASL and English, despite a lack of significant relationships with similar tasks using visuospatial stimuli.

Overall, the relationships between the Academic Fluency task and other Toolkit measures suggest that English skills, particularly reading comprehension and English reception, as well as all aspects of linguistic learning and memory, regardless of the language involved, are important for success on this measure. This is consistent with the recommendations by Wendling et al. (2007) that interventions targeted at improving performance on this task include language-rich environments, discussion of academic information, frequent reading, and direct instruction of vocabulary and related language skills.

7 Measures of Writing, Math, and General Academic Knowledge   133

Table 7.7 Rasch Analysis Person and Item Statistics: Woodcock-Johnson Academic Knowledge

	Persons	Items
Mean raw scores	58.6 (out of 78)	24.6 (out of 46)
SD of raw scores	7.3	15.7
Mean Rasch measures	0.32	0
SE of means (for measures)	0.23	0.42
Measure range	−2.14 to 4.12	−4.38 to 5.18
# with MSq out-fit >2.0	6	4
Reliability (KR-20)	0.89	

Rasch Analysis

(Note: a brief explanation of the Rasch analysis procedures used in this book is provided in Chap. 3, as an introduction to the discussion of the Rasch analysis conducted on the item data for the K-BIT2.)

Table 7.7 presents the Rasch statistics for the Woodcock-Johnson Academic Knowledge test (WJAK), and Fig. 7.1 presents the map of person ability and item difficulty logit scores for the WJAK. Figure 7.1 shows that there is a wide range of item difficulties, and a wide range of achievement levels among participants, although there are a large number of exceptionally easy test items for this group of participants. As noted in Table 7.7, items range in difficulty from −4.38 to 5.18 logits (a 9.56 point spread). Person abilities range from −2.14 to 4.12 logits (a smaller 6.26 point spread), which is also an indication of considerable range in ability. The mean Rasch measures for both persons and items are very close (0.32 for persons and 0 for items). With so many easy items, the proximity of the mean logit scores for persons and items is a little surprising, and it indicates that there are also a sizable number of very difficult items, which can be seen in Fig. 7.1 at the top of the vertical scale. In fact, six items on the test show item difficulty measures greater in value than the ability measure of the highest scoring participant.

The standard errors for the Rasch person and item measures are 0.23 and 0.42, respectively. These translate to 95 % confidence intervals of ±0.45 logits and 0.82, respectively, which, as with the other measures reported in this volume, are acceptable for an exploratory study (Linacre 1994). The wider confidence interval around item parameters may be due to the exceptionally wide spread of item difficulties and the clustering of items at both the very easy and very difficult ends of the scale, leading to greater instability of scaling. (Test item characteristics tend to be more stable around the midpoints of the scale.) Regarding the fit to the Rasch model, Table 7.7 shows that 6 (out of 46) participants and 4 (out of 78) items show patterns of responses that are "noisy" (i.e., participants who either made lucky guesses to difficult items, careless responses to easy items, or who demonstrated idiosyncratic response patterns). Additional analyses of these participants and items with large fit statistics are warranted.

Finally, the KR20 reliability coefficient for this test (for these participants) is 0.89 indicating a high level of internal test item consistency. In sum, the WJAK test

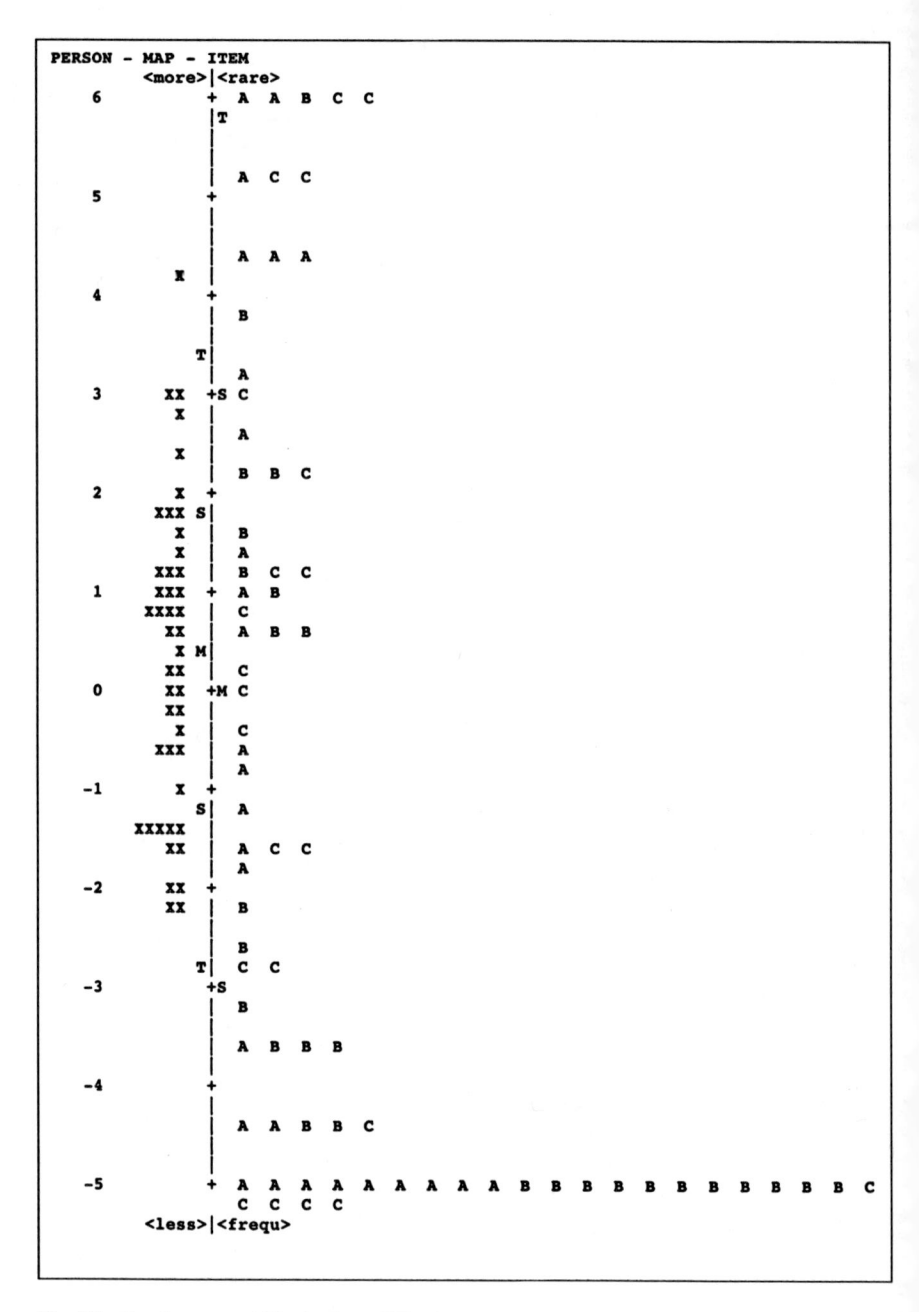

```
PERSON - MAP - ITEM
        <more>|<rare>
   6         +  A  A  B  C  C
             |T
             |
             |
             |  A  C  C
   5         +
             |
             |
             |  A  A  A
          X  |
   4         +
             |  B
             |
          T  |
             |  A
   3     XX +S  C
          X  |
             |  A
          X  |
             |  B  B  C
   2      X  +
        XXX S|
          X  |  B
          X  |  A
        XXX  |  B  C  C
   1    XXX  +  A  B
       XXXX  |  C
         XX  |  A  B  B
          X M|
         XX  |  C
   0     XX +M  C
         XX  |
          X  |  C
        XXX  |  A
             |  A
  -1      X  +
          S  |  A
      XXXXX  |
         XX  |  A  C  C
             |  A
  -2     XX  +
         XX  |  B
             |
             |  B
          T  |  C  C
  -3        +S
             |  B
             |
             |  A  B  B  B
  -4         +
             |
             |  A  A  B  B  C
             |
  -5         +  A  A  A  A  A  A  A  A  B  B  B  B  B  B  B  B  B  B  C
                C  C  C  C
        <less>|<frequ>
```

Fig. 7.1 Rasch person ability by item difficulty map: WJ-III Academic Knowledge

produced an acceptable array of Rasch statistics, both for persons and items. The clustering of items at the very easy and very difficult ends of the scale may result in some instability in parameter estimation and lead us to want to conduct further analysis of this test. As noted earlier, student performance on the Academic Knowledge test is quite low, indicating gaps in Academic Knowledge for this population of students. A study of the individual items at the top of the item scale (i.e., those that are very difficult) might help to identify academic areas that are particularly problematic for this population. Also, since deaf and hearing students are likely to come from very different educational backgrounds, a study that compares Rasch item characteristics for deaf students with those of hearing students would prove informative.

Summary

In contrast to the other academic achievement tasks, Math Fluency produced relatively limited correlations with other Toolkit measures. It should be noted that this task reflects only simple math calculation, and not word problems, which would be expected to have greater impacts of language skills. The relationships observed with this task focused primarily on cognitive flexibility and short-term/working memory.

Both Writing Fluency and Academic Knowledge produced significant correlations with a wide range of other skills and cognitive processes. This is consistent with previous research. For example, Schoonen et al. (2003) found that fluency measures correlated with writing skills in both languages for students bilingual in Dutch and English, but that language knowledge was the primary source of this association. Similarly, Sasaki and Hirose (1996) found that the largest component explaining English writing skills of college age Japanese students with an average of 6 years of English learning was proficiency in English, while Japanese writing skills represented the second most significant contributor. Similarly, Schoonen et al. (2010) concluded that while knowledge of grammar and processing speed are related to writing skills, it is the proficiency in the second language being written that is more important than proficiency in the writer's first language. This likely reflects limitations in the second language skills resulting in greater consumption of cognitive resources.

These studies are consistent with the current findings that while the writing and academic knowledge skills of the deaf students in the study, many of whom could be considered English Language Learners, are highly associated with their knowledge of English, they are also significantly associated with their ASL skills and general linguistic fluency. Further, consistent with the work of Adams et al. (2010), writing performance in adults is significantly associated with verbal short-term memory as reflected in the forward span tasks. It should be noted, however, that the current research used a writing task that required limited planning and should not involve revision, limiting the impacts of working memory which is thought to affect narrative writing (McCutchen 1996).

While the exact nature of the relationship is still a matter of discussion, the associations between WM tasks and writing are supported by a range of research (e.g., Hoskyn and Swanson 2003; Olive et al. 2008; Peverly 2006). McCutchen (1996) reviewed the related literature and concluded that, even for individuals writing in their first language, writing places demands on WM capacity and when language skills are more limited, the demands on cognitive capacity posed by writing result in more concrete, unplanned approaches to producing text. She suggested that the interaction between variations in WM capacity and language skills may account for the range of writing skills into adulthood. Olive et al. (2008) found that both visual and verbal WM are involved in writing; however, they differentiated visual and spatial WM, and found little involvement of spatial memory. The current results are consistent with the reported relationships between language skills, WM (both verbal and visual) and writing. While the current study did not distinguish visual and spatial WM, it is possible that the visuospatial nature of ASL may also increase the impact of spatial WM in this population.

McCutchen (2000) elaborated on her theory on the interaction between WM and writing, addressing the impact of demands for retrieval of information from long term memory (LTM), which must then be held in WM while text is conceptualized. This extended management of information during extended reasoning and conceptualization was labeled long term working memory (LTWM), and provides a link between information retrieved from LTM and information currently held in short-term WM (STWM). As in the model later developed (McCutchen 2011), linguistic skills and relevant knowledge are affected by the very limited STWM constraints, but as linguistic skills and knowledge increase, this gives way to the still constrained, but significantly greater LTWM. She noted that research has indicated that use of complex syntax and avoidance of common syntactic errors becomes more difficult as WM load increases due to factors such as lack of fluency. In contrast, those with greater relevant knowledge and linguistic competence will have increased LTWM capacity, making more complex and fluent writing possible.

These processes may interact in a complex manner. For example, as with the impact of developing graphomotor skills reported by Olive and Kellogg (2002), lack of fluency may cause increased cognitive resources to be focused on lower level processes, leaving fewer resources for higher order processes needed for advanced written composition. Thus, the associations between writing, academic knowledge, language, and linguistic fluency and memory seen in the current study are consistent with these lines of research.

References

Adams, A., Simmons, F., Willis, C., & Pawling, R. (2010). Undergraduate students' ability to revise text effectively: Relationships with topic knowledge and working memory. *Journal of Research in Reading, 33*(1), 54–76. doi:10.1111/j.1467-9817.2009.01432.x.

Hoskyn, M., & Swanson, H. L. (2003). The relationship between working memory and writing in younger and older adults. *Reading and Writing, 16*(8), 759–784.

Kelly, R. R., & Gaustad, M. G. (2007). Deaf college student' mathematical skills relative to morphological knowledge, reading level, and language proficiency. *Journal of Deaf Studies and Deaf Education, 12*(1), 25–37.

Kelly, R. R., Lang, H. G., & Pagliaro, C. M. (2003). Mathematics word problem solving for deaf students: A survey of practices in grades 6–12. *Journal of Deaf Studies and Deaf Education, 8*(2), 104–119.

Kritzer, K. L. (2009). Barely started and already left behind: A descriptive analysis of the mathematics ability demonstrated by young deaf children. *Journal of Deaf Studies and Deaf Education, 14*(4), 409–421.

Linacre, J. M. (1994). Sample size and item calibration stability. *Rasch Measurement Transactions, 7*(4), 328.

McCutchen, D. (1996). A capacity theory of writing: Working memory in composition. *Educational Psychology Review, 8*, 299–324.

McCutchen, D. (2000). Knowledge acquisition, processing efficiency, and working memory: Implications for a theory of writing. *Educational Psychologist, 35*, 13–23.

McCutchen, D. (2011). From novice to expert: Implications of language skills and writing-relevant knowledge for memory during the development of writing skill. *Journal of Writing Research, 3*(1), 51–68.

McGrew, K. S., Schrank, F. A., & Woodcock, R. W. (2007). *Technical manual, Woodcock-Johnson III normative update*. Rolling Meadows, IL: Riverside Publishing.

Mousley, K., & Kelly, R. R. (1998). Problem-solving strategies for teaching mathematics to deaf students. *American Annuals of the Deaf, 143*(4), 325–337.

Nunes, T., & Moreno, C. (2002). An intervention program for promoting deaf pupils' achievement in mathematics. *Journal of Deaf Studies and Deaf Education, 7*(2), 120–133.

Olive, T., & Kellogg, R. T. (2002). Concurrent activation of high- and low-level production processes in written composition. *Memory and Cognition, 30*(4), 594–600.

Olive, T., Kellogg, R. T., & Piolat, A. (2008). Verbal, visual, and spatial working memory demands during text composition. *Applied PsychoLinguistics, 29*, 669–687. doi:10.1017/S0142716408080284.

Peverly, S. T. (2006). The importance of handwriting speed in adult writing. *Developmental Neuropsychology, 29*(1), 197–216.

Sasaki, M., & Hirose, K. (1996). Explanatory variables for EFL students' expository writing. *Language Learning, 4*(1), 137–174.

Schoonen, R., Snellings, P., Stevenson, M., & van Gelderen, A. (2010). Towards a blueprint of the foreign language writer: The linguistic and cognitive demands of foreign language writing. In R. Manchon (Ed.), *Writing in foreign language contexts: Learning, teaching, and research* (pp. 77–101). Buffalo: Multilingual Matters.

Schoonen, R., van Gelderen, A., de Glopper, K., Hulstijn, J., Simis, A., Snellings, P., et al. (2003). First language and second language writing: The role of linguistic knowledge, speed of processing, and metacognitive knowledge. *Language Learning, 53*(1), 165–202.

Schrank, F. A., & Woodcock, R. W. (2007). *WJ III normative update compuscore and profiles program (Version 3.0) [Computer software].Woodcock-Johnson III*. Rolling Meadows, IL: Riverside.

Traxler, C. B. (2000). The Stanford Achievement Test, 9th Edition: National norming and performance standards for deaf and hard-of-hearing students. *Journal of Deaf Studies and Deaf Education, 5*, 337–348.

Wendling, B. J., Schrank, F. A., & Schmitt, A. J. (2007). *Educational interventions related to the Woodcock-Johnson III Tests of Achievement (Assessment Service Bulletin No. 8)*. Rolling Meadows, IL: Riverside Publishing.

Woodcock, R. W., McGrew, K. S., & Mather, N. (2001). *Examiner's manual. Woodcock-Johnson III tests of achievement*. Itasca, IL: Riverside Publishing.

Part IV
Linguistic Functioning

Language functioning is required for humans to function in the social world. It is necessary both in order to have the simplest of needs met and for every level of social, vocational, and academic functioning. For the VL2 Psychometric Toolkit study, both American Sign Language (ASL) and English skills (via print and indirect means) were measured in order to investigate the relative impacts of functioning in the two languages on academic skill outcomes. While standard measures were used when possible, some aspects of language functioning were, by necessity, evaluated using experimental or adapted measures. The linguistic skills measured include receptive ASL, "verbal" fluency, receptive fingerspelling, knowledge of English phonology and syntax, and speechreading skills.

This part covers the broad range of language functioning and contains five chapters: two chapters reflecting the assessment of expressive and receptive language functioning performed for the VL2 Toolkit project and three chapters discussing the assessment of ASL, fingerspelling, and speechreading skills in more depth.

Chapter 8
Measures of Expressive Language

Donna A. Morere, Gregory Witkin, and Leah Murphy

Expressive language is critical for the interaction of the individual with the environment. It represents the individual's ability to demonstrate knowledge and share information, make their needs and wants known, and share in social interactions. It also supports our executive functions, such as planning, organization, and self-control. Limitations in overall language functioning affect long-term academic outcomes, and expressive skills represent one component of this broad skill area (Young et al. 2002). While other tasks within the Toolkit also measure expressive skills (e.g., Writing Fluency), the focus of this chapter will be the measurement of linguistic fluency.

Linguistic Fluency

Category and letter naming tasks represent commonly used measures of semantic and phonological fluency. Recent research has suggested that these two types of tasks may be processed using a combination of shared and separate neural structures (Grogan et al. 2009). The ability to search, retrieve, and verbalize words quickly and fluently is governed by executive functioning, the self-regulatory, or control system that governs cognitive, behavioral, and emotional activity (Anderson 2008; Denckla 1996). The two tasks differ in that the words which begin with a specific letter on phonemic fluency tasks are not necessarily related, whereas category fluency accesses a sequence of related concepts, which are more quickly accessible (Schwartz et al. 2003). The single category presented on semantic fluency

---

D.A. Morere (✉) • G. Witkin • L. Murphy
Department of Psychology, Gallaudet University,
800 Florida Avenue, NE, Washington, DC 20002, USA
e-mail: Donna.Morere@Gallaudet.edu; Gregory.Witkin@Gallaudet.edu;
Leah.Murphy@Gallaudet.edu

tasks activates a network of multiple exemplars, the search of which is dependent on organization of semantic memory (Raboutet et al. 2010).

Verbal fluency as a whole reflects the manner in which we process previously learned information and the aspects of memory required to recall and retrieve that information at a later time. Memory studies often proceed with the assumption that while hearing individuals access verbal (or linguistic) memory through acoustic, phonological, and articulatory codes, deaf individuals function primarily through nonverbal (or nonlinguistic) memory (Marschark and Mayer 1998).

American Sign Language (ASL) is conveyed through a combination of facial expressions and other non-manual components, and manual signs involving configurational handshapes, spatial locations, and movements. It has been suggested that ASL may be processed and rehearsed using a sign-based "phonological loop" (or sign loop) analogous to the auditory memory-based loop used by hearing individuals (Wilson and Emmorey 1997).

Verbal fluency tasks, such as the Controlled Oral Word Association (COWA) test, are commonly used neuropsychological measures of executive function (Lezak et al. 2004). The COWA test measures the number of words an individual can report within a specified amount of time when prompted by a specific letter. A related task reflects semantic fluency, using the prompt of a general category. Thus, the two types of verbal fluency measures generally used involve lexical or phonemic fluency (words beginning with a specific letter, typically F, A, and S) and semantic, or categorical, fluency (words found in a specific category such as "animals" and "foods"). Both tasks involve the ability to spontaneously produce words within a 1-min time constraint (Bechtoldt et al. 1962; Benton 1967; Spreen and Benton 1969).

Verbal, or linguistic, fluency involves multiple cognitive processes, including (but not limited to) attention and initiation, short-term memory, cognitive flexibility, a range of vocabulary from which to access the responses, the linguistic search and retrieval skills to make use of this knowledge, and executive controls which allow for organization, decision-making, response inhibition, self-monitoring, and adherence to the rules of the task (Mitrushina et al. 2005; Ruff et al. 1997). Factors which have been shown to influence the individual's performance on a measure of verbal fluency include age, education, bilingualism, and disability (Kempler et al. 1998; Portocarrero et al. 2007).

Performance on verbal fluency measures generally increases during childhood, with relative stabilization during adolescence or early adulthood. This may in part relate to findings that word retrieval efficiency has been shown to increase with age (Cohen et al. 1999), with some studies showing that children reach adult levels of efficiency as early as age 10 (Regard et al. 1982) and others showing continued development into adolescence (Welsh et al. 1991). Within the adult population, mild declines in performance occur with age on measures of semantic fluency (Lezak et al. 2004). However, while some studies suggest a lack of age differences in performance among adults on phonemic fluency tasks (Axelrod and Henry 1992; Troyer et al. 1997), the meta-analysis by Rodríguez-Aranda and Martinussen (2006) indicates that these declines do occur, especially after age 40.

Ruff et al. (1997) presented multiple supports, including the impact of educational level on word fluency scores, for the contention that word knowledge is an essential component of verbal fluency, and that a larger pool of available words would lead to increased performance on word fluency. More recently, Luo et al. (2010) provided data supporting the direct impact of vocabulary on verbal fluency performance. The impacts of English vocabulary on performance on fluency tasks—particularly those based on English letters/phonemes—are especially relevant with people who are deaf or hard-of-hearing (D/HOH), as they typically have limited access to spoken language. Thus, they may not attain the same level of fluency expected of age- or education-matched hearing peers due to a more limited pool of available words.

It is important to analyze the effects of bilingualism on verbal fluency performance. While some debate exists about the definition of bilingualism, it is important to note that some D/HOH individuals use components of both English and ASL in their everyday lives. Communicating in more than one language, or language modality, may impact one's performance on verbal fluency tests. However, while bilingual children often have lower scores on vocabulary tests and other specialized language tests (Luo et al. 2010), this does not automatically lead to lower linguistic abilities in adulthood. Additionally, bilinguals are often slower at tasks requiring rapid lexical access, such as picture naming tasks, even if they are just as accurate as monolinguals (Costa 2005; Luo et al. 2010).

One theory proposes that there is a bilingual disadvantage for phonemic fluency tasks because such tasks consume more cognitive resources than category naming tasks, as words are typically stored semantically rather than lexically and cognitive associations and cognitive searches are typically based on categorical associations (Luo et al. 2010). Phonemic generation is not a common strategy in everyday word retrieval, making this type of task more dependent on executive control (Luo et al. 2010; Strauss et al. 2006). Further, interference from the person's "other" language (e.g., the language not targeted by the task) may slow the search, as the person may have to consider and reject phonemically appropriate responses from the "other" language. During categorical tasks, the person is searching by content, so there may be less lexical/phonological interference. Further, studies have found that fully bilingual people tend to have a reduced lexicon in each language compared to monolinguals, although there are no reductions in the overall corpus of vocabulary across languages (Bialystok et al. 2008; Oller and Eilers 2002).

Recent research has investigated individuals who are deaf and for whom ASL is a first language. Morford et al. (2011) found that deaf signers activated sign translations of the stimuli during a task involving reading English words, although the participants were not asked about ASL. Thus, the authors concluded that deaf readers activate ASL networks even on tasks that do not directly involve signs. While these types of activation may be occurring on the reading tasks, this raises the question of whether English demands will affect performance on tasks involving signed responses. The current study investigated linguistic fluency using three related tasks. First, in addition to the English-based phonemic fluency task using the standard F–A–S stimuli, a measure of fluency was developed based on the phonemes (or cheremes) of ASL related to handshapes. Second, semantic fluency was measured using categorical probes. In order to investigate the impact of priming in the two languages, the semantic tasks were administered twice, once after each of the two phonemic tasks. (Note that although technically the handshapes represent cheremes, since they are not sound based, the term phoneme will be used here as a generic term for the basic discernible units of both languages.)

The Linguistic Fluency Tasks

Phonemic Fluency: F–A–S and 5–1–U

The previously discussed COWA, or F–A–S, was used to measure English letter, or phonemic, fluency. The F–A–S task was selected due to its wide use, both clinically and in research. It is the most commonly used form of phonemic fluency (Barry et al. 2008), and is the form of the task used in the Delis–Kaplan Executive Function System (D-KEFS; Delis et al. 2001), a respected battery of executive functioning.

The 5–1–U was developed in-house to measure sign-based phonemic fluency. While the task administration may vary slightly, Strauss et al. (2006) report that on the F–A–S task, the hearing individual is given the spoken prompt of the letter and asked to produce as many words as possible which start with that letter within a 1-min time frame. Prior to being given the first prompt, the participant is provided with a model of an unrelated letter (e.g., "For example, if I were to say "G", you could respond with gum, go, gas, etc.") and is told that neither proper nouns (e.g., names of people and places, "you shouldn't say Greg or Georgia") nor multiple forms of the same word but with a different ending (e.g., run, running, runs) are allowed. These are standard rules for phonemic fluency tasks. After the first letter task is completed, the subsequent two letters are presented, one at a time. For the oral administration, the examiner typically writes down the participant's responses in the order they are given. This has the added advantage of allowing further analyses of constructs such as clustering (e.g., producing multiple words from a semantic group or subgroup) and switching (changing to a different word type).

For the current F–A–S task, the instructions were signed to the participant, who responded via sign. In addition to the examiner's writing down the responses, the participants' responses were videotaped, so that unclear or missed responses could be reviewed to ensure accurate scoring. While individual signs can represent multiple English words, credit for each sign was given if a standard or commonly used English interpretation of the sign began with the relevant letter.

As mentioned above, the 5–1–U is a sign-based task internally developed by Morere and members of the VL2 team specifically for this study. Based on a linguistic analysis, ASL has three main phonological criteria (Battison 1978; Stokoe 1960): handshape, location of the sign, and movement of the hands. While for spoken languages, the influence of phonologically, morphologically, or semantically related words stimulate a priming effect on target words (Hamburger and Slowiaczek 1996); ASL priming occurs based on the sign language phonemic domains of handshape, location, and movement (Corina and Emmorey 1993). As handshapes appear to be the parameter which exhibit categorical perception (Emmorey et al. 2003), the 5–1–U task focuses on the parameter of handshapes. This task requires the participant to generate signs that use specific handshapes. It was designed to recruit sign-based strategies comparable to those used on the letter-based task. The handshapes 5, 1, and U were selected and sequenced in an attempt to reflect the relative frequency of their occurrence in the ASL lexicon similar to the forms of commonly used phonemic frequency tasks. While few data are available related to the frequency of handshapes used in signs in ASL, the data from Morford and Macfarlane (2003) suggest that the 1 and 5 handshapes are used by the dominant, the nondominant, or both hands in the signs having the highest frequency, while the U represents a less frequent but not rare usage, presenting a somewhat more challenging task. These frequencies are supported by a more recent study (Chong et al. 2009). While the selection of the letters F, A, and S is less well defined—indeed Mitrushina et al. (2005) state that they were chosen at random—and all three letters are considered relatively easy, the other two most commonly used letter sets (CFL and PRW) were developed so that one letter had a very high frequency and the other two letters were selected for decreasing frequency in English words (Ruff et al. 1996). Although the latter tasks might be considered more difficult than the FAS, a meta-analytic study comparing the FAS and CFL forms found that while such a difference did occur, the effect size was small, suggesting that while norms for the two tasks should not be used interchangeably, performance by normal individuals was similar (Barry et al. 2008).

Although the current frequency data for ASL do not allow for precision, the general approach to item selection and sequencing used to develop the CFL and PRW was taken with the 5–1–U, with both the 5 and 1 handshapes having a reportedly high frequency in ASL, and the U being somewhat more moderate usage. As is suggested by the comparison of the FAS and CFL, even within a language direct comparison between independently developed forms of superficially identical tasks should be done with caution. As will be discussed below, even greater caution is advised when comparing tasks using not only different languages, but also different modalities

For the 5–1–U task, analogous to the F–A–S, participants were asked to come up with as many signs as possible that use the ASL manual alphabet/number handshapes representing the closed hand version of the number 5 (also referred to as an open B), the number 1, and the letter U. An English translation of the instructions follows: "I will show an ASL handshape. Then I want you to give me as many words (signs) that use that handshape as quickly as you can. For instance, if I use the handshape "K," you might give me "pink, plant, king..." I do not want you to use words that are proper nouns such as "Philadelphia" or namesigns like "Krystle." Any questions?" After a pause, the examiner would sign, "Begin when I show the handshape. You will have one minute for each handshape. The first handshape is 5. Go ahead."

Scoring also paralleled the standard phonemic fluency tasks, with proper names and repetition of the same sign with elaboration (e.g., grandfather and then great-grandfather only given one point, with the elaborative sign scored zero). One point was given for any sign which used a handshape which resembled the relevant handshape (e.g., 5, 1, or U). Additionally, if the concept presented was clearly differentiated, a score of one was given even when the sign was the same (analogous to giving points for homophones such as "see" and "sea" if the meaning is clarified).

As noted above, while this task was designed to emulate commonly used English phonemic fluency tasks, there are a number of issues which make direct comparison of the 5–1–U to the English-based tasks problematic. For one thing, as previously discussed, these tasks are affected by the range of the individual's vocabulary. While ASL is a rich language with the ability to offer detailed and complex information, since the signs are conceptual in nature, the overall number of signs in ASL is generally considered to be smaller than the number of words in English. Thus, even moderate impacts of vocabulary could limit the number of signs produced. Additionally, while handshapes represent one aspect of the basic units of ASL, they are only one component of the formational structure of signs, sharing this distinction with location, movement, and palm orientation. Thus, they are not directly analogous to speech-based phonemes. Even so, this task provides a potential tool for use in this population, both for the study of processing of ASL and for clinical use, although additional research would be required on broader populations prior to clinical application of this task.

Semantic Fluency: Animals and Foods

As previously discussed, the second general type of fluency task involves semantic fluency, for which the participant is asked to provide words belonging to a specific semantic category. Category fluency is generally considered to be a less difficult task than letter fluency (Lezak et al. 2004). While phonemic and semantic fluency tasks appear to tap somewhat different, although overlapping cognitive processes (Grogan et al. 2009), they are superficially fairly similar. While on the phonemic tasks, the participant is asked to produce as many words (signs) as possible within 1 min which begin with a certain letter or handshape, for the semantic tasks, they are asked to produce as many words as possible from within a specified category.

The most commonly used categorical task is to ask the participant to report the names of as many types of animal as they are able within the 1-min time constraint (Mitrushina et al. 2005; Strauss et al. 2006). This was selected for the first category used for the Psychometric Toolkit. The second measure was foods. This category is one which is used in various forms (e.g., foods; things you eat and drink; fruits and/or vegetables; things you find in a supermarket) in multiple studies and within various instruments, and represents a clear category of common items with which most people are familiar. It avoids the issues associated with using boys or girls names (e.g., unique namesigns and dependence on fingerspelling) and provides a wider range of potential responses than categories such as furniture and clothing.

As noted above, each categorical task was presented twice, once following the F–A–S task, and once after the 5–1–U task. The two trials were administered during separate testing sessions with an average of approximately 1 week between sessions. While both the order of the sessions (for example, half were administered 5–1–U on the first session and half F–A–S on the first session) and sequence of presentation of the Toolkit tasks were counterbalanced for the linguistic fluency tasks, the semantic task was always administered immediately following the phonemic fluency task, with foods administered followed by the animal category. As with the phonemic tasks, the instructions were signed to the participant and all responses were signed by the participants.

Results for Measures of Linguistic Fluency

Descriptive Statistics

Metanorms based on 32 studies of the F–A–S task by hearing participants indicate a mean of 43.51 and standard deviation of 9.44 for individuals below age 40 (Loonstra et al. 2001). The participants in the current study demonstrated a comparable standard deviation; however, their mean performance was more than one standard deviation below the performance of typical English-speaking young adults (Table 8.1). It should be noted that these participants were performing a task best approached using an English alphabetical search, but were required to respond using signs. Thus, the impact of both English proficiency and translation demands need to be taken into consideration. Furthermore, despite their status as college students, it is likely that their English vocabulary is lower than expectations for same age peers. With this in mind, while the two measures can only be compared in very general terms, it is notable that the performance on the sign-based task was approximately half of a standard deviation greater than that on the English-based task, although the ranges were still comparable. This suggests that the participants may have been better able to access a sign-based search than one based on English letters/phonemes. It is possible that the sign-based task was less resource-intensive, as it required only the retrieval and production of the signs, while responses on F–A–S required the student to search for the English word and then associate it with the relevant sign in order to respond. One possible future area of research would be to investigate the relative performance on this type of task when the responses were written or typed rather than signed for the speech-based task. While this may limit use of sign-based processing on the English fluency task, based on the work of Morford et al. (2011), it is possible that activation of signs will occur regardless of the modality of the task.

A meta-analysis of 11 studies of animal naming indicated that individuals between the ages of 25 and 29 are predicted to generate 24.28 words with a standard deviation of 4.65 (Mitrushina et al. 2005). The animal naming outcomes for the current group were consistent, with a mean which rounds to 21 and standard deviation of about 5. Indeed, this was true for both the animal and food tasks regardless of whether they were primed using the ASL- or English-based phonemic fluency task. The current

Table 8.1 F–A–S and 5–1–U—descriptive statistics

Language	Test/subtest	Range	N	Mean (SD)
English	F–A–S	13–58	49	30.08 (10.84)
	Animals	10–38	49	21.16 (5.03)
	Foods	9–35	49	20.69 (5.04)
ASL	5–1–U	15–57	48	35.00 (9.94)
	Animals	13–40	46	20.57 (4.75)
	Foods	13–36	46	21.20 (5.31)

data reflect outcomes that are below, but within one standard deviation of, the outcomes on the animal fluency task for hearing English speakers in previous studies. This is not surprising, as many signs represent broad categories of animals. For example, a hearing person might report salmon, trout, carp, and flounder. The sign for all of these is "fish" and in order to indicate the individual species of fish, the participant would have to fingerspell the English word. This would both slow down the response due to the time demands of fingerspelling and it would require activation of the English. This difference in the range of animal names directly available in ASL and English could account for some of the differences in the above scores. Even so, the mean performance of this group was within expectations on this task.

While metanorms were not available for the food category, and this category is often reported combined with other categories in a single score, a number of the studies presented by Mitrushina included categories such as items found in the supermarket, fruits, or vegetables in conjunction with animal naming. It appears that the broader category of items found in a supermarket generally produces a slightly larger set of responses than animal naming, while the more restrictive categories of either fruits or vegetables produce slightly fewer items than the animal category. Thus, the consistency between the relatively broad, but somewhat constrained categories of animals and foods appears to be appropriate. This is consistent with the results of Halperin et al. (1989), who found that children between the ages of 6 and 12 increased the number of words retrieved for the categories of animals and foods, but that the numbers for the two categories were within one item of each other for each 1-year age group. This again suggests that these are comparable semantic retrieval categories.

Overall, the descriptive data for these measures suggest that the deaf students in this study found the English-based phonemic fluency task more difficult than their hearing peers. They also found it to be more challenging than an analogous sign-based task as well as the semantic fluency tasks. There are multiple potential explanations for the difficulty observed with the F–A–S task relative to the other two types of tasks.

Correlational Relationships

Table 8.2 presents the significant correlations between the F–A–S and the other toolkit measures. Considering the need for English word knowledge and the ability to use English letter-based search strategies, it is not surprising that this task correlated moderately with all of the reading and writing tasks. This does not solely represent

Table 8.2 F–A–S—significant correlations

Test	r	N
WJ-III Reading Fluency	0.53**	46
WJ-III Writing Fluency	0.38**	46
WJ-III Academic Knowledge	0.41**	46
WJ-III Passage Comprehension	0.44**	47
PIAT Reading	0.36*	47
F–A–S Animals	0.46**	49
F–A–S Food	0.50**	49
5–1–U	0.43**	47
5–1–U Animals	0.47**	46
5–1–U Food	0.55**	46
ASL-SRT	0.47**	33
Fingerspelling Test Total Correct	0.50**	49
Fingerspelling Test Real Words Correct	0.50**	49
Fingerspelling Test Fake Word Correct	0.45**	49
TOSWRF	0.29*	46
TSA Percent Correct	0.44*	23
TSA Relativization Percent Correct	0.50*	23
Print Letter Forward Span	0.58**	36
ASL Letter Forward Span	0.39**	49
ASL Letter Backward Span	0.41**	49
ASL Digit Backward Span	0.37**	49

**Significance at $p<0.01$, *significance at $p<0.05$

the impacts of academic fluency, which would be assumed to be related to linguistic fluency, as the correlations with the untimed reading and academic knowledge tasks were similar to those on the two fluency tasks. Not unexpectedly, F–A–S correlated at moderate levels with the other linguistic fluency tasks, including the sign-based 5–1–U, suggesting that despite their differences, these measures do tap an underlying linguistic fluency process. Similarly, the ability to receive fingerspelling, whether real- or pseudo-words were used, is consistent with facility with English words and the ability to use an alphabetic search: individuals who are better able to read fingerspelling would be expected to have broader access to English words.

Moderate to strong correlations were also observed with the letter-based linguistic short-term/working memory tasks as well as one digit-based working memory task. This is consistent with the observation by Mitrushina et al. (2005) that a range of studies in hearing populations have revealed relationships between verbal fluency and digit span tasks. The moderate correlations between F–A–S and both of the scores on the Test of Syntactic Ability (TSA) support the contention that while the TSA does not target word knowledge, greater word knowledge would be expected to be associated with knowledge of English syntax. Perhaps the most interesting relationship was the moderate correlation with the ASL-SRT, a measure of receptive ASL skills. It is possible that this reflects an underlying effect of general language skill; however, overall it appears that the F–A–S measure tracks most closely with tasks reflecting English skills.

Table 8.3 5–1–U—significant correlations

Test	r	N
WJ-III Writing Fluency	0.29*	47
F–A–S	0.43**	47
5–1–U Animals	0.40**	46
5–1–U Food	0.41**	46
M-SVLT Cued Recall	0.32*	46
Fingerspelling Test Total Correct	0.39**	47
Fingerspelling Test Real Words	0.38**	47
Fingerspelling Test Fake Words	0.39**	47
Print Letter Forward Span	0.40**	36
Corsi Blocks Manual Backward Span	0.43**	47

**Significance at $p<0.01$, *significance at $p<0.05$

As can be seen in Table 8.3, a smaller set of measures produced significant correlations with the sign-based 5–1–U measure, which involved both measures which correlated with F–A–S and measures which did not produce significant correlations with the English-based task. As previously noted, a moderate correlation was observed between the 5–1–U and F–A–S measures, suggesting both shared and disparate processes in these two superficially similar tasks. Interestingly, while the F–A–S task correlated significantly with both the English- and ASL-primed semantic fluency tasks, 5–1–U correlated significantly only with the self-primed categorical tasks. This suggests that while, as noted above, the results for the differentially primed semantic fluency tasks appear to be consistent, there may be differences in the underlying search and retrieval processes involved in achieving those scores. As with the F–A–S, the 5–1–U task correlated moderately, and somewhat more highly, with the fingerspelling reception tasks. These moderate to high correlations indicate a relatively strong relationship between receptive signing and the ability to use handshape-based information to perform the linguistic search and retrieval process involved in the 5–1–U.

Despite the shared relationships between the two phonemic fluency tasks, the relationships seen between the speech-based task and the tasks reflecting English skills were notably absent in the 5–1–U correlations. While there was a relatively weak association with the Writing Fluency task, this could reflect underlying linguistic fluency and/or motor speed and dexterity which are involved in both writing and signing, rather than English skills. Perhaps the most surprising absence was the significant association with the ASL-SRT. While there was a moderate correlation which approached significance ($r=0.336$, $p=0.06$), a stronger relationship would have been expected between the measure of receptive ASL skills and the sign-based task than with the speech-based task. This is an area which deserves further investigation.

In addition to the limited shared relationships, 5–1–U produced some correlational relationships not evident with the speech-based fluency task. While both tasks correlated moderately with the forward print letter span task, only 5–1–U correlated significantly with any of the visuospatial working memory tasks. While it correlated significantly only with the manually administered reverse span task, this does support the involvement of visual working memory in the sign-based fluency task. This may represent similar relationship to that of the various linguistic short-term/working memory tasks in the processing of the F–A–S. Rende et al. (2002) found that hearing college students used a combination of visual and verbal (phonological) working memory on verbal fluency tasks, with greater involvement of verbal working memory for letter fluency and greater visuospatial working memory involvement for categorical fluency. It may be that the association seen with the visual working memory task suggests a shift towards the more visual working memory focus for the sign-based phonemic fluency task. It is also possible that the priming with the 5–1–U task encouraged an even greater use of this strategy with the categorical fluency tasks in this battery, resulting in the significant associations reported above. Another unique relationship seen with the 5–1–U was the low moderate correlation with the cued recall trial of the sign-based memory and learning task. This may reflect underlying sign-based memory and retrieval skills for both tasks, although the lack of significant correlations with the other SVLT scores suggests that this may represent a more specific relationship which is not clear.

Overall, while there are clearly some shared processes between the 5–1–U and its English phonemic fluency equivalent, the ASL-based task appears to involve a somewhat different set of processes, focusing more on the visuospatial and manual aspects of cognitive processing and having little, if any, involvement of speech-based phonology and language. This suggests that the shared processing may reflect the underlying linguistic organization and search processes which are then applied in quite different manners for the two related tasks, which differ in their sensory foundations as well as the language of the underlying task.

While the differential associations with the F–A–S and 5–1–U tasks suggest some degree of discrepancy in the underlying processes, in general the ASL- and English-primed semantic fluency tasks appeared to be quite similar. Thus, the two animal and food tasks will be discussed jointly. As can be observed in Tables 8.4 and 8.5, the relationships between the two animal fluency tasks and the other measures are quite similar. Both tasks produced moderate to strong correlations with a range of academic measures reflecting reading and writing skills. Not unexpectedly, the English-primed task produced somewhat higher correlations with these tasks and correlated with a slightly broader range of English reading and achievement measures. This pattern of slightly stronger correlations was also seen with the receptive fingerspelling measures, suggesting that the English basis of this task had a significant impact on these associations despite the manual spelling of the stimuli.

Both animal fluency tasks also correlated at strong to moderate levels with all of the other linguistic fluency tasks, with the stronger associations being with the other semantic fluency tasks, suggesting that these tasks do reflect a relatively cohesive process separate from the phonemic fluency tasks. Both animal fluency measures also correlated at moderate levels with a range of linguistic short-term/working memory tasks; however, once again the English-primed measure correlated with a broader range of these tasks. Furthermore, consistent with the results of the F–A–S and 5–1–U, while the ASL-primed task produced a moderate correlation with a visuospatial

Table 8.4 F–A–S Animals—significant correlations

Test	r	N
WJ-III Reading Fluency	0.55**	46
WJ-III Writing Fluency	0.54**	46
WJ-III Academic Knowledge	0.44**	46
WJ-III Passage Comprehension	0.51**	47
PIAT Reading	0.48**	47
F–A–S	0.46**	49
F–A–S Food	0.65**	49
5–1–U Animals	0.61**	46
5–1–U Food	0.45**	46
ASL-SRT	0.40*	33
Fingerspelling Test Total Correct	0.62**	49
Fingerspelling Test Real Words	0.59**	49
Fingerspelling Test Fake Words	0.64**	49
Print Letter Forward Span	0.38*	36
Print Digit Backward Span	0.31*	49
ASL Letter Backward Span	0.41**	49
ASL Digit Backward Span	0.37**	49

**Significance at $p<0.01$, *significance at $p<0.05$

Table 8.5 5–1–U Animals—significant correlations

Test	r	N
WJ-III Reading Fluency	0.52**	45
WJ-III Writing Fluency	0.32*	45
PIAT-Reading	0.31*	46
TOL Time Violations	0.32*	45
F–A–S	0.47**	46
F–A–S Animals	0.61**	46
F–A–S Food	0.63**	46
5–1–U	0.40**	46
5–1–U Food	0.66**	46
M-SVLT Cued Recall	0.33*	45
M-SVLT Recognition Number Correct	0.30*	44
ASL-SRT	0.48**	31
Fingerspelling Test Total Correct	0.53**	46
Fingerspelling Test Real Words	0.50**	46
Fingerspelling Test Fake Words	0.52**	46
TOSWRF	0.36*	45
Print Letter Forward Span	0.34*	45
Corsi Blocks Manual Backward Span	0.31*	46
ASL Letter Backward Span	0.39**	46

**Significance at $p<0.01$, *significance at $p<0.05$

working memory task, this was not the case with the F–A–S-primed task. This suggests that while Rende et al. (2002) found a greater focus on visual processing in semantic fluency tasks in the hearing students in their sample, it appears that priming with a speech-based task may elicit more linguistic analysis even on semantic fluency tasks in this population.

Perhaps one of the more interesting shared relationships for this task was the moderate correlations seen for both animal fluency measures with the receptive ASL measure. Just as the associations with the measures of English skills correlated more strongly with the F–A–S-primed trial, the 5–1–U-primed trial appeared to have a somewhat stronger relationship with the receptive ASL measure. These relationships support the importance of underlying language skills, regardless of the language, on this type of task. At the same time, the slight difference in balance of the relationships does suggest that there was some effect of priming on the manner in which the tasks were performed. Consistent with that contention, the final relationship observed for the animal fluency tasks was that of the ASL-primed task with two scores on the sign-based learning and memory task. While relatively low, these correlations again support the impacts of ASL priming on the participants' approach to this task.

While the correlations with the food-based tasks were similar to those for the animal category, this category appeared to tap a broader range of underlying processes (Tables 8.6 and 8.7). The correlations with the measures reflecting English literacy and academic knowledge were consistent across the two trials of this task, perhaps suggesting a greater influence of reading on knowledge of a variety of foods compared to animals. Furthermore, in addition to the intercorrelations with the other linguistic fluency tasks and the relationships with the fingerspelling, working memory, and receptive ASL measures, the two food fluency measures both produced significant correlations with other measures of executive functioning. Both correlated moderately with at least one score on the Wisconsin Card Sorting Test (WCST) as well as with the Towers of Hanoi.

The correlations between the fluency tasks and the WCST are consistent with the lesion study by Davidson et al. (2008), which found that these two tasks were both affected by lesions to the same frontal lobe structures, although a meta-analysis of lesion studies by Henry and Crawford (2004) suggested that the relationship between the WCST and phonemic fluency should be greater than that for semantic fluency despite conflicting data from some previous research. The fact that the two food fluency tasks both produced moderate, but significant, correlations with the WCST as well as other executive functioning measures suggests that perhaps there is a greater involvement of the executive control system for this type of semantic fluency task than is typical for this task as well as compared to the current animal fluency task. It is possible that this is related to the stronger relationships with the academic and English literacy measures seen with the food compared to the animal fluency task. Additional analysis of the current data might investigate the possibility that higher levels of fingerspelled responses, which might recruit more English-oriented strategies, were produced for this category than for the animal category. Clearly, while these tasks involve many shared cognitive processes and skills, they also tap unique aspects of cognitive functioning.

Table 8.6 F–A–S Food—significant correlations

Test	r	N
WJ-III Reading Fluency	0.55**	46
WJ-III Writing Fluency	0.52**	46
WJ-III Academic Knowledge	0.34**	46
WJ-III Passage Comprehension	0.48**	47
PIAT Reading	0.55**	47
WCST Total Correct	0.35*	35
WCST Categories Completed	0.42*	35
Towers of Hanoi	0.45**	43
F–A–S	0.50**	49
F–A–S Animals	0.65**	49
5–1–U	0.37*	47
5–1–U Animals	0.63**	46
5–1–U Food	0.64**	46
ASL-SRT	0.53**	33
Fingerspelling Test Total Correct	0.59**	49
Fingerspelling Test Real Words	0.57**	49
Fingerspelling Test Fake Word	0.57**	49
TOSWRF	0.39**	46
Print Letter Forward Span	0.39*	36
Print Digit Backward Span	0.31*	45
ASL Letter Forward Span	0.35**	49
ASL Letter Backward Span	0.39**	49
ASL Digit Backward Span	0.34**	49

**Significance at $p<0.01$, *significance at $p<0.05$

Summary of Linguistic Fluency

The measures of linguistic fluency correlated with a wide range of measures, with a primary focus on language (both English and ASL) and literacy related tasks. While the sign-based phonemic task correlated with a narrower range of measures than the English-based phonemic task and the semantic fluency tasks, it did correlate significantly with both the English word-based fingerspelling task and the writing measure, suggesting an underlying linguistic mechanism which can be accessed using either speech- or sign-based strategies. One of the more interesting outcomes was the apparent subtle impact of priming with either the speech- or sign-based phonemic tasks on the strategies used for the semantic fluency tasks. The outcomes were comparable for the two tasks, as reflected in the near identical means and standard deviations for the two administrations of both the food and animal fluency tasks. However, the correlations suggest somewhat more English-oriented associations with the tasks administered following the English-based F–A–S task, and more sign-oriented and visual associations with the semantic tasks administered immediately following the sign-based 5–1–U task. The equivalent outcomes suggest that the search strategies employed are equally effective for semantic searches. This is a fascinating outcome and is worthy of future investigation.

Table 8.7 5–1–U Food—significant correlations

Test	r	N
WJ-III Reading Fluency	0.64**	45
WJ-III Writing Fluency	0.51**	45
WJ-III Passage Comprehension	0.48**	44
PIAT Reading	0.50**	46
WCST Total Correct	0.37*	35
Towers of Hanoi	0.37*	42
F–A–S	0.55**	46
F–A–S Animals	0.45**	46
F–A–S Food	0.64**	46
5–1–U	0.41**	46
5–1–U Animals	0.66**	46
M-SVLT List B Recall	0.31*	46
M-SVLT Cued Recall	0.46**	45
M-SVLT Delayed List A Free Recall	0.41**	45
M-SVLT Recognition Number Correct	0.47**	44
ASL-SRT	0.55**	31
Fingerspelling Test Total Correct	0.55**	46
Fingerspelling Test Real Words	0.56**	46
Fingerspelling Test Fake Words	0.50**	46
TOSWRF	0.43**	45
Print Letter Forward Span	0.36*	35
Corsi Blocks Manual Backward Span	0.41**	46
ASL Letter Forward Span	0.33*	46
ASL Letter Backward Span	0.39**	46

**Significance at $p<0.01$, *significance at $p<0.05$

In addition to the language and literacy connection, the linguistic fluency tasks also produced consistent relationships with measures of short-term/working memory, especially the linguistic forms of these tasks. This is not surprising as the linguistic fluency tasks employ working memory during the search and retrieval process. Additionally, most of the tasks yielded significant correlations with one or more measures of executive functioning. This is consistent with the traditional use of verbal fluency tasks as measures of executive functioning and suggests that this relationship holds for this population.

While further work needs to be done, it appears that (1) signing deaf individuals will likely produce fewer words than their English-speaking hearing peers on measures of English phonemic fluency, (2) the sign-based phonemic fluency task shows promise as a more appropriate measure of overall phonemic fluency in signing deaf individuals, and (3) although the underlying strategies being used may vary, outcomes of semantic fluency tasks appear to be consistent regardless of whether they follow sign- or speech-based measures. While these data do not provide norms for clinical interpretation, they do provide guidance for clinicians who are aware of the issues related to working with deaf individuals and could be used as supportive data in careful clinical practice as well as research.

References

Anderson, P. (2008). Towards a developmental model of executive function. In V. Anderson, R. Jacobs, & P. J. Anderson (Eds.), *Executive functions and the frontal lobes: A lifespan perspective* (pp. 3–21). New York: Taylor and Francis.

Axelrod, B. N., & Henry, R. R. (1992). Age-related performance on the Wisconsin Card Sorting, Similarities, and Controlled Oral Word Association Tests. *The Clinical Neuropsychologist, 6*, 16–26.

Barry, D., Bates, M. E., & Labouvie, E. (2008). FAS and CFL forms of verbal fluency differ in difficulty: A meta-analytic study. *Applied Neuropsychology, 15*(2), 97–106.

Battison, R. (1978). *Lexical borrowing in American Sign Language*. Silver Spring, MD: Linstok Press.

Bechtoldt, H. P., Benton, A. L., & Fogel, M. L. (1962). An application of factor analysis in neuropsychology. *Psychological Record, 12*, 147–156.

Benton, A. L. (1967). Problems of test construction in the field of aphasia. *Cortex, 3*, 32–58.

Bialystok, E., Craik, F. I., & Luke, G. (2008). Lexical access in bilinguals: Effects of vocabulary size and executive control. *Journal of Neurolinguistics, 21*, 522–538.

Chong, A., Sankar, L. & Poor, H. V. (2009). Frequency of occurrence and information entropy of American Sign Language, archived draft arXiv:0912.1768; downloaded from http://arxiv.org/abs/0912.1768.

Cohen, M. J., Morgan, A. M., Vaughn, M., Riccio, C. A., & Hall, J. (1999). Verbal fluency in children: Developmental issues and differential validity in distinguishing children with attention-deficit hyperactivity disorder and two subtypes of dyslexia. *Archives of Clinical Neuropsychology, 14*(5), 433–443.

Corina, D., & Emmorey, K. (1993, November). *Lexical priming in American Sign Language*.

Costa, A. (2005). Lexical access in bilingual production. In J. F. Kroll & A. M. de Groot (Eds.), *Handbook of bilingualism: Psycholinguistic approaches* (pp. 308–328). New York: Oxford University Press.

Davidson, P. S. R., Gao, F. Q., Mason, W. P., Winocur, G., & Anderson, N. D. (2008). Verbal fluency, trail making, and Wisconsin Card Sorting Test performance following right frontal lobe tumor resection. *Journal of Clinical and Experimental Neuropsychology, 30*(1), 18–32. doi:10.1080/13803390601161166.

Delis, D. C., Kaplan, E., & Kramer, J. H. (2001). *Delis Kaplan executive function system (D-KEFS)*. San Antonio, TX: Psychological Corporation.

Denckla, M. B. (1996). A theory and model of executive function: A neuropsychological perspective. In G. R. Lyon & N. A. Krasnegor (Eds.), *Attention, memory, and executive function* (pp. 263–278). Baltimore, MD: Paul H. Brookes.

Emmorey, K., McCullough, S., & Brentari, D. (2003). Categorical perception in American Sign Language. *Language & Cognitive Processes, 18*, 21–45.

Grogan, A., Green, D. W., Ali, N., Crinion, J. T., & Price, C. (2009). Structural correlates of semantic and phonemic fluency ability in first and second languages. *Cerebral Cortex, 19*(11), 2690–2698. doi:10.1093/cercor/bhp023.

Halperin, J. M., Healey, J. M., Zeitchik, E., Ludman, W. L., & Weinstein, L. (1989). Developmental aspects of linguistic and mnestic abilities in normal children. *Journal of Clinical and Experimental Neuropsychology, 11*, 518–528.

Hamburger, M., & Slowiaczek, L. M. (1996). Phonological priming reflects lexical competition. *Psychonomic Bulletin and Review, 3*, 520–525.

Henry, J. D., & Crawford, J. R. (2004). A meta-analytic review of verbal fluency performance in traumatic brain injured patients. *Neuropsychology, 18*, 621–628.

Kempler, D., Teng, E. L., Dick, M., Taussig, I. M., & Davis, D. S. (1998). The effects of age, education, and ethnicity on verbal fluency. *Journal of the International Neuropsychological Society, 4*, 531–538.

Lezak, M. D., Howieson, D. B., & Loring, D. W. (2004). *Neuropsychological assessment* (4th ed.). New York: Oxford University Press.

Loonstra, A. S., Tarlow, A. R., & Sellers, A. H. (2001). COWAT metanorms across age, education, and gender. *Applied Neuropsychology, 8*(3), 161–166. doi:10.1207/S15324826AN0803_5.

Luo, L., Luk, G., & Bialystok, E. (2010). Effect of language proficiency and executive control on verbal fluency performance in bilinguals. *Cognition, 114*, 29–41. doi:10.1016/j.cognition.2009.08.014.

Marschark, M., & Mayer, T. S. (1998). Interactions of language and memory in deaf children and adults. *Scandinavian Journal of Psychology, 39*, 145–148.

Mitrushina, M., Boone, K. B., Razani, J., & D'Elia, L. F. (2005). *Handbook of normative data for neuropsychological assessment* (2nd ed.). NY: Oxford University Press.

Morford, J. P., & Macfarlane, J. (2003). Frequency characteristics of American Sign Language. *Sign Language Studies, 3*(2), 213–225.

Morford, J. P., Wilkinson, E., Villwock, A., Piñar, P., & Kroll, J. F. (2011). When deaf signers read English: Do written words activate their sign translations? *Cognition, 118*(2), 286–292. doi:10.1016/j.cognition.2010.11.006.

Oller, D. K., & Eilers, R. E. (Eds.). (2002). *Language and literacy in bilingual children*. Clevedon: Multilingual Matters.

Portocarrero, J. S., Burright, R. G., & Donovick, P. J. (2007). Vocabulary and verbal fluency of bilingual and monolingual college students. *Archives of Clinical Neuropsychology, 22*, 415–422.

Raboutet, C., Sauzeon, H., Corsini, M., Rodrigques, J., Langevin, S., & N'Kaoua, B. (2010). Performance on semantic verbal fluency task across time: Dissociation between clustering, switching, and categorical exploitation process. *Journal of Clinical and Experimental Neuropsychology, 32*(3), 268–280.

Regard, M., Strauss, E., & Knapp, P. (1982). Children's production on verbal and non-verbal fluency tasks. *Perceptual and Motor Skills, 55*(3), 839–844.

Rende, B., Ramsberger, G., & Miyake, A. (2002). Commonalities and differences in the working memory components underlying letter and category fluency tasks: A dual-task investigation. *Neuropsychology, 16*(3), 309–321. doi:10.1037/0894-4105.16.3.309.

Rodríguez-Aranda, C., & Martinussen, M. (2006). Age-related differences in performance of phonemic verbal fluency measured by Controlled Oral Word Association Task (COWAT): a meta-analytic study. *Developmental Neuropsychology, 30*(2), 697–717.

Ruff, R. M., Light, R. H., & Parker, S. B. (1996). Benton controlled oral word association test: Reliability and updated norms. *Archives of Clinical Neuropsychology, 11*(4), 329–338.

Ruff, R. M., Light, R. H., Parker, S. B., & Levin, H. S. (1997). The psychological construct of word fluency. *Brain and Language, 57*, 394–405.

Schwartz, S., Baldo, J., Graves, R. E., & Brugger, P. (2003). Pervasive influence of semantics in letter and category fluency: A multidimensional approach. *Brain and Language, 87*(3), 400–411.

Spreen, O., & Benton, A. L. (1969). *Neurosensory center comprehensive examination for aphasia: Manual of directions*. Victoria, BC: Neuropsychology Laboratory, University of Victoria.

Stokoe, W. C. (1960). *Sign language structure. Studies in linguistics*. Buffalo, NY: University of Buffalo Press.

Strauss, E., Sherman, E. M., & Spreen, O. (2006). *A compendium of neuropsychological tests: Administration, norms, and commentary* (3rd ed.). New York: Oxford University Press.

Troyer, A. K., Moscovitch, M., & Winocur, G. (1997). Clustering and switching as two components of verbal fluency: Evidence from younger and older healthy adults. *Neuropsychology, 11*(1), 138–146.

Welsh, M. C., Pennington, B. F., & Groisser, D. B. (1991). A normative-developmental study of executive function: A window on prefrontal function in children. *Developmental Neuropsychology, 7*, 131–149.

Wilson, M., & Emmorey, K. (1997). Working memory for sign language: A window into the architecture of the working memory system. *Journal of Deaf Studies and Deaf Education, 2*(3), 121–130.

Young, A. R., Beitchman, J. H., Johnson, C., Douglas, L., Atkinson, L., Escobar, M., et al. (2002). Young adult academic outcomes in a longitudinal sample of early identified language impaired and control children. *Journal of Child Psychology and Psychiatry, 43*(5), 635–645. doi:10.1111/1469-7610.

Chapter 9
Measures of Receptive Language

Donna A. Morere and Daniel S. Koo

Reception of American Sign Language

As will be discussed in more depth in a later chapter in this volume, there is a dearth of instruments designed to measure skills in American Sign Language (ASL). The current study employed a measure, the American Sign Language Sentence Reproduction Test (ASL-SRT; Hauser et al. 2008) developed for VL2, which will also be discussed in more detail in the chapter on the assessment of ASL. While this instrument continues to be experimental in nature and has undergone some modifications in scoring since the data collection for this project, it does provide a reflection of the skills of the participant in what the majority of students reported was their primary mode of communication. Hauser and colleagues noted that, based on pilot data with deaf native signing children, the 39 item test was reordered so that examinees are presented with sentences representing a developmental sequence of increasing complexity. The original instrument was found to differentiate both hearing and deaf adult native signers and deaf native and nonnative signers. While the original ASL-SRT had 39 items, a shortened version with 20 items was used for the current study. The 20 item version scored in a manner consistent with the current study was used by Freel et al. (2011).

While the response of the participant is signed, the response is fully dependent on the ability of the participant to accurately receive linguistically accurate ASL; thus, it is considered a receptive measure for the purposes of this study. The task involves computer-administered signed sentences presented by deaf native signers. The participant must reproduce each sentence from memory. The stimuli were accessed through a secure, password-protected online interface housed on a server at the National Technical Institute for the Deaf (NTID) and the responses are captured

D.A. Morere (✉) • D.S. Koo
Department of Psychology, Gallaudet University,
800 Florida Avenue, NE, Washington, DC 20002, USA
e-mail: Donna.Morere@Gallaudet.edu; Daniel.Koo@Gallaudet.edu

Table 9.1 American Sign Language Sentence Reproduction Test (ASL-SRT)—descriptive statistics

Test	Scale	Range	N	Mean (SD)
ASL-SRT	Total Correct	1–17	33	8.97 (4.33)

by a webcam and returned to NTID where the responses were scored by deaf native signers at the Deaf Studies Lab headed by Peter Hauser, Ph.D.

While future iterations of this test may use modified scoring, for the current study, a strict scoring paradigm was used, which required the exact reproduction of the sentence as it was signed. Alterations in the sign production resulted in a score of zero for the sentence even if the meaning of the utterance was retained. Scoring of the original 39 item test using this method was reported to yield adequate inter-rater reliability ($r=0.83$, $p<0.01$), although one of the two raters apparently used a higher criterion for the scoring (Hauser et al. 2008). However, there are two concerns related to this method of scoring. First, it relies on subjective ratings which, according to Hauser et al., even in the pilot study produced significant differences in the mean scores generated by the two highly trained deaf native signers. Second, the reliance on exact reproduction raises the question of the relative importance of ASL skills versus visual memory, since it is possible that an individual with strong ASL skills might repeat the meaning of the sentence, but slightly alter the production, resulting in an error, while someone with lower ASL fluency but high levels of visuospatial memory might depend on their retention of the visuospatial sequence and provide an accurate reproduction despite a less clear understanding of the meaning of the item. While it is assumed that linguistic mediation of the more skilled signer would decrease the load on visual memory, this possibility must be considered.

Results of the ASL-SRT

As seen in Table 9.1, despite the presence of a relatively high proportion (44%) of participants with deaf parents, suggesting a relatively high proportion of native signers in the group, not only did no participant achieve a perfect score, they did not approach the 19 correct seen in the study by Freel et al. (2011). While the mean scores of the current sample are slightly below those of Freel and colleagues (mean 10.70, SD 4.42), they are not inconsistent and could be explained by differences in the samples.

As can be seen in Table 9.2, a broad range of the Toolkit measures produced significant correlations with the ASL-SRT. The moderate to strong correlations with measures of reading and writing are consistent with those of Freel et al. (2011), who used the ASL-SRT and the WJ-III Passage Comprehension tests with a sample similar to the current study and found that performance on the two measures correlated significantly (r (53)=0.48, $p<0.001$). This supports the contention that a strong language base is important for literacy and academic success regardless of whether it is English or ASL. Moderate to strong correlations were also obtained with the three receptive fingerspelling tasks, with the higher correlations appearing to reflect

Table 9.2 American Sign Language Sentence Reproduction Test (ASL-SRT)—significant correlations

Test	r	N
MRT Short Form A	0.60*	15
WJ-III Reading Fluency	0.45**	32
WJ-III Writing Fluency	0.60**	31
WJ-III Passage Comprehension	0.39*	33
PIAT-Reading	0.56**	32
TOSWRF	0.41*	31
WCST Perseverative Errors	−0.43*	23
K-BIT2 Matrices	0.35*	32
F–A–S	0.46**	33
F–A–S Animals	0.40*	33
F–A–S Food	0.53**	33
5–1–U Animals	0.48**	31
5–1–U Food	0.55**	31
M-SVLT Cued Recall	0.44*	33
Fingerspelling Test Total Correct	0.52**	33
Fingerspelling Test Real Words	0.53**	33
Fingerspelling Test Fake Words	0.46**	33
Print Letter Forward Span	0.45*	24
ASL Letter Forward Span	0.43*	33
ASL Letter Backward Span	0.45**	33
ASL Digit Backward Span	0.35*	33

**Significance at $p<0.01$, *significance at $p<0.05$

the participant's use of English vocabulary to support their responses, again suggesting an interaction between the two languages used by these participants. The relationships with the Fingerspelling Tests also likely involve visual short-term and working memory, as both tasks require visual reception and retention of transient visuospatial stimuli. This is also reflected in the moderate relationships observed with the ASL letter and digit span tasks, as well as the visually presented Print Letters Forward. Visual and linguistic working memory would be expected to be involved in the visual retention and reproduction of signed sentences.

The moderate to large correlations obtained for the linguistic fluency tasks again support the relationships between language functioning and linguistic fluency. Although the work of Luo et al. (2010) focused on the impact of English vocabulary on verbal fluency performance, it is reasonable to suppose that skill with ASL could also affect linguistic fluency performance. Thus, the outcomes of these studies appear to be consistent. This is further supported by the moderate correlation with the cued recall trial of the sign-based list learning task.

In addition to the relationships with academic, linguistic, and memory tasks, the ASL-SRT produced significant correlations with the measure used to estimate general cognitive abilities. While this correlation may in part reflect an underlying association between intelligence and language skills, in this case, there is also the impact of visual perception and analysis on both tasks, since the cognitive measure used for this study involves visual reasoning and ASL is a visuospatial language.

Thus, the relationship between these two measures likely reflects a combination of general cognitive abilities and visuospatial functioning. The interaction between the ASL-SRT and visuospatial abilities is more apparent in the strong correlation obtained between this test and the mental rotation task. This is consistent with previous research which has indicated a significant relationship between ASL skills and mental rotation abilities, with long-term users of ASL demonstrating enhanced mental rotation skills (Emmorey 2002; Emmorey et al. 1998; Marschark 2003). One additional correlation was the negative correlation with perseverative errors on the Wisconsin Card Sorting Test. It is unclear why perseveration would correlate even moderately with sign skills, and further exploration of this relationship is warranted.

Fingerspelling

Fingerspelling represents the use of the manual alphabet to represent English words. As will be discussed in a later chapter, there are multiple forms of the manual alphabet which are used with different languages and are used to represent the letters used in the relevant languages. However, it should be noted that just because two groups use the same spoken language does not mean that they will use the same manual alphabet. This is reflected in the difference between the one-handed manual alphabet associated with ASL and the two-handed manual alphabet associated with British Sign Language (BSL) despite the fact that the spoken language used in both countries is English. Fingerspelling represents a bridge between the spoken and signed languages, as the manual letters are generally considered to be a part of the signed language, but they are used to depict words from the spoken languages. Typically, fingerspelling is used to represent words which have no direct signed equivalent as well as names and nonwords (e.g., nonsense words used for rhyming in Dr. Seuss books) or slang. Fingerspelling has also been used as a route to access reading of English (Haptonstall-Nykaza and Schick 2007). One unique aspect of the relationship between English and ASL related to fingerspelling is the conversion of fingerspelled words to signs; some words that are commonly signed become incorporated into ASL and become more sign-like, or lexicalized (Valli et al. 2005). These fingerspelled loan signs may differ significantly from their precisely fingerspelled equivalents, and appear to be received as signs rather than as fingerspelled words. As will be discussed in the later chapter, recent research which has indicated that, at least for native signers of BSL, while both signs and fingerspelling share areas of brain activation, additional areas are recruited in the processing of fingerspelling compared to signs (Waters et al. 2007).

Table 9.3 Fingerspelling Test—descriptive statistics

Test	Scale	Range	N	Mean (SD)
Fingerspelling Test (raw scores)	Total Correct	29–69	49	52.90 (10.00)
	Real Words correct	19–45	49	33.92 (6.57)
	Pseudo-words Correct	10–25	49	18.98 (3.71)

The Fingerspelling Test

The Fingerspelling Test was developed for this study based on two subtests from the Woodcock Johnson Tests of Academic Achievement, Third Edition (WJ-III; Woodcock et al. 2001): Spelling and Spelling of Sounds. The former task uses real words while the latter uses pseudo-words. These were intermingled for the current task so that the participants would focus on the fingerspelled letters and be less able to depend on their English vocabulary to support their reception. The participants were presented with fingerspelled words using video clips presented on an iMac computer. The test was designed for the responses to be written verbatim; however, responses can be either written or fingerspelled and videotaped. As deaf individuals are exposed to English vocabulary through fingerspelling in addition to print, the accuracy of their reception of such input could significantly impact English vocabulary skills. Additionally, the relative performance on real words compared to the pseudo-words may reflect the ability of participants to use vocabulary knowledge to support reception. This will be discussed further in a later chapter. There were a maximum of 45 real words and 25 pseudo-words.

Fingerspelling Test Results

On average, the participants correctly received and reported 75% of both the real (75.4%) and pseudo-words (75.9%) on the Fingerspelling Test (Table 9.3). The fact that there was no difference between the performances on real versus pseudo-words suggests that the ability to visually receive and decode fingerspelling may be more dependent on visual reception of the letters than knowledge of English vocabulary. It should be noted, however, that the fact that the pseudo-words were intermingled with the real words may have artificially focused the participants' reception on the individual letters. In everyday use, where both context and the expectation of real words would be present, the use of vocabulary to support reception would be more likely.

As can be seen in Tables 9.4–9.6, all three scores derived from the Fingerspelling Test correlated with a wide range of measures, with nearly identical correlations being observed with most other measures. Thus, the three sets of correlations will be discussed together. As expected, the three Fingerspelling scores were highly intercorrelated, suggesting that the real and fake word portions tap highly related sets of cognitive processes. Strong relationships were also observed with all mea-

Table 9.4 Fingerspelling Test Total Correct—significant correlations

Test	r	N
WJ-III Reading Fluency	0.68**	46
WJ-III Writing Fluency	0.60**	46
WJ-III Academic Knowledge	0.49**	46
WJ-III Passage Comprehension	0.55**	47
PIAT Reading	0.61**	47
WCST Total Score	0.35*	35
WCST Categories Completed	0.36*	35
K-BIT2 Matrices	0.41**	47
F–A–S	0.50**	49
F–A–S Animals	0.62**	49
F–A–S Food	0.59**	49
5–1–U	0.39**	47
5–1–U Animals	0.53**	46
5–1–U Food	0.55**	46
M-SVLT List A Total Recall	0.29*	49
M-SVLT Cued Recall	0.29*	48
M-SVLT Delayed Cued Recall	0.31*	47
ASL-SRT	0.52**	33
Fingerspelling Test: Real Words	0.99**	49
Fingerspelling Test: Fake Words	0.95**	49
TOSWRF	0.53**	46
Print Letter Forward Span	0.46**	36
Print Digit Backward Span	0.31*	45
Corsi Blocks Manual Backward Span	0.29*	49
ASL Letter Forward Span	0.44**	49
ASL Letter Backward Span	0.45**	49

**Significance at $p<0.01$, *significance at $p<0.05$

sures of reading and writing. This supports the contention that fingerspelling can serve as a bridge to print. This is supported by the moderate positive correlation with Academic Knowledge observed for all three tasks. It is likely that in practice the relationship between reading and fingerspelling is interactive: increased use of both receptive and expressive fingerspelling likely enhances reading and writing skills and vice versa.

The next highest correlations were with the measures of linguistic fluency. All three of the Fingerspelling Test scores produced moderate to strong correlations with both the semantic and phonemic (ASL and English) fluency tasks, with the stronger relationships generally occurring with the semantic fluency tasks despite the fact that the two phonemic tasks would be expected to recruit aspects of fingerspelling (e.g., the letters for F–A–S and handshapes representing the letters for 5–1–U). Interestingly, the relationships with F–A–S were generally stronger, supporting an effect of alphabetic knowledge on both tasks.

Table 9.5 Fingerspelling Test Real Words Correct—significant correlations

Test	r	N
WJ-III Reading Fluency	0.69**	46
WJ-III Writing Fluency	0.60**	46
WJ-III Academic Knowledge	0.48**	46
WJ-III Passage Comprehension	0.54**	47
PIAT Reading	0.61**	47
WCST Total Correct Raw Score	0.36*	35
WCST Categories Completed	0.40*	35
K-BIT2 Matrices	0.43**	47
F–A–S	0.50**	49
F–A–S Animals	0.59**	49
F–A–S Food	0.57**	49
5–1–U	0.38**	47
5–1–U Animals	0.50**	46
5–1–U Food	0.56**	46
M-SVLT List A Total Recall	0.28*	49
M-SVLT Cued Recall	0.29*	48
M-SVLT Delayed Cued Recall	0.30*	47
ASL-SRT	0.53**	33
Fingerspelling Test Total Correct	0.99**	49
Fingerspelling Test Fake Words	0.89**	49
TOSWRF	0.54**	46
Print Letter Forward Span	0.46**	36
Corsi Blocks Manual Backward Span	0.29*	49
ASL Letter Forward Span	0.47**	49
ASL Letter Backward Span	0.48**	49
ASL Digit Backward Span	0.29*	49

**Significance at $p<0.01$, *significance at $p<0.05$

Moderate to strong correlations were also observed with the ASL-SRT. While this task involves signs rather than fingerspelling of English words, it is a measure of dynamic visual reception of language, and it could be expected that more fluent signers would also be more skilled in the use of fingerspelling (receptively as well as expressively). Additionally, as noted above, the two tasks involve shared cognitive processing despite some differences in brain activation. Despite the relatively strong relationships with sentence level ASL reception, performance on the sign-based list learning task was correlated at only moderate to weak levels with the fingerspelling scores. While these measures both require linguistic reception and recall, the Fingerspelling Test uses the manual modality to represent English while the SVLT is purely sign based. Additionally, while the former task requires ordered reproduction of the letters, recall of the list of signs on the latter is not order dependent. Thus, the weak to moderate relationships observed likely reflect underlying facility with language and memory rather than a direct relationship.

Moderate to weak correlations were observed between the fingerspelling tasks and the linguistic working memory tasks. In general, the stronger relationships were with the letter span tasks, again supporting the impact of alphabetic

Table 9.6 Fingerspelling Test Fake Words Correct—significant correlations

Test	r	N
WJ-III Reading Fluency	0.61**	46
WJ-III Writing Fluency	0.54**	46
WJ-III Academic Knowledge	0.47**	46
WJ-III Passage Comprehension	0.53**	47
PIAT-Reading	0.58**	47
K-BIT2 Matrices	0.34*	47
F–A–S	0.45**	49
F–A–S Animals	0.64**	49
F–A–S Food	0.57**	49
5–1–U	0.39**	47
5–1–U Animals	0.54**	46
5–1–U Food	0.50**	46
M-SVLT List A Total Recall	0.28*	49
M-SVLT Delayed Cued Recall	0.31*	47
ASL-SRT	0.46**	33
Fingerspelling Test Total Correct	0.95**	49
Fingerspelling Test Fake Words	0.89**	49
TOSWRF	0.48**	46
Print Letter Forward Span	0.44**	36
Print Digit Backward Span	0.32*	45
ASL Letter Forward Span	0.36*	49
ASL Letter Backward Span	0.35*	49

**Significance at $p<0.01$, *significance at $p<0.05$

knowledge in addition to the impacts of working memory on the Fingerspelling Test, which required the participants to hold the fingerspelled words in short-term/working memory for reproduction. Indeed, in the absence of the support of vocabulary and the rules of spelling, this could be considered a forward span task with the letters produced at a somewhat faster rate than the digit and letter span tasks. Each fingerspelling score also correlated at moderate to low levels with one reverse digit span task, and overall score and real word score correlated weakly, but at significant levels, with the manually administered reverse spatial span task, again supporting the impact of working memory on this task.

Overall the relationships between the measure of fingerspelling and the other Toolkit tasks support a strong relationship between English skills and receptive fingerspelling as well as an underlying effect of basic linguistic skills regardless of language. The impact of memory was also apparent, particularly linguistic short-term/working memory. Further investigation of fingerspelling both as a tool for accessing literacy and as an aspect of ASL in daily communication is warranted.

English Phonological Knowledge in Deaf Populations

Historically, deaf children have lagged behind their hearing peers in literacy levels (Karchmer and Mitchell 2003; Traxler 2000). One explanation for this discrepancy is that deaf children lack access to spoken phonology (Shankweiler et al. 1979; Perfetti and Sandak 2000) and by extension, the use of phonological strategies during reading—most notably phonetic encoding in working memory, phonological awareness, and phonetic recoding in lexical access. This argument has been supported by a substantial body of literature indicating a strong correlation between phonological skills and literacy development (Adams 1990; Bradley and Bryant 1985; Ehri and Sweet 1991; Goswami & Bryant 1992; Olson et al. 1994; Snow et al. 1998; Torgeson et al. 1994; Wagner and Torgeson 1987). As a result, the role of phonology in deaf students vis-à-vis reading outcomes has been a subject of great interest to scholars and educators. Previous studies have shown that even with limited exposure to the speech sounds of language, deaf individuals are able to utilize phonological codes during language-related tasks (Hanson 1989; Hanson and Lichtenstein 1990; Hanson and Fowler 1987; Leybaert 1993; Conrad 1979; LaSasso et al. 2003). Many of these studies have used tasks of rhyme recognition or generation (as rhyming is seen as one indicator of phonological awareness). While there are other measures of phonological awareness used in hearing populations (e.g. Rosner Test of Auditory Analysis Skills, the Lindamood Auditory Conceptualization Test, or the Comprehensive Test of Phonological Processing), these tests require the stimuli to be verbally presented or mandate oral responses from subjects, which raises questions about test validity for deaf subjects who do not speech-read or use speech to communicate.

Koo Phoneme Detection Test (Koo PDT)

In order to remove communication barriers, a computer-based test called the Phoneme Detection Test (PDT) was developed to directly measure phonemic awareness in deaf populations (Koo et al. 2008). The use of visually presented stimuli (using Presentation version 0.81, http://www.neurobs.com) and keyboard responses eliminated undesirable confounds from subjects' different communication and language backgrounds and allowed between-group comparisons of accuracy and reaction time. In this test, participants were asked to detect the presence of a single phoneme in 150 words with multiple orthography-to-phonology correspondences (i.e. 'c' maps to /s/ and /k/ phonemes such as 'cent' and 'call'); visually presented words were divided into five target-phoneme sets: /s/, /g/, /j/, and /k/ (each repeated two times). Half the items contained target phonemes appearing in initial, medial, or word-final positions and the other half served as orthographic foils in which an alternate grapheme-to-phoneme correspondence was used. Subjects were instructed to respond as quickly and accurately as possible with keyboard buttons indicating "Yes" or "No" if an item contained the target phoneme. Explicit instructions and

Table 9.7 Koo Phoneme Detection Test (Koo PDT)—descriptive statistics

Test	Scale	Range	N	Mean (SD)
Koo Phoneme Detection Test	Total Score	70–145	47	94.36 (18.93)
	/k/ in C Score	11–29	47	19.57 (5.27)
	/s/ in C Score	14–30	47	20.49 (4.42)
	/j/ in G Score	8–29	47	19.23 (5.05)
	/g/ in G Score	6–29	47	16.11 (5.07)
	/k/ in CH Score	7–30	47	19.55 (5.66)

examples were given at the beginning of the test to ensure subjects understood that the task was not to detect orthographic units, but phonemic units. In addition, each set was preceded by a four-item practice session. The order of set presentation was counterbalanced across subjects

Koo Phoneme Detection Test Results

The results of the PDT showed considerable variability in total raw scores ($M=94.36$; $SD=18.93$). This represents an accuracy rate of approximately 63%, consistent with the 65% for deaf users of ASL in the study by Koo et al. (2008) and well below their other samples both hearing (signers and nonsigners) and deaf (oral and Cued Speech). The range of the scores on this test suggests that while some participants have negligible skills with English phonemes, others are quite skilled, with some participants achieving a near perfect performance (145/150). This suggests that while it is possible for deaf to access English phonology, not all do. Considering the range of educational and linguistic backgrounds of the participants in this study, it is possible that further investigation of the demographic characteristics as they relate to performance on this task may help to clarify the factors affecting this skill (Table 9.7).

In comparing the PDT with other Toolkit measures, consistent with the results of Koo et al. (2008), Pearson's correlation revealed no significant correlation between the PDT and standard scores from TOSWRF ($r=-0.09$; $p>0.05$). This is interesting because it shows how sight word recognition (as measured by TOSWRF) occurs independently of phonological awareness, at least for this group. Similarly, no significant correlation was detected between the PDT and language sub-scores of the WJ-III, including the Reading Fluency ($r=0.10$; $p>0.05$) and Writing Fluency standard scores ($r=-0.03$; $p>0.05$). In addition, WJ-III Passage Comprehension subscore was not significantly correlated with PDT ($r=0.20$; $p>0.05$). This latter differed from the results of the Koo et al. study, which found a positive, if somewhat weak, correlation between the PDT and Passage Comprehension. Somewhat surprising is the weak correlation between phonological knowledge and Reading/Writing Fluency or Passage Comprehension but considering the unique linguistic profile of this population and the results of the TOSWRF, the correlation outcomes further support the premise that the reading skills of deaf individuals are independent of phonological skills. However, there was significant positive correlation between the total raw score of the PDT and WJ-III Academic Knowledge Standard

Table 9.8 Koo PDT Total Score (Koo Test)—significant correlations

Test	r	N
MRT Short Form A	−0.40*	24
WJ-III Academic Knowledge	0.44**	46
Tower of London Timed Violations	−0.38*	45
M-SVLT List A Free Recall	0.31*	46
Lip Reading Percent Sentences Correct	0.62**	24
Print Digit Forward Span	0.33*	44

**Significance at $p<0.01$, *significance at $p<0.05$

Score ($r=0.41$; $p<0.05$) which is essentially an oral inquiry into subject's knowledge of academic content such as sciences and humanities. This indicates that despite the lack of association with the literacy measures, academic performance is significantly predicted by phonological awareness (Table 9.8).

The strongest relationship seen with the PDT was that with the Lipreading Screening Test (LST). This is not surprising, as speechreading is a significant source of information about English phonology, and individuals skilled in speechreading would be expected to have greater access to such information. This result is consistent with the finding of Koo et al. (2008) that the two orally oriented groups of deaf participants, who would be expected to be highly skilled in speechreading, performed in a manner consistent with hearing participants on the PDT. The other relationships observed with the PDT were all weak to moderate, although the moderate correlation with the forward print digit span task is consistent with previous research suggesting associations between verbal sequential processing and speech-based phonological awareness (Baddeley and Wilson 1985; Madigan 1971).

One interpretation from the above seemingly contradictory correlations is that while deaf people apparently do not need phonological skills to read, phonological awareness may prove to be an essential cognitive tool that facilitates later academic performance. In other words, a reading strategy that depends on sight word recognition may be sufficient for broad reading skills such as letter and word identification. But the use of phonological skills and strategies may be critical for higher level reading skills such as comprehension of increasingly difficult passages and decoding of novel print words encountered in academic settings. Moreover, the sight word strategy may be insufficient to handle the cognitive demands of retention and recall of increasingly complex words particularly in the face of increased vocabulary sizes and considerable orthographic similarities in the lexicon (Rack 1985).

Knowledge of English Syntax

Reading is more than single word decoding; it is a complex task requiring a range of skills in addition to decoding, including retrieval of concepts from long-term store, analysis of the grammar and syntax of the sentence, and the use of the reader's fund of information to use for top-down analysis to arrive at an understanding of the writers' intent Kelly (2003a). Understanding individual words will leave a reader with the ability to parrot the sentences without understanding the content. Knowledge of syntax resulting in automaticity of this analysis becomes increasingly important as the complexity of the text increases (Kelly 2003b). Thus, skill with English syntax would be expected to have an impact on the academic success of deaf students.

Test of Syntactic Ability

The Test of Syntactic Ability (TSA) (Quigley et al. 1978) evaluates syntactic knowledge of written English. The TSA Screening Test, which was used in this study, consists of 120 items in four-alternative, multiple-choice format. Participants are asked to detect errors in English syntactic structure and to identify the meaning of sentences that differ in syntactic construction. It provides a relatively quick and reliable assessment of a participant's general knowledge of written English syntax and pinpoints overall strengths and weaknesses in individual syntactic structures. The individual structures of syntax include: Negation, Determiners, Question Formation, Nominalization, Verb Processes, Complementation, Pronominalization, Conjunction, and Relativization. Test materials include norms for deaf children between 10 and 18 years of age.

Test of Syntactic Ability Results

Data from the TSA indicate that, while there are some participants who struggle with the task, the vast majority of the participants were highly skilled in recognizing accurate English structures. Even so, a subset of the participants struggled with this task, achieving less than 50% correct on the overall test, and with performance on some aspects of the test below chance levels. While most participants were able to recognize the structures tested, this test does not reflect automaticity with these skills or the students' ability to apply this knowledge in either writing or the reading of extended text. Since most of the scores approached the test ceiling, the correlational analyses will be limited to the Total Test Score and two sub-scores: Pronominalization and Relativization (Table 9.9).

Table 9.10 presents the significant correlations between the TSA Total Test Score, and the other Toolkit measures. Not surprisingly, moderate to strong correlations were observed with both of the other TSA scores as well as with most measures of reading and writing. The lack of a significant correlation with the WJ-III Reading Fluency supports the range of complexity on the TSA, as Reading Fluency consists entirely of sentences with very simple structure. Performance on the two tasks requires divergent skills: knowledge of increasingly complex sentences demonstrated without time constraints and the ability to quickly and accurately read and make decisions about a series of very simple sentences. All of the other reading tasks require some degree of facility

9 Measures of Receptive Language

Table 9.9 Test of Syntactic Ability (TSA)—descriptive statistics

Test	Scale	Range	N	Percent Correct (SD)
Test of Syntactic Ability (TSA)	**Total Test Score**	**43.33–99.17**	**40**	**89.15 (9.82)**
	Negation	62.50–100.00	40	97.50 (7.60)
	Determiners	57.14–100.00	40	93.39 (9.89)
	Question Formation	18.18–100.00	40	93.18 (15.09)
	Nominalization	15.79–100.00	40	86.18 (17.05)
	Complementation	44.44–100.00	40	89.86 (12.19)
	Pronominalization	**50.00–90.00**	**40**	**79.25 (9.97)**
	Conjunction	54.55–100.00	40	94.55 (11.24)
	Relativization	**36.84–100.00**	**40**	**82.63 (15.32)**
	Verb Processes	60.00–100.00	40	92.75 (9.87)

Tests in bold were included in the other analyses.

Table 9.10 TSA Total Test Score—significant correlations

Test	r	N
WJ-III Writing Fluency	0.47*	22
WJ-III Passage Comprehension	0.45*	22
PIAT Reading	0.55**	22
TOSWRF	0.46*	22
WCST Total Correct	0.50*	17
WCST Categories Completed	0.57*	17
F–A–S	0.44*	23
TSA Pronominalization Percent Correct	0.54**	40
TSA Relativization Percent Correct	0.85**	40
Print Digit Backward Span	0.48*	22
Corsi Blocks Computer Backward Span	0.59**	22
ASL Letter Forward Span	0.59**	23
ASL Letter Backward Span	0.49*	23
ASL Digit Backward Span	0.44*	23

**Significance at $p<0.01$, *significance at $p<0.05$

with increasing levels of syntactic complexity. The moderate to strong relationships with the WCST, a measure of executive functioning, may relate to the need for cognitive flexibility and executive control required for the careful analysis of the items on the test, a demand which would increase with the difficulty of the items. This may tap a similar process to that responsible for the moderate relationship between the TSA Total Test Score and the measure of English-based phonemic fluency (F–A–S). The underlying skills in English would contribute to both, and executive control is also important for the performance of these tasks.

Perhaps the most interesting set of correlations is that between this score and the measures of working memory, including one representing visual working memory. As the sentences become increasingly complex, it is necessary to hold the content in working memory as it is being analyzed. Kelly (2003b) noted that automaticity with basic reading processes, including syntax, interacts with working memory

Table 9.11 TSA Pronominalization Score—significant correlations

Test	r	N
WJ-III Academic Knowledge	0.51*	22
M-SVLT Delayed List A Free Recall	0.53**	23
TSA Total Correct	0.54**	40
TSA Relativization Percent Correct	0.41**	40
Corsi Blocks Computer Backward Span	0.44*	22

**Significance at $p<0.01$, *significance at $p<0.05$

capacity to affect reading outcomes. On the other hand, greater working memory capacity would allow for more analysis of the sentences with more complex structure. The relatively strong correlation with the measure of visual working memory may reflect students' use of visualization to analyze the sentences, either visualization of the meaning or visualizing the sentences for cognitive analysis. Further investigation of these relationships could clarify the relationships between linguistic knowledge and working memory.

In contrast to the overall test score, the TSA Pronominalization score correlated with relatively few measures in addition to the other TSA scores (Table 9.11). Instead of the reading and writing measures, this score correlated strongly with the WJ-III Academic Knowledge subtest, which reflects the student's learning of subject related content and vocabulary through reading and academic exposure as well as the delayed recall trial of the sign-based list learning task. These two measures reflect the individual's ability to retain information over time and may represent the impact of linguistic memory, regardless of language modality, on their understanding and facility with English. In ASL pronouns are typically indicated through pointing and spatial referents rather than multiple signs, whereas in English pronouns can be confusing even for native speakers of the language (e.g., "Joe and me" versus "Joe and I"). Additionally, as with the overall test score, there was a significant correlation with a visual working memory task, again possibly reflecting the use of visualization to analyze the sentences. This might have particular relevance for participants using a sign-based analysis of the sentences involving spatially placed referents for the pronouns.

Comprehension of relative clauses has long been seen as an area of difficulty for deaf readers (Kelly 2003b; Quigley et al. 1974); thus, it is not surprising that strong correlations were observed between this score and all of the reading measures—even Reading Fluency, which does not contain any such structures in the stimuli (Table 9.12). This latter is likely related to the impact on automaticity of basic reading skills required for the rapid, accurate reading required for this task. As indicated by Kelly, automaticity with basic structures is important for freeing cognitive resources for higher levels of analysis. Although the correlation is only moderate, the relationship with Academic Knowledge suggests that competence with complex syntax such as relative clauses on the learning of academic content. Furthermore, as with the previous discussions, the strong to moderate correlations with a range of linguistic working memory tasks is consistent with the interaction between the cognitive load associated with the degree of automaticity of basic reading and linguistic skills and the working memory capacity of the reader. This interaction is an important area for further research, since there are multiple areas of potential intervention which may arise from such research.

Table 9.12 TSA Relativization Score—significant correlations

Test	r	N
WJ-III Reading Fluency	0.51*	22
WJ-III Writing Fluency	0.50*	22
WJ-III Academic Knowledge	0.44*	22
WJ-III Passage Comprehension	0.61**	22
PIAT-Reading	0.61**	22
WCST Categories Completed	0.50*	17
F–A–S	0.50*	23
M-SVLT Delayed List A Free Recall	0.46*	23
TSA Percent Correct	0.85**	40
TSA Pronominalization Percent	0.41**	40
Print Digit Backward Span	0.45*	22
ASL Letter Forward Span	0.58**	23
ASL Letter Backward Span	0.57**	23
ASL Digit Backward Span	0.51*	23

**Significance at $p<0.01$, *significance at $p<0.05$

Visual Reception of Spoken Language

Regardless of the beliefs about the desirability of oral skills or the capacity of individuals to develop these skills, use of lipreading, or speechreading, is common among both deaf and hearing individuals to support their reception of spoken language to varying degrees, depending on the availability and clarity of the auditory signal (for a recent review, see Woodhouse et al. 2009). Furthermore, skill with speechreading has been associated with reading skills (Harris and Moreno 2006). However, Musselman (2000) noted that while previous research has suggested that speechreading skills are associated with use of phonological code, the accessible visual information is ambiguous, with multiple phonemes having similar oral configurations. Thus, even highly skilled speechreaders are able to accurately identify only about 48–85% of words in sentences (Bernstein 2006), although Auer and Bernstein (2007) found that individuals with early onset deafness who depended on oral skills for communication had significantly enhanced speechreading skills compared to hearing individuals. This raises the question of the importance of speechreading on linguistic, cognitive, and academic functioning within the current sample, which overwhelmingly identifies ASL as their primary mode of communication.

The Lipreading Screening Test

The LST, developed by Auer and Bernstein (2007), measures the individual's ability to accurately perceive a spoken sentence based on visual reception, without auditory support. Although this is commonly referred to as lipreading, Bernstein (2006)

noted that while information in and on the mouth and lips is important, research has demonstrated that visual speech perception also involves visual cues on the cheeks, jaw, and other areas of the lower face. Thus, the term speechreading more accurately reflects the full range of information involved in visual reception of spoken language.

The LST consists of 30 sentences, 15 spoken by an adult female and 15 spoken by an adult male. The faces of the two talkers are displayed on a monitor screen and responses (words understood) are typed on a keyboard by the participant after each sentence is displayed. The sentences range in length from 3 to 12 words, and the topics cover a variety of everyday events, e.g., parking, pets, food, and activities. The test is challenging because no context is provided; the sentences are not related to each other, and each sentence is displayed only once. Two scores are generated: the number of words correct in each sentence and the number of sentences that are semantically correct. The number of sentences correct refers to the number of sentences in which the participant correctly understands the semantic meaning of the sentence. In other words, for the sentence-correct score the sentence "Don't close the door" could be correctly interpreted as "Don't shut the door" or "leave the door open" while the sentence "Close the door" would be incorrect.

Auer and Bernstein found that early deafened individuals with a history of oral education and English as their first language achieved a mean of 43.55% of words correct (standard deviation 17.48), while hearing participants achieved only a mean of 18.57 (SD 13.18). As noted above, previous research has suggested that even highly skilled deaf speechreaders achieve approximately 48–85% accuracy of identifying words in sentences (Bernstein 2006).

Lipreading Screening Test Results

While the mean performance of the participants in this group was lower than that of the participants in the Bernstein (2006) study, participants in the current study included a significant number of individuals whose primary mode of communication is ASL, and who would therefore be expected to have less experience with speechreading compared to oral deaf individuals. Thus, the speechreading skills of this population appear to be appropriate considering their preferred communication mode. Furthermore, the range of skills varied from those who essentially had no speechreading skills, to those who are among the highly skilled speechreaders reported by Bernstein. Although only a small percentage of the sentences were correctly reported, these are sentences out of context, and in typical receptive situations, it would be expected that the communication success would be higher than that reflected by these scores (Table 9.13).

As seen in Tables 9.14 and 9.15, the two speechreading measures correlated quite highly with each other, and both the Speechreading Test Percentage of Words Correct and Speechreading Test Percentage of Sentences Correct produced strong correlations with the Koo PDT, supporting the research cited by Musselman (2000)

9 Measures of Receptive Language

Table 9.13 Lipreading Screening Test—descriptive statistics

Test	Subtest	Range	N	Mean (SD)
Lipreading Screening Test	Words Correct (raw score)	0–172	45	56.58 (42.10)
	Percent Correct Words	0–72.27	45	23.77 (17.69)
	Sentences Correct (raw score)	0–15	45	3.67 (3.60)
	Percent Correct Sentences	0–50.00	45	12.22 (12.00)

Table 9.14 Lipreading Screening Test Percent of Words Correct—significant correlations

Test	r	N
WJ-III Academic Knowledge	0.43*	24
WJ-III Passage Comprehension	0.44*	22
PIAT Reading	0.44*	24
Tower of London Time Violations	−0.56**	24
M-SVLT List A Free Recall	0.41*	24
M-SVLT Delayed List A Free Recall	0.46*	24
Koo Phoneme Detection Test	0.62**	24
Lip Reading Sentences Correct	0.94**	45

**Significance at $p<0.01$, *significance at $p<0.05$

Table 9.15 Lipreading Screening Test Percent of Sentences (Semantic Meaning) Correct—significant correlations

Test	r	N
WJ-III Academic Knowledge	0.42*	24
WJ-III Passage Comprehension	0.44*	22
PIAT Reading	0.48*	24
Tower of London Time Violations	−0.58**	24
Koo Phoneme Detection Test	0.62**	24
Lip Reading Percent Words Correct	0.94**	45

**Significance at $p<0.01$, *significance at $p<0.05$

suggesting that speechreading is associated with use of a phonological code. Both were also moderately correlated with measures of reading and academic knowledge, suggesting that while speechreading skills may not be a primary component of reading and academic achievement, it may support their development. Additionally, both scores correlate negatively with the scores on Time Violations on the Tower of London test, which reflects the ability to solve problems in a timely manner. It is unclear why this would produce a negative correlation with these measures, since speechreading requires rapid analysis of the speech movements and consideration of the member of the set of likely words being represented. Thus, this relationship deserves further investigation.

In addition to the shared relationships, the number of words correctly reproduced also correlated significantly with the two main free recall trials of the sign-based list learning task. Despite their foundations in different languages, both of these tasks depend on a combination of attention, language reception in the visual mode, and vocabulary in the relevant languages in addition to linguistic memory and retrieval. Thus, the moderate associations between the two tasks make sense despite the language differences involved. Furthermore, the lack of significant association between the SVLT scores and the LST score reflecting retention of meaning rather than precise words suggests that the latter task may depend more on integrative language abilities rather than retention of linguistic details. Overall, while speechreading is clearly associated with academic success, at least for a subset of the sample, it is one of many processes affecting literacy and academic achievement.

Summary of Linguistic Measures

As a whole, the measures of linguistic functioning appear to be highly interactive. One interesting observation is the fact that many of these measures produced significant correlations with multiple measures of working memory, particularly linguistic working memory. As this is an area of cognitive processing that has consistently demonstrated lower scores in deaf signers compared to typical hearing populations, these outcomes suggest that approaches to ensure optimal development of working memory may enhance language outcomes.

A second observation is the wide-ranging associations of fingerspelling not only with other language measures, but also with linguistic memory (regardless of language), literacy, and academic achievement. These data suggest that fingerspelling should be introduced early and used often, as it appears to contribute to a wide range of skills important for academic, as well as social and vocational, success.

This provides a segue into the third observation; in general, language functioning in one language appears to contribute to language functioning in the other language. For example, sign-based linguistic memory performance was correlated with a wide range of literacy and academic achievement scores as well as awareness of English phonology and reception and reproduction of both speechreading and fingerspelling. While bilingual exposure from an early age would be ideal, the interaction of language processes observed in these data suggests that some form of early accessible language may be more important than *which* language is accessed. If a strong first language is developed, these data suggest that it can be used to enhance functioning in the second language.

References

Adams, M. (1990). *Beginning to read: Thinking and learning about print*. Cambridge, MA: MIT Press.

Auer, A. T., & Bernstein, L. E. (2007). Enhanced visual speech perception in individuals with early-onset hearing impairment. *Journal of Speech, Language, and Hearing Research, 5*(5), 1157–1165.

Baddeley, A. D., & Wilson, B. A. (1985). Phonological coding and shortterm memory in patients without speech. *Journal of Memory and Language, 24*, 490–502. doi:10.1016/0749-596-X(85)90041-5 DOI:10.1016%2F0749-596X%2885%2990041-5.

Bernstein, L. E. (2006). Visual speech perception. In E. Vatikiotis-Bateson, G. Bailly, & P. Perrier (Eds.), *Audio-visual speech processing*. Cambridge: MIT Press.

Bradley, L., & Bryant, P. (1985). *Rhyme and reason in reading and spelling (IARLD Monographs, No. 1)*. Ann Arbor, MI: University of Michigan Press.

Conrad, R. (1979). *The deaf school child*. London: Harper and Row.

Ehri, L., & Sweet, J. (1991). Fingerpoint-reading of memorized text: What enables beginners to process the print? *Reading Research Quarterly, 24*, 442–462.

Emmorey, K. (2002). The impact of sign language use on visuospatial cognition. In *Language, cognition and the brain: Insights from sign language research*. Mahwah, NJ: Lawrence Erlbaum Associates.

Emmorey, K., Klima, E., & Hickok, G. (1998). Mental rotation within linguistic and non-linguistic domains in users of American Sign Language. *Cognition, 68*(3), 221–246.

Freel, B., Clark, D., Anderson, M., Gilbert, G., Musyoka, M., & Hauser, P. (2011). Deaf individuals' bilingual abilites: American sign language proficiency, reading skills, and family characteristics. *Psychology, 2*(1), 18–23.

Goswami, U., & Bryant, P. (1992). Rhyme, analogy, and children's reading. In P. B. Gough, L. C. Ehri & R. Treiman (Eds.), *Reading Acquisition* (pp. 49–64). Hillsdale, NJ: Lawrence Erlbaum Associates.

Hanson, V. (1989). Phonology and reading: Evidence from profoundly deaf readers. In D. Shankweiler & E. Y. Liberman (Eds.), *Phonology and reading disability: Solving the reading puzzle* (pp. 67–89). Ann Arbor, MI: University of Michigan Press.

Hanson, V., & Fowler, C. (1987). Phonological coding in word reading: Evidence from hearing and deaf readers. *Memory and Cognition, 15*, 199–207.

Hanson, V., & Lichtenstein, E. (1990). Short-term memory by deaf signers: The primary language coding hypothesis reconsidered. *Cognitive Psychology, 22*, 211–224.

Haptonstall-Nykaza, T. S., & Schick, B. (2007). The transition from fingerspelling to English print: Facilitating English decoding. *Journal of Deaf Studies and Deaf Education, 12*(2), 172–183.

Harris, M., & Moreno, C. (2006). Speech reading and learning to read: A comparison of 8-year-old profoundly deaf children with good and poor reading ability. *Journal of Deaf Studies and Deaf Education, 11*(2), 189–201.

Hauser, P. C., Paludnevičiene, R., Supalla, T., & Bavelier, D. (2008). American Sign Language-Sentence Reproduction Test: Development and implications. In R. M. de Quadros (Ed.), *Sign Language: Spinning and unraveling the past, present and future* (pp. 160–172). Petropolis, Brazil: Editora Arara Azul.

Karchmer, M. A., & Mitchell, R. E. (2003). Demographic and achievement characteristics of deaf and hard-of-hearing students. In M. Marschark & P. E. Spencer (Eds.), *Deaf studies, language, and education* (pp. 21–37). New York: Oxford University Press.

Kelly, L. (2003a). Considerations for designing practice for deaf readers. *Journal of Deaf Studies and Deaf Education, 8*(2), 171–186.

Kelly, L. (2003b). The importance of processing automaticity and temporary storage capacity to the differences in comprehension between skilled and less skilled college-age deaf readers. *Journal of Deaf Studies and Deaf Education, 8*(3), 230–249.

Koo, D., Crain, K., LaSasso, C., & Eden, G. (2008). Phonological awareness and short-term memory in hearing and deaf individuals of different communication backgrounds. *Annals of the New York Academy of Sciences, 1145*, 83–99.

LaSasso, C., Crain, K., & Leybaert, J. (2003). Rhyme generation in deaf students: The effect of exposure to cued speech. *Journal of Deaf Studies and Deaf Education, 8*(3), 250–270.

Leybaert, J. (1993). Reading in the deaf: The roles of phonological codes. In M. Marcshark & M. Diane (Eds.), *Psychological perspectives on deafness* (pp. 269–309). Hillsdale, NJ: Lawrence Erlbaum Associates.

Luo, L., Luk, G., & Bialystok, E. (2010). Effect of language proficiency and executive control on verbal fluency performance in bilinguals. *Cognition, 114*, 29–41. doi:10.1016/j.cognition.2009.08.014.

Madigan, S. A. (1971). Modality and recall order interactions in short-term memory for serial order. *Journal of Experimental Psychology, 87*, 294–296.

Marschark, M. (2003). Cognitive functioning in deaf adults and children. In M. Marschark & P. Spencer (Eds.), *Oxford handbook of deaf studies, language, and education* (pp. 464–477). New York: Oxford University Press.

Musselman, C. (2000). How do children who can't hear learn to read an alphabetic script? A review of the literature on reading and deafness. *Journal of Deaf Studies and Deaf Education, 5*(1), 9–31.

Olson, R., Forsberg, H., Wise, B., & Rack, J. (1994). Measurement of word recognition, orthographic, and phonological skills. In R. G. Lyon (Ed.), *Frames of reference from the assessment of learning disabilities* (pp. 243–277). Baltimore: Brooks.

Perfetti, C., & Sandak, R. (2000). Reading optimally builds on spoken language: Implications for deaf readers. *Journal of Deaf Studies and Deaf Education, 5*(1), 32–50.

Quigley, S. P., Smith, N. L., & Wilbur, R. B. (1974). Comprehension of relativized sentences by deaf students. *Journal of Speech and Hearing Research, 17*, 325–341.

Quigley, S. P., Steinkamp, M. W., Power, D. J., & Jones, B. W. (1978). *Test of syntactic abilities—A guide to administration and interpretation*. Oregon: Dormac Inc.

Rack, J. P. (1985). Orthographic and phonetic coding in developmental dyslexia. *British Journal of Psychology, 76*(3), 325–340.

Shankweiler, D., Liberman, I. Y., Mark, L., Fowler, C., & Fischer, F. (1979). The speech code and learning to read. *Journal of Experimental Psychology: Human Learning and Memory, 5*, 531–545.

Snow, C., Burns, S., & Griffin, P. (Eds.). (1998). *Preventing reading difficulties in young children*. Washington, DC: National Academy Press.

Torgeson, J. K., Wagner, R. K., & Rashotte, C. A. (1994). Longitudinal studies of phonological processing and reading. *Journal of Learning Disabilities, 27*(5), 276–286.

Traxler, C. B. (2000). The Stanford Achievement Test, 9th Edition: National norming and performance standards for deaf and hard-of-hearing students. *Journal of Deaf Studies and Deaf Education, 5*, 337–348.

Valli, C., Lucas, C., & Mulrooney, K. J. (2005). *Linguistics of American Sign Language: An introduction* (4th ed.). Washington, DC: Gallaudet University Press.

Wagner, R. K., & Torgeson, J. K. (1987). The nature of phonological processing and its causal role in the acquisition of reading skills. *Psychological Bulletin, 101*(2), 192–212.

Waters, D., Campbell, R., Capek, C. M., Woll, B., David, A. S., McGuire, P. K., et al. (2007). Fingerspelling, signed language, text and picture processing in deaf native signers: The role of the mid-fusiform gyrus. *NeuroImage, 35*, 1287–1302.

Woodcock, R. W., McGrew, K. S., & Mather, N. (2001). *Woodcock-Johnson III Tests of Achievement*. Itasca, IL: Riverside Publishing.

Woodhouse, L., Hickson, L., & Dodd, B. (2009). Review of visual speech perception by hearing and hearing-impaired people: Clinical implications. *International Journal of Language & Communication Disorders, 44*(3), 253–270.

Chapter 10
Fingerspelling

Donna A. Morere and Rachel Roberts

The use of manual alphabets dates back centuries, and historically was not restricted to use within the deaf community. Bragg (1997) noted that manual alphabet systems have been in existence since at least 1592, when the first such alphabet was memorialized in print. Many of these early forms were developed within monasteries to allow for communication while maintaining a vow of silence (Padden and Gunsauls 2003). Fingerspelling as it is used today is a component of signed languages such as American Sign Language (ASL), and involves the use of handshapes to represent the letters of the print forms of spoken languages.

Although it is common to consider the representations used in fingerspelling as letters, or the manual alphabet, Valli et al. (2005) argue that linguistically they should be considered signs. However, consistent with common usage, in this chapter the ASL signs used to represent letters will be labeled manual (or ASL) letters and the set of manual letters representing the alphabet as the manual alphabet. Manual letters are unusual in that they are a representation of a representation, twice removed from their linguistic source. That is, they are signed representations of the orthographic representations of the spoken language (Paul 2009). The discussion for this chapter will focus on the form of fingerspelling used in ASL. Forms of fingerspelling are, however, associated with many signed languages, although the degree and manner of use varies among the languages (Padden and Gunsauls 2003). Padden and Gunsauls noted that the use of fingerspelling within ASL is considered relatively high. In contrast, use of fingerspelling in Italian Sign Language is relatively limited, as it is used primarily to represent words from foreign languages. Italian words are represented by a related sign combined with mouthing of the spoken Italian word.

The form of the manual letters used in signed languages varies as well. Some, such as that associated with ASL use one hand per manual letter, while other

D.A. Morere (✉) • R. Roberts
Department of Psychology, Gallaudet University,
800 Florida Avenue, NE, Washington, DC 20002, USA
e-mail: Donna.Morere@Gallaudet.edu; Rachel.Roberts@Gallaudet.edu

languages, such as British Sign Language (BSL), use two-handed letters. The divergence of the forms of these two manual alphabets representing written English highlights the fact that fingerspelling is a part of the signed language, not the spoken language, despite its use to represent the orthography of the spoken language. Indeed, there can be variability in the representation of printed letters within a signed language. For example, in New Zealand, while the BSL alphabet is officially used, aerial writing, or writing with the forefinger in the air, is reportedly commonly used by many deaf adults to convey English words for which there is no sign (Forman 2003). Thus, the manual representation of print appears to be widespread as a means of representing print in through-the-air communication. However, as discussed below, its use is not restricted to simple representation of spoken words with no signed equivalents.

Fingerspelling in American Sign Language

While typical use of fingerspelling has been to represent names, places, and words that have no sign equivalent, it is also used for emphasis in discourse (Akamatsu and Stewart 1989), to signify distinctions in meaning for signs (Padden and Gunsauls 2003), and in both home and school settings to introduce English vocabulary. It has been used even more extensively in some settings. Indeed, in the late nineteenth century a school for the deaf in Rochester, New York implemented a communication method in which speech or mouth movements were accompanied by fingerspelling of everything that was said: the Rochester Method (Moores 1970; Padden and Gunsauls 2003; Paul 2009). This method was intended to replace signed communication and provide a direct route to English, but it was too cumbersome for most people. Thus, while it was used in deaf education programs during the 1950s and 1960s, and continued to be used in some schools into the 1970s, today the Rochester Method represents more of a historical footnote than a communication method (Paul 2009).

Padden and Gunsauls (2003) suggest that while the Rochester Method has generally been abandoned by deaf education, the more than seven decades of its use may have spurred greater use of fingerspelling in ASL within the deaf community in America. However, they also note that the expanded use of fingerspelling within ASL may also have been due to the access to education through Gallaudet University and the establishment of many schools for the deaf during the same period, resulting in increased literacy among deaf Americans. It was also suggested that fingerspelling may have been seen as a means of defending against the push for oralism which was co-occurring. Regardless of the source, fingerspelling became integrated into ASL, and appears to be widely used among the signing American deaf population.

Padden and Gunsauls noted that Americans fingerspell about 10–15% of the words in typical signed output, and that the proportion of fingerspelling varies depending on the topic and context. They analyzed a large database of videotaped conversations of American signers compiled in 2001 and found that while the grammatical category of words most frequently fingerspelled involved nouns, both common and proper, a wide range of grammatical structures were represented, including adjectives, verbs, and occasional adverbs, conjunctions, and articles. Among their analyses of variability in the use of fingerspelling among the participants, they found that native signers fingerspelled approximately 18% of their utterances, while nonnative signers' fingerspelling was closer to 15%. About half of the native signers fingerspelled 20% or more of their output, while a portion of the nonnative signers made little use of fingerspelling. Thus, while fingerspelling appears to be relatively heavily used in ASL compared to some sign languages, its use varies somewhat within the population.

With respect to the use of fingerspelling as a signifier, Padden and Gunsauls (2003) noted that it can be used to both signify the words which have no sign equivalents and to signify differences in meaning for words which do have sign equivalents. They provided an example of a teacher using fingerspelling to signify the difference between the word "problem" as it refers to a difficult situation and its use in the scientific sense. This type of use allows both the expansion of the depth of English vocabulary (providing multiple meanings for the same word) and the connection of previously understood concepts to new, in this case more analytical, concepts. Similarly, fingerspelling can be used for emphasis, as in the case of an adolescent using emphatic movements marching across the signing space in front of her fingerspelling B-I-G to emphasize the excessive size of something she had seen. This type of use is seen in both conversational signing, as in the above sample, and in academic and professional settings, as when it is used to emphasize specific aspects of content in a lecture. Padden and Gunsauls also noted that American signers continue to fingerspell many words in daily use which do have sign equivalents, as well as many words which, in other sign languages, have developed signed representations over the years, such as names of brands or famous people. Thus, fingerspelling appears to be an integral part of ASL as a form of communication and not simply a manual representation of print. Indeed, some frequently fingerspelled English words become converted into signs. This process of lexicalization involves changes to the fingerspelling which render it more sign-like (Valli et al. 2005). These fingerspelled "loan signs" may have letters omitted; there may be changes in shape, location, movement, or orientation of the hand, or a second hand added, rendering a lexicalized sign which may be significantly different from the original fingerspelled word. This can be a rich source of new vocabulary for the living language of ASL.

Use of the Manual Letters in ASL

The ASL manual alphabet includes both manual letters which are also used as handshapes in signs (e.g., the handshape used for the letter H or U—depending on the orientation—is also used in the signs for "train" and "egg") and those which are rarely, if ever, used as formational components of ASL signs (e.g., M). Manual letters are used in a variety of ways in ASL, though. Name signs typically use the initial letter of the individual's name in some manner and state names are routinely represented through abbreviated spelling. There is also a subset of two-letter fingerspelled abbreviations which have been incorporated into ASL, such as F-B for feedback and W-D for withdraw. Padden (1998) notes that these abbreviations differ from loan signs in that they tend to use the first and middle letter of the words instead of the first and last letters, which are most commonly retained in loan signs. Some ASL signs incorporate manual letter handshapes to represent aspects of words as components of the signs themselves, as in the signs for colors such as blue, yellow, and green. In general, though, initialization (representation of a related English word through use of the manual letter as the first handshape for the sign) was apparently not common in ASL until the advent of English sign systems.

While Padden (1998) suggests that it grew concurrent with the professional deaf middle class, who required more technical vocabulary, initialization appears to have flourished with the advent of manually coded English forms, particularly Signing Exact English which used initialization of signs to clarify their English translations (e.g., use of C handshape for the sign "person" to represent "client"). When possible, natural ASL signs were retained for the most commonly used word in a word family, and then the first letters of related English words were added to create synonyms (Paul 2009). Thus, Padden indicated that the defining characteristic of initialized signs is that they represent semantic groups of signs which vary along a semantic dimension. Thus, while some sign families represent a core sign which varies only by its initialized sign (e.g., the initialized variants of person, group, and science), other groups may be represented by different signs, each of which is initialized (e.g., colors). According to Padden, "Initialization is one of the most productive of word-building processes in ASL, used widely for technical or professional purposes" (p. 46).

Development of Fingerspelling Skills

While fingerspelling is used to represent words in a manner similar to print, its introduction and development diverges significantly from typical development of reading and writing skills. Although use with their children varies, in deaf families who use ASL for the language of the home, fingerspelling may be introduced quite early and may be used as a means of representing English words (Padden 1991). This may be more common in households placing a high value on literacy, and Padden noted that some parents in her study reported actively encouraging attempts to make associations between fingerspelling and print with children as young as 2 years old. However, even for these highly motivated families, fingerspelling reportedly comprised 10% or less of their communication. Furthermore, Padden reported that despite comprehension and use of fingerspelling at younger ages, the children observed did not appear to make even limited associations between the print and manual letters until about age 3.

Early readers depend on the visual features of words before they develop the alphabetic skills to decode print (Scott and Ehri 1990). As noted above, deaf children appear to use a similar logographic strategy with fingerspelling, seeing the fingerspelled words simply as complex signs. The transition between this more holistic reception of fingerspelling and the alphabetic approach appears to develop during the preschool years with deaf children provided with rich signing environments incorporating fingerspelling (Padden 1991). She noted that while children varied in their age of understanding, between the latter part of the second year and the fourth year, children demonstrated an understanding that signs and fingerspelling were different and are used in different contexts (e.g., fingerspelled names versus signed labels). Expressively, early attempts at fingerspelling may be rough approximations or simple mimicking of hand/finger movements. Anderson and Reilly (2002) noted that parents reported that their children were able to fingerspell words well before they produced individual letters, suggesting that they are also producing the words as complex signs rather than spelling in an alphabetic manner. Akamatsu and Stewart (1989) suggest that while it may be adequate to process fingerspelled words as gestalt in conversation, for the development of literacy and English vocabulary, they need to analyze the alphabetic components of the words.

In addition to the holistic reception of fingerspelling, preschoolers may confuse the hand configurations used in signs with manual letters, and even numbers (Akamatsu and Stewart 1989). Anecdotally, even hearing children in a signing environment can demonstrate such confusions, as in the case of a child, who, when asked the first letter of the word "father" responded "5"—the handshape with which the sign is made—and then looked confused, knowing that could not be right. This can actually be an effective strategy for initialized signs, but problematic for many natural signs; however, as they learn to read, these types of confusions typically resolve.

Fingerspelling as a Bridge to Literacy

Fingerspelling is considered by many to be an important component of the development of English literacy by deaf students (Akamatsu and Stewart 1989; Grushkin 1998; Haptonstall-Nykaza & Schick 2007; Hirsh-Pasek 1987; Humphries & MacDougall 1999/2000). While Mayberry et al. (2011) found only a weak positive relationship between reading skills and fingerspelling in their meta-analysis of studies of deaf readers, their study selection focused on phonology rather than fingerspelling.

Padden and Ramsey (2000) found a moderate correlation between receptive fingerspelling (writing down a word seen fingerspelled in a sentence) and reading comprehension, and a strong correlation between the ability to spell the words represented by initialized signs and reading comprehension in a sample of deaf school children. They also found that performance on measures of receptive and expressive ASL competence and memory for ASL sentences, rather than having deaf parents, was significantly correlated with fingerspelling and initialized sign skills. However, the authors note that the relationship between reading and fingerspelling is not unidirectional. While deaf children can understand and use fingerspelling before they learn to read, their use of fingerspelling to depict new words appears around the time they learn to read, when they begin to transition from the perception of the gestalt to the alphabetic analysis of the words. While the assumption that deaf children who develop early fingerspelling skills will naturally transfer those skills to reading may not be accurate, techniques have been used to enhance English skills using fingerspelling and Padden and Ramsey suggest that deaf children should be taught to exploit the information contained in fingerspelling and initialized signs to enhance their reading skills. This is consistent with the finding of Hirsh-Pasek (1987), who found that training deaf children in strategies such as segmenting the fingerspelled words in their lexicons and encouraging the use of fingerspelling as a strategy for decoding enabled them to improve their performance of word recognition tasks.

One method of enhancing the associations between signs, fingerspelling, and print is the technique of "chaining" described by Humphries & MacDougall (1999/2000) and observed by Padden and Ramsey (1998) in classrooms of teachers who often used fingerspelling. They noted that this system highlights the relationships between the languages and texts, and that similar associations between signing and fingerspelling are observed in parents of deaf children, who may accompany such pairings with pointing to the object of the sign. These types of use of fingerspelling and signs which provide clues to print can support both linguistic competence and literacy. Multiple approaches to using fingerspelling as a means of enhancing literacy have been developed over the years, and the data from the Toolkit study suggest that further investigation of such techniques may support increased literacy access for deaf children in the future.

Reception and Expression of Fingerspelling

While many new signers struggle to understand fingerspelling, skilled signers can receive fingerspelling at an impressive rate. By artificially increasing the rate of fingerspelling through altering the rate of playback on videotaped fingerspelled sentences, Reed et al. (1990) documented 50% accuracy at two to three times the normal speed of fingerspelling production (accelerated rates of 12–16 letters per second). They note that their study suggests that receptive capacity is comparable to that of aural reception even though expressive fingerspelling is limited by the constraints of manual production (about one manual letter per 150–200 ms, or about 5–6 letters per second). This latter is consistent with previous research cited by Akamatsu and Stewart (1989) which reported expressive fingerspelling speeds of fluent signers of about 170 ms per letter. Akamatsu and Stewart suggested that such speeds would influence the recipient to process the fingerspelled words as gestalts rather than a series of individual letters. Based on previous research by Akamatsu, they suggested that the fluent signers reading fingerspelled words look for a pattern of finger configuration which Akamatsu labeled the "movement envelope" rather than focusing on the individual manual letters. This would argue for a more "sign-like" reception rather than letter decoding.

Receptively, Waters et al. (2007) found that native signers of BSL recruited additional areas of the brain when processing fingerspelled words compared to signs, but that both signs and fingerspelling share areas of brain activation, providing some support for sign-like reception. However, the participants appeared have increased involvement of both mid-fusiform gyri, an area generally considered to be involved in processing orthographic stimuli, during the fingerspelling reception task compared to the sign reception task. Thus, this study could support an integrative process combining both a more holistic, sign-like analysis and an orthographically based analysis during receptive fingerspelling. Despite the differences in cognitive resources recruited for the tasks, the participants' accuracy was comparable for reception of signs, fingerspelling, print, and pictures, although the responses for the fingerspelled items were significantly slower, likely due differences in articulation time. The participants included in their study had mean receptive fingerspelling accuracy of 21/25 fingerspelled words using a video clip task. They noted that individuals with a score lower than 17/25 were not included in the study, but provided no information on the number individuals so excluded.

Expressive fingerspelling also appears to involve both shared and separate cognitive processes compared to signing. Emmorey et al. (2003) found that while deaf native signers retrieving signs for expressive naming activated similar brain regions to hearing participants during retrieval of words, use of fingerspelling activated additional regions involved in motor planning and sequencing. This was thought to be due to the requirement of sequential production of the manual letters for fingerspelling compared to the relatively constrained sequences involved in production of individual signs.

In general, more appears to be known about the brain regions involved in processing fingerspelling than its relationships with cognitive and achievement outcomes. While fingerspelling is clearly important both as a component of ASL and as the intersection between ASL and English, its relationships with underlying cognitive processes and academic and linguistic outcomes are not well understood. Additionally, little work has been done focusing on measurement of fingerspelling skills, suggesting the need for a standard instrument which can be used in multiple settings. The Fingerspelling Test was included in the VL2 Psychometric Toolkit in order to address these needs.

Measurement of Fingerspelling Reception

Many of the above cited studies used some form of estimate of fingerspelling skills, such as having students write words that had been fingerspelled in sentences. Other studies have had the participants fingerspell expressively as a means of evaluating competence with fingerspelling. However, little has been done to develop a standardized measure of fingerspelling skills. If the relationships between fingerspelling and literacy and academic competence are to be studied in a systematic manner, there is a need for a measure that can be used with multiple studies and which is applicable to participants with a wide range of skills. That was the goal of developing the measure reported in Chap. 9.

The Finger Spelling Test

As noted in the chapter on linguistic functioning, the Fingerspelling Test was developed for this study based on two subtests from the Woodcock Johnson Tests of Academic Achievement, Third Edition (WJ-III; Woodcock et al. 2001): Spelling and Spelling of Sounds. The former task uses real words while the latter word uses pseudo-words. A total of 45 real words and 25 pseudo-words were intermingled, beginning with items at the early elementary school level and becoming increasingly difficult as the task progressed. The participants were presented with the fingerspelled words using video clips presented on a computer. The test was designed for the responses to be written verbatim; however, responses can be either written or fingerspelled and videotaped to ensure accurate scoring. In no case should an attempt be made to have the participants fingerspell their responses and have the examiners write down their responses and/or score them in real time.

As deaf individuals are exposed to English vocabulary through fingerspelling in addition to print, the accuracy of their reception of such input could significantly affect the development of their English vocabulary skills. While reception of conversational fingerspelling would be expected to benefit from the recipient's knowledge of English vocabulary, the development of new vocabulary would depend more on accurate reception of the letter sequences. Thus, the mixture of real and pseudo-words was used, so that while word knowledge could certainly support the participants' reception of the fingerspelled words, they would have to attend carefully to the stimuli. As noted in Chap. 6, the participants responded correctly to about 75% of both the real and pseudo-words on the Finger Spelling Test. The comparable performances on real versus pseudo-words suggest that in the context of mixed real and pseudo-words the ability to visually receive and decode fingerspelling was more dependent on visual reception than knowledge of English vocabulary. This is consistent with the observation on other Toolkit measures, such as the F-A-S and 5–1–U, that the task demands of adjacent stimuli can influence the strategies used to complete tasks.

Although the types of interpretation of the scores on this measure and their relationships with other Toolkit measures such as those offered above and in Chap. 9 offer a rich source of further investigation, review of the responses and the relative performances of individual participants suggested that there was a wealth of information from this measure that went well beyond the participants' scores.

Beyond the Fingerspelling Scores

While the number correct on the Fingerspelling Test and its component scores for the real and fake word tasks produced an impressive range of associations with measures of linguistic skills (English and ASL) and literacy, the errors provide additional clues to the underlying processes involved in the performance of these tasks. The initial plan to code the errors as representing English phonemic, dactylic, or orthographic errors proved untenable, as it quickly became evident that (1) often it was impossible to tell which type of error had occurred and (2) most errors represented either omission of letters, insertion of letters, or sequencing errors. It was anticipated that real word substitutions might be made for the pseudo-words, and this did happen occasionally (e.g., "fridge" and "fudge" for "flidge"); however, substitutions also occurred for real words, although the substituted word was not always accurately spelled. The most frequent of these was a reflection of the population being investigated; the word "congenial" was frequently replaced with various clear attempts to spell "congenital". Six participants, or 12% of the 49 participants who completed the test, and 22% of those who missed that word made this type of error. Another context-related substitution was the not infrequent replacement of "syllable" with "syllabus". One common (12%) letter substitution which appeared to be dactylic was the replacement of the "L" in "glounder" with an "R".

Twenty one, or 43%, of the participants made fewer than two errors on the first 41 items on the test, reflecting accurate reception of at least eighth grade spelling words. While most of those students missed at least 1/3 or more of the remaining 29 items, 1 participant missed only 1 item—a pseudo-word, and 2 more missed fewer than 6 items, equivalent to postbaccalaureate level performance on the WJ-III Spelling subtest. Ten (20%) of the participants received scores on the Real Word Test reflective of late college level spelling. Of those participants, the most common errors were omissions of one or more letters, and while the numbers were too small for quantification, there appeared to be a trend of fewer omissions per word as the total number of spelling errors declined, suggesting stronger working memory capacity in the better spellers. This is consistent with the moderate correlations between the fingerspelling tasks and the linguistic working memory tasks on the toolkit. On the other hand, the words on this measure could not have been retained adequately by simply retaining a sequence of letters. Working memory spans for the Toolkit tasks ranged from three to nine letters or digits. Fully half a dozen real words on the Fingerspelling Test had ten or more letters. Thus, strong performance on this task appears to represent a combination of strong linguistic working memory and high levels of English vocabulary.

Of the students who missed large numbers of early items (more than 6 of the first 41), most tended to simplify the stimuli, either substituting simple real words for the real or pseudo-words or omitting letters. The pseudo-word "gat" was replaced by "get" or "jong" by "jog". While omissions were common in both strong and weak receptive fingerspellers, those who missed few items tended to omit one letter in longer words, while low scorers tended to omit one or more letters even in common, simple words, such as "house" or "second" and two or more letters on longer words. Some participants either omitted responses or provided one to three letters on some later items. Interestingly, as with reports of preschool fingerspellers, almost all items to which the participants responded had the first letter correct. Additionally, while to a much lesser extent than the initial letters, the majority of completed words had the final letter correct. This suggests that these participants are depending on relatively weak verbal sequential memory, with relatively little support from their English vocabulary.

There was one participant who differed from this pattern. That participant's errors were heavily loaded with real word substitutions which did not suggest the simplification seen with other weak performers on this task. For example, "floor" was replaced by "flower" and "cough" by "couch" and later "inflammation" was replaced by "information." However, on later items, while the initial letters were retained, some spellings had little relation to the stimulus. One could speculate that this person has an adequate vocabulary, but has limited receptive fingerspelling skills. Investigation of performance of beginning fingerspellers compared to fluent fingerspellers on receptive fingerspelling tasks could help to define the types of performances to be expected on this type of task.

Other potential studies would include investigation of the impacts of vocabulary support on performance by administering alternate forms of the test, one with the real- and pseudo-words intermingled, as on this test, and the other with them separated, and the participants informed of the type of stimulus they were to receive. While there are further questions to be answered, this task provides a measure which clearly separates individuals who struggle with receptive fingerspelling form those who are highly skilled at this task. However, advanced performance on this task clearly requires a combination of strong fingerspelling reception combined with high levels of English vocabulary and linguistic working memory. The Toolkit data suggest that early intervention to enhance all three of these areas could support higher levels of literacy and academic achievement.

References

Akamatsu, C. T. & Stewart, D. A. (1989). *Fingerspelling within the context of simultaneous communication.* Occasional paper no. 128. Retrieved from the Michigan State University Institute for Research on Teaching website: http://education.msu.edu/irt/PDFs/OccasionalPapers/op128.pdf.

Anderson, D., & Reilly, J. (2002). The MacArthur communicative development inventory: Normative data for American Sign Language. *Journal of Deaf Studies and Deaf Education, 7*, 83–106.

Bragg, Lois. (1997). Visual-kinetic Communication in Europe before 1600: A survey of sign lexicons and finger alphabets prior to the rise of deaf education. *Journal of Deaf Studies and Deaf Education, 2*, 1–25.

Emmorey, K., Grabowski, T., McCullough, S., Damasio, H., Ponto, L. L. B., Hichwa, R. D., et al. (2003). Neural systems underlying lexical retrieval for sign language. *Neuropsychologia, 41*, 85–95.

Forman, W. (2003). The ABCs of New Zealand Sign Language: Aerial spelling. *Journal of Deaf Studies and Deaf Education, 8*(1), 92–96.

Grushkin, K. A. (1998). Why shouldn't Sam read? Toward a new paradigm for literacy and the deaf. *Journal of Deaf Studies and Deaf Education, 3*(3), 199–203.

Haptonstall-Nykaza, T. S. & Schick, B. (2007). The transition from fingerspelling to English print: Facilitating English decoding. *Journal of Deaf Studies and Deaf Education, 12*(2), 172–183.

Hirsh-Pasek, K. (1987). The metalinguistics of fingerspelling: An alternative way to increase vocabulary in congenitally deaf readers. *Reading Research Quarterly, 22*, 455–474.

Humphries, T., & MacDougall, F. (1999/2000). 'Chaining' and other links: making connections between American Sign Language and English in two types of school settings. *Visual Anthropology Review, 15*(2), 84–94.

Mayberry, R. I., del Giudice, A. A., & Lieberman, A. M. (2011). Reading achievement in relation to phonological coding and awareness in deaf readers: A meta-analysis. *Journal of Deaf Studies and Deaf Education, 16*(2), 164–188.

Moores, D. F. (1970). Psycholinguistics and deafness. *American Annals of the Deaf, 115*(1), 37–48.

Padden, C. (1991). The acquisition of fingerspelling by deaf children. In P. Siple & S. Fischer (Eds.), *Theoretical issues in sign language research* (Psychology, Vol. 2, pp. 193–210). Chicago: University of Chicago Press.

Padden, C. A. (1998). The ASL lexicon. *Sign Language and Linguistics, 1*(1), 39–60.

Padden, C. A., & Gunsauls, D. C. (2003). How the alphabet came to be used in a sign language. *Sign Language Studies, 4*(1), 10–33.

Padden, C., & Ramsey, C. (1998). Reading ability in signing deaf children. *Topics in Language Disorders, 18*, 30–46.

Padden, C., & Ramsey, C. (2000). American Sign Language and reading ability in deaf children. In C. Chamberlain, J. Morford, & R. Mayberry (Eds.), *Language acquisition by eye* (pp. 165–189). Mahwah, NJ: Lawrence Erlbaum & Associates.

Paul, P. V. (2009). *Language and deafness* (4th ed.). Boston: Jones & Bartlett.

Reed, C. M., Delhorne, L. A., Durlach, N. I., & Fischer, S. D. (1990). A study of the tactual and visual reception of fingerspelling. *Journal of Speech and Hearing Research, 33*, 786–797.

Scott, J. A., & Ehri, L. C. (1990). Sight word reading in prereaders: Use of logographic vs. alphabetic access routes. *Journal of Literacy Research, 22*, 149. doi:10.1080/10862969009547701.

Valli, C., Lucas, C., & Mulrooney, K. J. (2005). *Linguistics of American Sign Language: An introduction* (4th ed.). Washington, DC: Gallaudet University Press.

Waters, D., Campbell, R., Capek, C. M., Woll, B., David, A. S., McGuire, P. K., Brammer, M. J., & MacSweeney, M. (2007). Fingerspelling, signed language, text and picture processing in deaf native signers: The role of the mid-fusiform gyrus. *NeuroImage, 35*, 1287–1302.

Woodcock, R. W., McGrew, K. S., & Mather, N. (2001). *Examiner's manual. Woodcock-Johnson III Tests of Achievement*. Itasca, IL: Riverside Publishing.

Chapter 11
Issues and Trends in Sign Language Assessment

Raylene Paludneviciene, Peter C. Hauser, Dorri J. Daggett, and Kim B. Kurz

Issues and Trends in Sign Language Assessment

Valid and reliable sign language assessments are essential for researchers, educators, and service providers who work with sign language users. They would be central, for example, in the documentation of deaf students' sign language competency for educational planning/placement purposes [as required by the Individualized Educational Program in the USA and similar programs elsewhere] or in sign language rehabilitation for deaf individuals who do not have age-appropriate sign language fluency.

Sign language assessment is an essential component of a variety of academic disciplines, including education, psychology, and linguistics. In education, graduate-level teacher training programs for bilingual deaf education require valid assessments of the communication skills of their trainees, and schools for deaf children need to assess the signing skills of both students and personnel. In psychology, valid sign language assessments are required to assess the impact of signing on a wide variety of brain and cognitive functions.

R. Paludneviciene, (✉) • D.J. Daggett
Department of Psychology, Gallaudet University,
800 Florida Avenue, NE, Washington, DC 20002, USA
e-mail: raylene.paludneviciene@gallaudet.edu; Dorri.Daggett@Gallaudet.edu

P.C. Hauser
Deaf Studies Laboratory, National Technical Institute for the Deaf,
Rochester Institute of Technology, 52 Lomb Memorial Drive,
Rochester, NY, 14623, USA
e-mail: pchgss@rit.edu

K.B. Kurz
American Sign Language and Interpreting, National Technical Institute for the Deaf,
Rochester Institute of Technology, 52 Lomb Memorial Drive,
Rochester, NY 14623, USA
e-mail: kbknss@rit.edu

In linguistics, analyses of the results of sign language tests could contribute to the evolution of linguistic theory.

Recently, researchers have been using sign language assessments developed in their labs to measure their deaf participants' sign language fluency in order to study the effects of sign language skill on a variety of outcome measures. For example, studies by Morford et al. (2011) and Kubus et al. (2010) employed newly developed strategies for assessing sign skill in their investigations of crosslinguistic activation of signed words while their participants were reading written words. Corina et al. (2011) used similar strategies in their investigation of neurobiological activation of signed and written words. These new strategies have enabled researchers to move beyond the tradition of using deaf children of deaf adults (assumed to be native signers) and deaf children of hearing adults (assumed to be less skillful) as a means for testing the effects of sign language competency on different cognitive functions. They have also allowed researchers to treat sign language fluency as a continuous variable rather than a grouping variable (e.g., Allen et al. 2009).

Unfortunately, in spite of their importance, most sign language assessments are not widely available at the present time. One of the few commercially available signed language assessment tests is the *Assessing BSL Development-Receptive Skills Test* (BSL-RST; Herman et al. 1999), developed in the UK for the assessment of British Sign Language (BSL). This assessment is used for children aged 3–11 years old and measures syntactic and morphological aspects of BSL through a video-based receptive test. Currently, efforts are underway to translate this test into American Sign Language (ASL) (Enns and Herman 2011; Haug and Mann 2008).

There has been ongoing work on developing sign language tests in research laboratories, some of which have resulted in working prototypes (see Haug 2008; Singleton & Supalla 2011 for reviews). Still, the insufficient number of readily available tools prevents test developers worldwide from having models on which to develop and norm new instruments for distribution on a broader scale. Ideally, those who are interested in sign assessment would be able to have access to a toolkit of a variety of tests assessing sign language proficiency. With such a toolkit, deaf educators and language specialists would be able to utilize the results of these tests to develop appropriate curriculum materials tailored to specific levels of language competency. Researchers would be able to use the same set of tests across different studies. Organizations that involve working with deaf students, patients, or customers could use such tests for hiring and promotions purposes.

Fortunately, the Science of Learning Center on Visual Language and Visual Learning (VL2) at Gallaudet University is developing just such a toolkit that will combine a group of new tests that have been developed to advance the Center's research agenda. It will be distributed widely to researchers, educators, and clinicians to help propel further the practice of ASL assessment.

Creating such a collection of tests for distribution presents many challenges to substantiate any claim that the tests are reliable and valid for their stated purposes. The remainder of this chapter will discuss these challenges.

Apples and Oranges: Spoken and Signed Languages

In order to develop a robust test of sign language competence, one needs first to understand differences between languages in the spoken and signed modalities. Since the formal study of sign language began relatively recently, there is much that we still do not know about the formal structure of sign languages and how they are processed in the brain. Understanding these differences will greatly facilitate the construction of appropriate measurements. For example, simply understanding that signed languages require visuospatial abilities as well as linguistic abilities alters our approaches to conceptualizing the domains of competence that need to be assessed, changes our understanding of what constitutes a test item, requires us to be clever in how we present the test and score the responses, and presents huge challenges in standardizing the scoring and interpreting the results.

Sign languages are complex. Since the beginning of the linguistic investigation of sign languages in the 1960s, linguists have provided ample evidence demonstrating that the structure of signed languages is equally as complex as the structure of spoken languages. Arguably, it is more complex, since it involves both spatial and temporal characteristics, includes (in addition to sign vocabulary) grammatical elements that are depicted through the embodiment of meaning and the positioning of the signer and her facial and body expressions, and has no written form. Linguists are only now beginning to unravel and describe this complexity, even decades after Stokoe's (1960) seminal work.

Issues with Translating Existing Spoken Language Tests

A naïve individual might assume that any spoken language fluency test can be simply translated into sign language. This assumption would be incorrect even if the test administrator were fluent in a specific sign language and had made faithful translations of each of the test items. Administering language assessments through direct translation jeopardizes test validity (see Haug and Mann 2008 for discussion). To illustrate, consider how an ASL translation of Peabody Picture Vocabulary Test (PPVT; Dunn and Dunn 1997) might be administered in ASL to a deaf test-taker. The PPVT was developed to measure English vocabulary knowledge. To administer the PPVT, a test administrator shows four pictures from a booklet, and upon hearing an English word spoken, the examinee determines which of the four pictures best represents the spoken word. This test is widely used in psycho-educational and neuropsychological evaluations of hearing children and adults. The issues associated with a direct translation of this test into ASL will be discussed below. An ASL version of the PPVT (*American Sign Language Vocabulary Test*, Schick 1997) was developed in a lab; however, to date it is not available for use outside of research labs. There are no published studies reporting on this test's validity and reliability.

One critical issue in translating tests of language fluency pertains to differences in the frequency of a test word in the original language and the frequency of its translation in the translated language. Since word-frequency is important in both the construction of vocabulary tests and in their scoring and interpretation, disparities in word frequencies may invalidate the scores of the translated tests.

Another issue is that many words and phrases in a language may not have equivalents in the translated language. This may lead a test administrator to fingerspell a word (or phrase) rather than attempt to translate it outright. This strategy clearly alters the content of the test, as it requires that fingerspelled words be recognized as English words. For the PPVT, measurement is clearly jeopardized. The PPVT is not a reading test; it is a spoken English receptive vocabulary test.

Finally, the norms for tests such as the PPVT were developed on samples of hearing individuals. Applying these norms (i.e., conversions of raw scores to standard scores) to the raw scores of deaf individuals (who are taking the test in a different language and in a different modality) will likely result in scores that are not interpretable.

When test items are sentences rather than words, several other translation issues arise. For example, the *Test of Adolescent and Adult Language* (TOAL-3), *Speaking/Grammar Subtest* (Hammill et al. 1994) requires the examinee to listen to a sentence such as "A blue bird flies over the sunset" and then repeat it back verbatim. This example is likely to be considered to be a relatively simple sentence. The naïve test administrator might assume that an ASL translation of this simple test item would also be a single, simple ASL sentence. This is not necessarily the case. In the sample sentence, a spatial relationship between two objects, one moving (the blue bird) and one static (the sunset) is conveyed. Rather than use word-for-word sign translations of the English words, ASL is likely to use a depicting verb to describe this relationship (e.g., Dudis 2004, 2008). A depicting verb incorporates, into the sign itself, additional information about the verb, such as size, direction, activity, or location. Thus, depicting verbs may be more complex than nondepicting verbs, and therefore require different levels of skills in processing and interpreting than their English counterparts (when administered to hearing examinees.)

Also, note that the English sentence has no explicit mention of the perspective taken from among the many possible locations, from which the situation can be viewed. Information about perspective may be necessary as the translator not only needs to select a location, but also decide on one of several possible "viewing modes" (e.g., Liddell 2003). Multiple viewing modes are possible, some in which the signer becomes part of the scene, and some in which he does not. For example, to use Langacker's (1991) stage model, the signer might be offstage relative to the depiction of the bird's flight. Thus, test item translators must make decisions with respect to the perspectives represented in each sentence, potentially rendering the translated items nonequivalent to the original English.

Another translation concern pertains to the explicit mention of the prominent entities within the sentence, such as the bird and the sunset. By itself, the depiction of the bird's flight is a perfectly good ASL expression. In ASL, however, depending on the context, it would be appropriate to not specify what the moving object and the static object are, particularly if the bird and the sunset have been previously introduced. This expression might be considered to be a simple sentence (and thus a more equivalent translation), compared with the more complex alternatives.

Since the TOAL3 sentences are not provided in context, translators are left to make decisions with respect to each of these depictive aspects. This is particularly problematic, as, without context, it is not possible to provide sufficient discourse to allow for naturalistic depiction to occur. Thus, decisions will be arbitrary, again leading to difficulties in interpreting test performance.

A final illustration of how difficult it is to translate tests of language fluency from English into ASL concerns test items that use numbers and space in varying formats. The example below is a typical word problem in English that requires the test-taker to mentally compute the correct answer:

Ahmad has four green paper clips, ten red paper clips, seven blue paper clips. How many red and green paper clips does Ahmad have?

ASL translations of this test item would likely utilize space as part of the description of the problem. If the use of space is avoided, the resulting expression is likely to be stilted, and perhaps more seriously, the expression would not reflect ordinary, conventional usage in the community of sign language users. One conventional expression has each of the three number-color groupings represented in front of the signer. The question itself would then involve pointing to the relevant groups. Since this use of space facilitates memory of number-color groupings, signers then have an advantage over English speakers who are not likely to utilize space in the same fashion. It appears safe to say that the way sign language typically and frequently produces spatial representations of entities, both physical and abstract, not only sets the two languages apart but also poses difficulties for test translation efforts.

To summarize, a full and complete sign language translation of a spoken language test is impossible without first making significant changes to test structure and content. These changes may inevitably alter the purpose of the test and what it measures. The significant degree to which spoken and signed languages differ warrants caution when developing sign language tests, whether they are translations or original. Constructing tests in sign language requires an appropriate degree of familiarity of sign language linguistics and expertise in the theories and principles of test construction. It also requires the participation and consultation of deaf native sign language users who have appropriate background and training. Test developers or administrators should be wary of attempts to directly translate spoken language tests into tests of signed languages.

Development of Tests Directly in Sign Language

While newly developed tests using spoken languages typically include many language conventions that have been validated in previous tests using spoken languages, there are no established conventions for tests incorporating sign language linguistics. Indeed, the study of sign language linguistics is in its infancy, and there are currently disagreements among linguists about the grammar of signed languages at all levels, including phonology, morphology, syntax, and discourse. Thus, using ASL as the primary language for assessment involves considerable risk. As already noted, test developers must make decisions with respect to the depiction of test items (such as the use of depicting verbs and perspective), the morphological complexity of the signs used, and establishing semantic contexts within which signed items are presented.

Additionally, the test developer must articulate the characteristics of those who will take the test. Tests of sign language fluency are administered to test-takers with skills ranging from those who have had no exposure to a signed language to native users of sign language. In addition to language fluency, test-taking skills of test-takers as a group may vary widely from those with excellent metalinguistic skills to those without the appropriate educational background and practice with tests in general. If tests are not targeted to the general ability levels of the intended examinees, measurement is undermined.

Since signed languages are not often formally taught in schools, most deaf signers have never studied sign language formally. Over the past decade, there have been a growing number of schools offering sign language specialists, tutors, and curricula to deaf students. As discussed later in this chapter, there are no widely accepted standards for sign language instruction. Therefore, the sign vocabulary and grammar taught to 8-year olds at one school might be different from that of 8-year olds in another school. Also, sign models for deaf children are usually teachers and parents, who are often not native signers, so sign variation is widespread. This variation poses a challenge for developing appropriate test items for this age group.

As with spoken language variation, sign language variation, with respect to factors such as region, age, culture, ethnicity, and gender, needs to be taken into consideration (e.g., Haug and Mann 2008; Lucas et al. 2005). The majority of the frequently used signs are the same across different regions of the USA (Lucas et al. 2005) and test developers should limit item development to these signs. In the UK, as a response to the sign variation problem, two different versions of the receptive skills test referenced above (Herman et al. 1999) were developed, taking into account the regional variation of signs found in the northern and southern part of the country.

Given the wide range of considerations that we have discussed regarding the development of tests *in* a signed language (and *of* a signed language fluency), and the relative infancy of the field of sign language linguistics, it is inevitable that test developers will make decisions based on linguistic assumptions that may not be universally accepted. These decisions are apt to be subject to more criticism than are decisions made in the development of tests in spoken languages. However, the need for new tools is so great that test developers should not be dissuaded. It is necessary to start somewhere. True, it will also be necessary for new tests to be developed as new understandings of signed language are achieved.

Item Development, Selection, and Piloting

When developing a new test for a specific signed language, it is necessary first to create a large number of items. After pilot testing these items with signers of varying levels of fluency, many items will be omitted or revised after careful analysis. This often involves having sign language linguists and native signers providing input on the face validity of the items.

It is general practice in test development to utilize experts to assist with the identification of appropriate items for tests (Freidenberg 1995). For sign language tests, native signers are utilized during this process to assist with the development of appropriate test items. The *Test of American Sign Language* (Prinz et al. 1994), *American Sign Language Comprehension Test* (ASL-CT; Hauser et al. 2010), and the *American Sign Language Sentence Reproduction Test* (ASL-SRT; Hauser et al. 2008) are examples of tests that utilized native signers during the test development phase. These native deaf signers served as principal investigators and consultants for item development and as models for test items.

Native deaf signers are those who were exposed to a sign language since birth, often with deaf parents who themselves are native signers. Typically, the native deaf signer is a "24/7" user of sign language, which means that she uses sign language everyday at all times. We argue that *deaf* native signers will contribute greater levels of expertise in the test item development process than will hearing native signers, as there is some evidence that they possess higher levels of sign language fluency (Hauser et al. 2008). Also, we urge test developers to ensure that their native deaf collaborators have a history of exposure to the highest quality of sign language throughout their lives. Evidence for this might be that they attended a self-contained school for deaf students for most of their schooling, or that they maintain frequent contacts with the deaf community.

Ideally, a team of sign language linguists, native deaf signers, and test developers work together to create test items for new test development projects. In fact, more than one native signer is preferable in this stage since two or more native signers can serve as validity checks for each other. For example, a native signer could sign a possible item and the other native signers could provide a response. If the response is correct, then the item would be validated for pilot testing. If the response is incorrect, then the team would work to modify or delete that item from the pool of potential test items.

In the subsequent pilot testing, linguists and native signers should be consulted for their opinion on the items' relevance to the construct being measured (for example, vocabulary items for a test measuring vocabulary knowledge). During the development of items for a test, sign language linguists and native signers would provide input on the appropriateness of the item (signs or sentences) as a measure of sign language and for the construct (i.e., sign competency, sign fluency, and vocabulary knowledge) the test is intended to measure. The process itself also involves providing feedback on what might be considered unacceptable variations that might threaten the validity of the test.

After a large pool of items has been developed, these items need to be piloted with a small sample to get immediate feedback and to investigate unexpected patterns of errors. Through this process, items will be omitted, modified, and/or added. The process of removing items with poor validity and reliability often involves several rounds of pilot testing with groups of examinees with varying levels of fluency and careful statistical analyses of the data from these groups. The final set of items would have robust validity and reliability and would be those items best able to discriminate among groups known to have different levels of fluency.

After the items have been selected and a working test created, it needs to be administered to a large sample to establish its psychometric validity. This might involve testing different groups of examinees with known and divergent levels of fluency. While this would be a challenge, given a dearth of available measures, it would be possible to use extant groups of examinees about which we might assume different levels of fluency (e.g., native versus non-native signers; signers at different ages; etc.)

Sign language tests typically are developed for use with different groups of signers including hearing signers and deaf non-native signers, but it is important for tests to be validated first with native signers. This is common practice among those who develop tests of spoken language fluency; they use native speakers of that language to develop and screen out inappropriate items. If native speakers of that language do not do well on a test measuring fluency in that language, then the problem lies with the test items or the test itself, not with the speaker of that language. Native speakers are used to establish a baseline, and will help ensure that the test measures language fluency. Spoken language assessments are usually developed based on trials with native speakers of that language, as well as feedback received from native speakers of the language of interest.

For an individual to be considered a native user of a language he must have been exposed to that language from birth in a home environment. Hearing children of deaf adults are sometimes wrongly assumed to be fluent native signers. This is comparable with children from Chinese or Spanish speaking families who were raised in the USA, many of whom do not achieve fluency in their parents' native language (Newman et al. 2003; Newport 1990).

Hearing native signers are different from deaf native signers, given their immediate access to both spoken and visual language modalities. For example, if the paper clip math item mentioned earlier in the chapter is presented to a fluent hearing native signer, she might be able to take advantage of the use of space when the item is presented in ASL, and then translate the item to a spoken language to take advantage of the larger short-term memory capacity for auditory-based information (see Emmorey 2002). One advantage that bimodal bilinguals (those who are fluent in a sign language and a spoken language) have is that they are able to translate items to the language that holds the most cognitive advantage. For the paper clip item example, the bimodal bilingual test-taker would be able to retain memory of groupings based on use of space in sign language, and translate the numbers into spoken English to assist with the memorization of numbers.

When developing a test that measures language competency in a signed language, the impact of a test-taker's native fluency, and her use of languages in other modalities (spoken languages) would have to be taken into consideration during pilot testing (and also when developing scoring guidelines). It might be possible to use separate norming samples for different groups so that scores can be interpreted in the context of the individual's language history. This would require including, during pilot testing, test-takers from varying backgrounds and levels of fluency.

Test Design and Format

Tests developed to measure language proficiency come in many forms, each measuring a particular domain of a language and each having a set of advantages and disadvantages. Interview-based tests, for example, are more difficult to score than true–false or multiple-choice tests. While a test that is easy to score might be more reliable (i.e., lead to consistent results upon repeated administrations), it might also be more restricted in the range of the skills that can be measured. It may be more difficult to establish the reliability of tests that require rater judgments of interview protocols during the scoring process, but the information they provide about a particular test-taker is potentially richer. Interviews also require considerably more time to administer and score, require both skilled interviewers and skilled raters, and are more expensive both to administer and to score.

In the sections that follow, we discuss different test formats in more detail, and provide examples of each that are currently available or under development.

Proficiency Interviews

The *Sign Language Proficiency Interview* (SLPI, Caccamise et al. 1983) was created using the Foreign Language Oral Proficiency Assessment (Liskin-Gasparro 1982) as a model. SLPI measures a person's functional sign communication skills, which means that the test does not measure ASL skills, per se. It basically measures how well a person communicates using signs. The SLPI is a test of competence in the continuum of contact signing (Lucas and Valli 1992), which makes scoring more flexible. Knight (1983) illustrated a concern that the lack of a native ASL signer and a clear "anchor" in ASL would compromise the validity of the scoring scale. In the SLPI, fluency is assessed based on functional features, such as ease of communication about different topics, rather than specific grammatical features of ASL. However, it is unclear as to how grammatical features of contact signing can be measured, as this variation in signing is not standard and its "appropriateness" depends on who is in the situation (see Lucas and Valli 1992). The rating scales for the SLPI include superior, advanced, intermediate, survival, and novice. Raters for the SLPI are selected based on their proficiency in signing, knowledge of regional signs, and personality, and raters can include both hearing and deaf persons (Caccamise et al. 1983). The interview itself is 20–30 min and is rated by "highly skilled, knowledgeable native-like signers" (Newell et al. 1983, p. 5). The validity and reliability of the SLPI was based on its face validity and evidence showing consistency in ratings among three independent raters (Caccamise et al. 1988).

The SLPI was the only test available to measure sign communication skills for a long time, until it became more widespread to use the *American Sign Language Proficiency Interview* (ASLPI; see Singleton and Supalla 2011 for discussion. The ASLPI measures ASL skills that an individual has at a given point. The rating is based on ASL grammar, vocabulary, accent/production, fluency, and comprehension. Like the SLPI, the ASLPI involves trained interviewers and raters for each person being measured. The interviewer will ask questions to elicit responses from the interviewee, with hopes that the responses will provide information about comprehension of questions, range of vocabulary, etc. Upon completion of the interview, raters watch a video of the interview and take notes on a standardized form. Then the raters independently assign a score of 0–5 to the interviewee, and three raters' scores will become the interviewee's final interview score.

Using the ASLPI to measure ASL fluency resolved some of the issues associated with the SLPI; however, many challenges remain. For example, training raters to provide consistent judgments using unambiguous criteria is a difficult process. Also, over time, ratings can "drift". That is, a holistic rating of *Superior* today may be assigned to an interview that would only have been rated *Advanced* in the past. These drifts in ratings may be the result of differences among different raters, a tendency for ratings to become less rigorous over time, or changes in a linguistic community's understanding of what constitutes different levels of performance. Agencies that conduct proficiency interviews such as the ASLPI must be vigilant about monitoring these drifts, must continually retrain raters to make sure that they continue to utilize consistent rating criteria, and engage in continual assessments of reliability.

Another related challenge for interview-based assessments is the application of a common understanding of what constitutes performance at different levels. This, in turn, requires a common understanding of critical aspects of the language that are germane to the demonstration of expertise. As we have noted previously in this chapter, our understanding of what these aspects are is evolving (and indeed are in an early stage of evolution). Thus, the quality of assessments is evolving as well, and achieving a common understanding of what, specifically, constitutes a rating of a particular numerical value will not be perfectly achievable until we know considerably more about the structure and expression of ASL.

A final challenge worth mentioning pertains to scoring. When three raters independently rate an interview, they will often not all agree. Procedures for resolution of disagreements are critical, and none of the procedures currently used is completely satisfactory. They range from averaging (a practice that is almost never warranted given that rating scores are ordinal measures that are based on categorical criteria of performance), to negotiation among raters (a practice that will give undue weight to the rater who may have the strongest personality rather than the greatest skill in rating), to re-rating with different raters (a practice that does not alleviate the fact that there were disagreements to begin with). The best solution to this challenge is to minimize disagreements from the start through clarifying the rating criteria and training raters to follow them. Certainly, when language proficiency tests are used in high stakes decisions (for example personnel decisions), achieving scoring agreement rates of 80–90% is mandatory.

Behavior Checklists

Some sign language assessments provide a list of behaviors that are to be observed within the performance of the individual. If the individual is seen performing the behavior, then the evaluator checks that item on the list. Evaluators can be comprised of trained professionals, teachers, or parents. The *MacArthur Communicative Development Inventory for American Sign Language* (ASL-CDI; Anderson and Reilly 2002) uses the checklist method on which parents evaluate their children's language development. The ASL-CDI can be used with children aged 8–36 months to measure their early expressive ASL vocabulary. This inventory consists of 537 signs in 20 semantic categories such as animals, people, action words, descriptive signs, etc. If the child is observed producing one of the signs on the list, the evaluator checks the item on the inventory. When using parents as evaluators, a common question is whether or not they have the ability to assess language; however, Anderson and Reilly report high levels of test–retest reliability for parent raters, indicating that parents are applying consistent criteria in their observations of their childrens' use of sign vocabulary.

The *Signed Language Development Checklist* (Mounty 1993, 1994) was developed to assess expressive ASL skills. In this checklist, the expressive skills are broken down into three domains: (1) overall language ability (communicative competence), (2) linguistic use, e.g., formational aspects (i.e., phonology), morphology, syntax, perspective (role-play), and (3) creative use of the language. The pilot version has not been tested with a large sample yet and no psychometric properties are available (Haug 2005). Again, the consistency among different individuals who complete the checklist may vary widely.

Performance-Based Tests on Targeted Linguistic Aspects of ASL

This type of test elicits ASL production on the part of an examinee with prompts that are targeted toward specific skills. Responses made by the test-taker are controlled and are dictated by the test instructions. An example of this type of test is the *American Sign Language Proficiency Assessment* (ASL-PA; Maller et al. 1999). The ASL-PA is intended for children aged 6–12 and includes assessments of how well examinees use eight identified ASL linguistic structures that are developmentally ordered: (1) one-sign/two-sign utterances; (2) nonmanual markers; (3) deictic pointing (real world and abstract indexing); (4) referential shifting; (5) verbs of motion incorporating the use of classifiers; (6) aspects and number; (7) verb agreement; and (8) noun–verb pairs. In order to assess language competence, three language samples are collected from each examinee through an interview, peer interaction, and story retelling. The interview is a set of questions designed to elicit detailed responses, similar to the SLPI and ASLPI. The peer interaction involves a conversation between the test-taker and a friend. In story-retelling task, a child is shown a brief cartoon with no linguistic content, after which the child is asked to reenact the story using different items such as figurines and miniature settings. After successfully completing the reenactment, the child is then asked to sign the whole story.

After the three language samples are collected, the videotapes are reviewed by a rater and partially crosschecked by a second rater for coding accuracy. The ASL-PA requires that the rater have native or near-native ASL skills as well as some knowledge of ASL linguistics. Protocols are given points for each observed target feature and are then assigned an ASL proficiency level based on the total score. Reliability of the ASL-PA is acceptable (Maller et al. 1999); preliminary validity was established by comparing the performances of Deaf Children of Deaf Parents with those of Deaf Children of Hearing Parents (DCHP) who used ASL and DCHPs who used manually coded English.

Two other examples of tests that rely heavily on ratings of examinees' ASL performances on tasks with targeted language skills are: the *Test Battery for American Sign Language Morphology and Syntax* (Supalla et al. 1995), and the *American Sign Language Assessment Instrument* (Hoffmeister et al. 1990).

A unique newly developed test, the ASL-SRT (Hauser et al. 2008), contains 20 ASL sentences of increasing complexity. Rather than soliciting ASL performance samples via interviews, peer interactions, or targeted prompts, the ASL-SRT utilizes discrete items presented via video that are scored as correct–incorrect. Thus, the ASL-SRT is both easier to administer and easier to score. In the ASL-SRT, test-takers are asked to view an ASL sentence on a video and then to reproduce the sentence from memory. They are awarded one point for every sentence they reproduce correctly. The ASL-SRT test design was based on the TOAL-3 (Hammill et al. 1994) Speaking/Grammar Subtest described briefly above in our discussion about the challenges involved in translating proficiency tests from a spoken language to a signed language. The ASL-SRT has been shown to have high inter-rater reliability using native signing deaf raters (Hauser et al. 2008). The test successfully distinguishes between native deaf signers born to deaf signing parents from non-native deaf signers, and it also successfully discriminates between young and older deaf signers.

The ASL-SRT relies on the premise that a less fluent signer would perform less well than a fluent signer because of the greater memory load required to reproduce sentences from memory for individuals who may not grasp the meaning of the stimulus sentences automatically. In general, if something is meaningful, then it is easier to memorize. By implication, higher scores are taken to be indicators of greater proficiency.

Based on extensive item analysis, the ASL-SRT has been modified since the publication of its preliminary results (Hauser et al. 2008). A final version of the test contains 20 items; these have been administered to over a 1000 hearing and deaf children and adults, including the VL2 Toolkit participants. (Statistical results for these participants are presented in Chap. 9 of this volume.) A refined rating protocol has been developed and tested, including lists of acceptable variations. A report on the validity and reliability of this final version of the ASL-SRT is forthcoming.

Objective Tests

Tests that do not involve the use of raters avoid certain kinds of problems found in such tests, such as inconsistency among raters and the time consuming and costly processes of interviewing, observing, and rating. In objective tests, scores are based on whether or not the test-taker makes a correct response, such as pointing to a picture that correctly represents an ASL utterance that has been presented.

The first standardized test of any sign language was the *Assessing* BSL-RST (Herman et al. 1999), developed in the UK for the assessment of BSL. The test was used as a template for the *German Sign Language Receptive Skills Test* (DGS RST; Haug 2011). Enns and Herman (2011) adapted the BSL-RST for use in the assessment of ASL, called the *American Sign Language Receptive Skills Test* (ASL RST). It consists of a 20-word vocabulary check, 3 practice items, and 42 test items. The vocabulary words are given at the beginning of the test to ensure that the child knows the signs used in the test. After passing the vocabulary check, practice items and test items are presented by video. The child watches a deaf adult who explains the test procedure and presents the test items. The child must watch the adult signing and then point to the picture, from four options, that best corresponds with the signed item. There are eight different grammatical categories assessed with the ASL RST, including spatial verbs, negation, size/shape specifiers, etc., and the child receives one point for every correct answer. Several studies are currently underway to provide normative and psychometric data for the ASL RST, including the VL2 Early Education Longitudinal Study of a national sample of deaf children who were aged 3–5 in the first wave of the 3-year project.

Recent cognitive linguistic studies propose a typology of depiction based in part on a larger inventory of "devices," including the body and space (Dudis 2004, 2008), that may be used to create imagistic items. The ASL-CT (originally known as *Depiction Comprehension Test*; Hauser et al. 2010) is an objective multiple-choice measure of a person's ASL depiction comprehension abilities. The test is used to assess knowledge of the varying types of depiction used in ASL as an indicator of proficiency. The ASL-CT currently contains 3 practice items as well as 65 test items presented through a computerized program. Each of the items was developed by a team of linguists, psychologists, and deaf native signers. In the test, the examinee is presented with a visual stimulus (video, still photograph, or line drawing) to represent depiction, and is required to manually select the correct answer from four possible choices. One point is assigned for each correct response, and the raw score is used as an indicator of performance. Although early in its development, pilot data suggest that the ASL-CT is sensitive to differences in deaf and hearing individuals' comprehension of ASL (Hauser et al. 2010).

Sign Language Standards

In addition to a need for new, validated tests of ASL proficiency, there is also a need for ASL standardization, both for deaf signers, and for hearing individuals who are learning to sign. Specific standards for ASL provide roadmaps for what students should learn in their lessons, defining what most language-learning experts agree on prior to language course delivery. Setting standards leads to effective training by guiding educators in the development and selection of curricula and in the adoption of assessment strategies that will inform students when the standards have been met.

In other words, setting standards implies setting the end-state of instruction *before* developing curricula or assessments. This "backward design model" (Tomlinson and McTighe 2006; Tyler 1949) outlines three steps for effective instructional design. The first step is to identify the desired results, i.e., the standards and their corresponding measurable outcomes. The second step would be to develop assessments that constitute evidence that the standards have been achieved. Finally, the third step is to plan instructional activities that will bring students to these competencies.

At this point in time, there are no formalized published national ASL standards, making the development of ASL assessments more challenging. One might question whether such standards are even possible, given widespread variation in ASL due to regional, ethnic, gender, age, and educational differences in what constitutes fluent ASL. If national standards of ASL skills were to be developed and used as the basis for developing effective assessments of those skills, who would make the decisions regarding the above noted variations?

Fortunately, there are current efforts being undertaken to address this problem. For example, the Laurent Clerc National Deaf Education Center is coordinating a national effort to develop ASL standards for P-12 education. Additionally, the *Standards for Learning American Sign Language in the 21st Century* (Ashton et al. 2012) was recently published through a collaboration between the American Sign Language Teachers Association (ASLTA) and the National Consortium of Interpreter Education Centers, with the encouragement and additional financial support of the American Council on the Teaching of Foreign Languages (ACTFL).

In the Spring of 2007, the American Sign Language National Standards committee was established comprised of ASL teachers, curriculum designers, and consultants who work at every level of ASL instruction from P-12 to postsecondary level. This committee drafted a set of proposed standards and sent them out for review by

ASLTA members and other ASL content specialists and teachers in 2008. After receiving extensive feedback from the field, a final set of standards were completed in 2012 and are currently under review by the Standards Collaborative Board, a reviewing board which is affiliated with ACTFL

Standards, in and of themselves, do not prescribe a curriculum or syllabus. The standards reflect the framework of communicative modes as established by ACTFL and incorporate the goals of the "5 C's" of foreign language instruction—Communication, Cultures, Connections, Comparisons, and Communities. Using a spiraling methodology, topics and skills are visited and revisited with increasing complexity in order to encourage learners to develop greater proficiency at each level.

Once standards are adopted, educators will have to develop specific curricula and indicators of progress. The ASLTA standards themselves include benchmarks for knowledge and performance of ASL learning at grade levels K, 4, 8, 12, and 16. Some activities are underway to translate these benchmarks into practical strategies. For example, a guide, *Learning Outcomes for American Sign Language Skills Levels 1–4* (Kurz and Taylor 2008), includes a comprehensive listing of measurable learning outcomes for each of the ASL levels. Organized around the "5 C's", this guide provides specific descriptions of what students should be able to demonstrate at each of the levels.

Conclusion

As this chapter has documented, there are a number of ASL tests being developed and should be readily available in the near future. The enterprise of developing sign language assessment instruments is still new. Researchers and test developers are learning the best ways to measure a visual language. Even when such tests become available for widespread use, there will continue to be a need to develop new tests that incorporate new avenues of knowledge and a greater understanding of the structure of ASL and how it develops in young children. With groundbreaking work being done in developing standards and specifying outcomes for ASL, in conducting linguistic research on the structures of ASL at different linguistic levels from phonological to semantic, and in developing tests suitable for a wide number of purposes, we are very optimistic about the future for ASL assessment and its role in education, clinical practice, and research.

Acknowledgements The authors wish to acknowledge Paul Dudis for his contributions to this chapter. This project was partially supported by the Gallaudet University Priority Grant to RP and PH, NSF Science of Learning Center grant # SBE-0541953 to PH and RP and NIH/NIDCD grant # RO1 DC004418-06A1 to PH. Special thanks to the assistants at the Deaf Studies Laboratory at the National Technical Institute for the Deaf at Rochester Institute of Technology for help with the preparation of this chapter

References

Allen, T. E., Hwang, Y., & Stansky, A. (2009). *Measuring factors that predict deaf students' reading abilities: The VL2 Toolkit-Project design and early findings*. Paper presented at the 2009 Annual Meeting of the Association of College Educators of the Deaf and Hard of Hearing, New Orleans.

Anderson, D., & Reilly, J. (2002). The MacArthur Communicative Development Inventory: Normative data for American Sign Language. *Journal of Deaf Studies and Deaf Education, 7*(2), 83–106.

Ashton, G., Cagle, K., Kurz, K., Newell, W., Peterson, R., & Zinza, J. (2012). Standards for Learning American Sign Language (ASL) in the 21st century. In *Standards for Foreign Language Learning in the 21st century*. Yonkers, NY: National Standards in Foreign Language Education Project.

Caccamise, F., Newell, W., Fennell, D., & Carr, N. (1988). The Georgia and New York State Programs for assessing and developing sign communication skills of vocational rehabilitation personnel. *Journal of the American Deafness and Rehabilitation Association, 21*, 1–14.

Caccamise, F., Newell, W., & Mitchell-Caccamise, M. (1983). Use of the Sign Language Proficiency Interview for assessing the sign communicative competence of Louisiana School for the Deaf dormitory counselor applicants. *Journal of the Academy of Rehabilitative Audiology, 16*, 283–230.

Corina, D. P., Lawyer, L., Hirshorn, E., & Hauser, P. C. (2011, April). *Functional neuroanatomy of skilled and non-skilled deaf readers: Data from implicit word recognition*.

Dudis, P. (2004). *Depiction of events in ASL*. Unpublished doctoral dissertation, University of California at Berkeley

Dudis, P. (2008). Types of depiction in ASL. In R. M. de Quadros (Ed.), *Sign Language: Spinning and unraveling the past, present and future* (pp. 159–190). Florianópolis, SC, Brazil: Editora Arara Azul. http://www.editora-arara-azul.com.br/Livros.php.

Dunn, L. M., & Dunn, L. M. (1997). *Examiner's manual for the PPVT-III: Peabody Picture Vocabulary Test* (3rd ed.). Circle Pines, MN: American Guidance Service.

Emmorey, K. (2002). *Language, cognition, and the brain: Insights from sign language research*. Mahwah, NJ: Lawrence Erlbaum Associates, Inc.

Enns, C. J., & Herman, R. C. (2011). Adapting the assessing British Sign Language Development: Receptive skills test into American Sign Language. *Journal of Deaf Studies and Deaf Education, 16*(3), 362–374.

Freidenberg, L. (1995). *Psychological testing: Design, analysis, and use*. Needham Heights, MA: Allyn and Bacon.

Hammill, D., Brown, V., Larsen, S., & Wiederholt, J. L. (1994). *Test of adolescent and adult language* (3rd ed.). Austin, TX: PRO-ED, Inc.

Haug, T. (2005). Review of sign language assessment instruments. *Sign Language & Linguistics, 8*, 59–96.

Haug, T. (2008). Review of signed language assessment instruments. In A. E. Baker & B. Woll (Eds.), *Sign language acquisition* (pp. 51–86). Philadelphia: John Benjamins Publishers.

Haug, T. (2011). Approaching sign language test construction: Adaptation of the German Sign Language Receptive Skills Test. *Journal of Deaf Studies and Deaf Education, 16*, 343–361.

Haug, T., & Mann, W. (2008). Adapting tests of sign language assessment for other sign languages—A review of linguistic, cultural, and psychometric problems. *Journal of Deaf Studies and Deaf Education, 13*, 138–147.

Hauser, P. C., Paludneviciene, R., Dudis, P., Riddle, W., Daggett, D., & Freel, B. (2010, September). *The Depiction Comprehension Test in American Sign Language*.

Hauser, P. C., Paludnevičiene, R., Supalla, T., & Bavelier, D. (2008). American Sign Language-Sentence Reproduction Test: Development and implications. In R. M. de Quadros (Ed.), *Sign Language: Spinning and unraveling the past, present and future* (pp. 160–172). Petropolis, Brazil: Editora Arara Azul.

Herman, R., Holmes, S., & Woll, B. (1999). *Assessing BSL development—Receptive skills test*. Coleford, UK: The Forest Bookshop.

Hoffmeister, R., Bahan, B., Greenwald, J., & Cole, J. (1990). *American Sign Language Assessment Instrument (ASLAI)*. Unpublished test, Center for the Study of Communication and the Deaf, Boston University.

Knight, D. (1983). Comment on Newell et al. Adaption of the Language Proficiency Interview (LPI) for assessing sign communicative competence. *Sign Language Studies, 41*, 311–352.

Kubus, O., Rathmann, C., Morford, J. P., & Wilkinson, E. (2010, September). *Effects and non-effects of sign language knowledge on word recognition: A comparison of ASL-English and DGS-German bilingual adults*. Paper presented at the 10th Theoretical Issues in Sign Language Research Conference, West Lafayette, IN.

Kurz, K., & Taylor, M. (2008). *Learning outcomes for American Sign Language levels 1–4*. Raleigh, NC: Lulu Publishing Company. www.lulu.com.

Langacker, R. W. (1991). *Foundations of cognitive grammar, Volume 2: Descriptive application*. Stanford, CA: Stanford University Press.

Liddell, S. K. (2003). *Grammar, gesture, and meaning in American Sign Language*. New York: Cambridge University Press.

Liskin-Gasparro, J. (1982). *ETS oral proficiency test manual*. Princeton, NJ: Educational Testing Service.

Lucas, C., & Valli, C. (1992). *Language contact in the American Deaf Community*. Washington, DC: Gallaudet University Press.

Lucas, C., Valli, C., & Mulrooney, K. J. (2005). *Linguistics of American Sign Language: An introduction*. Washington, DC: Gallaudet University Press.

Maller, S. J., Singleton, J. L., Supalla, S. J., & Wix, T. (1999). The development and psychometric properties of the American Sign Language Proficiency Assessment (ASL-PA). *Journal of Deaf Studies and Deaf Education, 4*, 259–269.

Morford, J. P., Wilkinson, E., Vilwock, A., Piñar, P., & Kroll, J. F. (2011). When deaf signers read English: Do written words activate their sign translations? *Cognition, 118*, 286–292.

Mounty, J. (1993). *Signed language development checklist—Training manual*. Princeton, NJ: Educational Testing Service.

Mounty, J. (1994). *Signed language development checklist*. Princeton, NJ: Educational Testing Service.

Newell, W., Caccamise, F., Boardman, K., & Holcomb, B. R. (1983). Adaption of the Language Proficiency Interview (LPI) for assessing sign communicative competence. *Sign Language Studies, 41*, 311–352.

Newman, A.J., Waligura, D.L., Neville, H.J., & Ullman, M. T. (2003). Effects of late second language acquisition on neural organization: Event-related potential and functional magnetic resonance imaging evidence. *Cognitive Neuroscience Society Abstracts, 11*.

Newport, E. L. (1990). Maturational constraints on language learning. *Cognitive Science, 14*, 11–28.

Prinz, P., Strong, M. & Kuntze, M. (1994). *The Test of ASL*. Unpublished test. San Francisco: San Francisco State University, California Research Institute.

Schick, B. (1997). *American Sign Language Vocabulary Test*. Unpublished test, University of Colorado, Boulder.

Singleton, J., & Supalla, S. (2011). Assessing children's proficiency in natural signed languages. In M. Marschark & P. E. Spencer (Eds.), *Oxford handbook of deaf studies, language and education* (2nd ed., pp. 306–319). New York: Oxford University Press.

Stokoe, W. C. (1960). Sign language structure: An outline of the visual communication system of the American deaf. In *Studies in linguistics: Occasional papers (No. 8)*. Department of Anthropology and Linguistics, University of Buffalo: Buffalo, NY.

Supalla, T., Newport, E., Singleton, J., Supalla, S., Coulter, G., & Metlay, D. (1995). *An overview of the Test Battery for American Sign Language morphology and syntax*. Paper presented at the Annual Meeting of the American Educational Research Association (AERA), April 20, 1995, San Francisco, CA.

Tomlinson, C. A., & McTighe, J. (2006). *Integrating differentiated instruction and understanding by design*. Alexandria, VA: Association for Supervision and Curriculum Development.

Tyler, R. W. (1949). *Basic principles of curriculum and instruction*. Chicago: University of Chicago Press.

Chapter 12
Analysis of Responses to Lipreading Prompts as a Window to Deaf Students' Writing Strategies

Corine Bickley, Mary June Moseley, and Anna Stansky

Background

There is a long-standing interest in the reading and writing abilities of deaf students. Although reading has received the majority of researchers' and teachers' attention over the years, writing has also been mentioned frequently; for recent discussions, see Cheng and Rose (2008), Paul (2009), and Marschark and Hauser (2012). All students, including deaf students, need to write for academic and professional achievement (Nichols and Moseley 1996; Paul 2009). Debates about the most effective ways to teach writing to deaf students and the associated need to test the ability of deaf students to write have been discussed for many years among researchers, teachers, and clinicians. The consequences of weak writing skills are serious in terms of access to education as well as well-paying, respected vocations. As clinical researchers, we are most interested in questions about testing the writing ability of deaf students, particularly as those testing methods might lead to insights for interventions by teachers and clinicians to improve the abilities of deaf student to write. Researchers' and educators' interest in the writing abilities of deaf students is part of a wider interest in the academic abilities of deaf students (for a recent summary, see Qi and Mitchell 2011).

Deaf students come to any testing experience with a variety of family and educational experiences, as well as differences in their psychological, intellectual, linguistic, and audiological characteristics. Because of this variability, Marschark and Hauser (2012) argue that deaf children are not simply hearing children who cannot hear. Their varied backgrounds necessitate unique strategies for supporting their growth and development. Early intervention, through effective parenting and early childhood education programs, has been shown to be important in developing

---

C. Bickley (✉) • M.J. Moseley • A. Stansky
Department of Hearing, Speech, and Language Sciences, Gallaudet University,
800 Florida Avenue, NE, Washington, DC 20002, USA
e-mail: corine.bickley@gallaudet.edu; maryjune07@comcast.net; anna_stansky@hotmail.com

written English skills among deaf students, but educational placement has not (Yoshinago-Itano 2003). Furthermore, Singleton et al. (2004) point out that the assessment of literacy among deaf students is far more complicated than simply the language and modality of the assessment strategy.

Many approaches to evaluating writing by deaf students have been used over the years using different kinds of prompts and different scoring rubrics (e.g., Birnbaum et al. 2006; Bochner et al. 1992; Carrow-Woolfolk 1995). For example, in many tests of writing, the requirement is to write one or more English sentence(s) in response to stimuli. Sentences have been elicited by tasks such as: asking the examinee to write a sentence using a group of words as in the Woodcock-Johnson III NU Tests of Achievement (WJIII), or requiring the examinee to write a sentence about a picture (WJIII) or supply a missing word to complete a sentence. The ability to write a coherent group of sentences, i.e., a paragraph, has been tested by tasks such as describing a picture or sequence of pictures and writing to communicate information on a topic.

The task of writing short stories or essays has been used to elicit longer samples of written material and to convey an idea or express an opinion: for example, writing about an incident or a memory, an experience in the dorm, or a story or an essay about an experience.

Recognizing correct English grammar, as opposed to writing grammatically, is a related skill that has been tested for several decades with the Test of Syntactic Abilities (TSA) (Quigley et al. 1978). The TSA test was included in the VL2 Toolkit set of tests, as was the WJIII; the responses of a subset of VL2 participants to the TSA diagnostic test were reported by Allen et al. (2009). The ability to recognize a correctly written sentence in contrast to writing syntactically correct sentences will be discussed below for each of the single case study participants in this report.

A Different Way of Judging Writing

Some tools require written responses, although the assessments themselves are not explicitly tests of writing. The Lipreading Screening Test (LST, Auer and Bernstein 2007) is one such test. This test was included in the battery of tests used in the VL2 Toolkit. During the process of collecting responses to the LST for analysis we noticed that the examinees differed considerably in the length and completeness of their written responses. These differences intrigued us. We became even more interested in this issue when we noticed that some of the most prolific writers were poor lipreaders, but they wrote many syntactically correct sentences in response to viewing the moving faces on the screen. What were the characteristics of the strings of words they wrote? The study reported here is an attempt to answer that question.

Although responses to a lipreading test are not usually scored as samples of writing, these responses do provide a unique window into a participant's knowledge of English syntax. The written responses to this lipreading test provide data that can be analyzed in terms of syntactic structures used, the words used, and the syntactic errors in sentences written. We undertook analyses of the responses to this lipreading test in order to answer the following questions:

1. What vocabulary was used in the responses?
2. What syntactic structures were used?
3. What error patterns were found?
4. What background characteristics of the participants might explain their vocabulary and syntactic choices as well as their errors in writing?

Lipreading in Deaf Education

Lipreading is a skill that has a long history in the education of deaf students (Auer and Bernstein 2007; Bally 1996; Berger 1972; Bernstein et al. 1998, 2011; Bunger 1932; DeLand and Montague 1968; Hazard 1971; Kaplan 1996; O'Neill and Oyer 1961; Paul 2009). As is well known, spoken English can be perceived visually; however, spoken English is seldom perceived easily or completely through vision alone. Although the terms "lipreading" and "speechreading" have often been used synonymously, the task of understanding speech (a spoken sentence or conversation) involves more than just watching the lips move, or even just watching the lips, jaw, and tongue move, and the body language used. For a deaf person to communicate with another person, hearing or deaf, by speech alone it is necessary to use conversational skills of maintaining a conversation and responding in sensible ways (Bally 1996). In addition to communication skills, knowledge of English words and syntax influence the success of visual communication using spoken English. Some English words are more predictable visually than others (e.g., question words because of their corresponding facial expressions) and other words are more predictable because of preceding words in a sentence (Kalikow et al. 1977). Also, some words are more common in everyday speech than others and more likely to be spoken in certain situations (e.g., the words "and cream in" are likely to be understood if a person recognizes the words "I take sugar" and "my coffee").

Even without the support of conversational context, speechreading can be enhanced by knowledge of English syntax and morphology (Carlisle 1996), including understanding appropriate grammatical markers (Kaplan 1996). Some English grammatical markers of tense and agreement are visually salient in written English but are not easy to discern on the face of a speaker of English, such as the present tense marker "s" in the written word "cheers" (realized as a final /z/ sound when spoken). In the sentence "Music always cheers me up," "cheers" is likely to be understood rather than "cheer" if a person knows the rules of English syntax. In some dialects such as African-American English (Craig and Washington 1994), English verb forms differ from standard English (e.g., deleted copulas), but we will not discuss these variations here, as we do not know which dialects our participants were raised in.

For deaf students, as well as for second-language learners, a variety of tests have been used, and often the results are variable and subject to the effects of small sample sizes. As pointed out by Bernstein et al. (2000), participants exhibit a wide range of skills in a task like lipreading, which is a task that is developed in a family, educational, and community environment of needing to communicate with many persons in many ways. Conclusions are difficult to draw that would guide educational policy and clinical practice. Because of these obstacles, we feel that an interpretive investigation of single case studies has relevance when examining the skills in written English shown by deaf students. We hope to contribute a useful addition to both the research literature and the evidence for clinical practice through an analysis of the written responses, the scores obtained on a TSA, and the background characteristics of four deaf college students. We hope that such a broad view of these single case study participants will illustrate the usefulness of careful examination of individual responses to a test as a means for assessing writing.

Method

Participants

The participants in our study were a subset of those who participated in the VL2 Toolkit Project that is the focus of this volume. (See Chap. 2 for a description of the project methodology.) The four VL2 Toolkit participants who completed the LST and who wrote the greatest number of sentences (i.e., responses with both a subject and a verb) were selected for our study. Coincidentally, these four participants exhibited a range of word accuracy in lipreading. Accuracy of lipreading was not a selection criterion. Our participant group consisted of individuals whose lipreading word accuracy covered a wide range: 75% of the 256 stimulus words, 56%, 19%, and 7%. Bernstein et al. (1998, p. 213) observed and reported a wide range of speechreading skills among deaf college students.

Some participants did not respond at all to many of the lipreading stimuli; others responded minimally. These responses for these participants are not useful for our syntactic analyses because we are primarily interested in the kinds of sentences deaf students write and the kinds of syntactic errors they make. Therefore, they were not selected for our case studies. We cannot guess whether these participants were not interested in the lipreading task, whether they found the lipreading task too difficult, whether they might have had trouble seeing the screen clearly, or whether they encountered other complications that prevented them from responding.

Materials

Our materials consisted of the:

- Lipreading Screening Test (Auer and Bernstein 2007)
- Test of Syntactic Abilities (Quigley et al. 1978)
- Portions of the Toolkit Background Questionnaire

The LST consists of high-quality video-only recordings of 30 English sentences (Auer and Bernstein 2007, used with permission of the authors). This lipreading test utilizes a subset of the CID (Central Institute for the Deaf) everyday sentences (Davis and Silverman 1970), which have been used for many years in research and in aural rehabilitation with deaf and hard-of-hearing persons. These sentences were designed to be representative of the vocabulary and syntactic structures of everyday spoken American English.

The TSA was developed to assess a deaf student's ability to recognize correct syntactic forms in English (Quigley et al. 1978). The test focuses on syntactic ability of nine of the major syntactic structures of English: negation, determiners, question formation, verb processes, pronominalization, relativization, complementation, and nominalization. We used only the screening test of the TSA in this study. The TSA Screening Test is comprised of 120 multiple choice items that provide a relatively quick and reliable assessment of a participant's general knowledge of English syntax and to pinpoint overall strengths and weaknesses in individual syntactic structures.

The Toolkit Background Questionnaire. The demographic questionnaire was designed to provide background information on study participants. We examined the responses of our participants to questions that concern their language development and experiences.

Procedures

After completing the Background Questionnaire, each participant who agreed to participate in the lipreading testing was first asked to read the test instructions and the informed consent form. A researcher or research assistant fluent in ASL then asked each participant if they understood and agreed to participate. Questions about the procedure were answered as needed by the researcher or assistant. Participants were tested individually with the LST, in a visually quiet room, using similar equipment to that used by Auer and Bernstein. Participant responses to the test items were also recorded using the same protocol as that used by Auer and Bernstein (2007). The participants sat approximately 0.5 m from a 14-in Trinitron monitor. Participants were instructed to watch the screen and then type on a computer keyboard the words they understood. The participants were told that they would watch the images one sentence at a time and that the sentences were about everyday topics, 15 spoken by a woman and 15 spoken by a man. They viewed each sentence only once and then typed the words they remembered on a computer keyboard positioned next to the video monitor. They were asked to make a best guess or make up a spelling if they were unsure of a word. Later, one of the researchers checked the files for typographic and spelling errors (such as "teh" for "the") and corrected the files before further analysis.

After the LST was completed, participants were asked to provide feedback about the process on a separate form that did not contain any identifying information. The computer program that administered the LST saved each response file with a unique numeric code that was not linked to a participant's personal information or to comments about the process.

The participants were next asked to complete the TSA. Some participants were able to complete the TSA at that time; others chose to return later for the TSA; some did not return to complete the TSA.

For the purposes of the study reported in this chapter, all responses to the LST were analyzed in detail by first sorting each response word into a word class, whether or not the sequences of words written conformed to grammatical rules for English sentences, or whether or not they contained words that matched the stimuli. We counted the vocabulary items in each word class. The word classes of noun, verb, adjective, function word (as used in Singleton et al. 2004), and wh-word were used in our analysis. Function words defined as words that convey grammatical meaning, such as pronouns, articles, prepositions, auxiliary verbs, and adverbs. We looked for syntactic patterns used by the participants in their responses. We were interested in identifying correct syntactic patterns and word usage. In this report, we did not utilize a words correct score (other than as an indicator of a range of skills in lipreading among our participants).

Our approach to analyzing the responses made by participants in this study has much in common with the methods of Grounded Theory (Strauss and Corbin 1990); that is, we collected as much data as possible related to the reasons why the participants might have written the sentences they wrote. We combined their test responses with information provided on the Background Questionnaire for details about their experiences related to language and to writing. We looked at their comments about their parents' encouragement, or not, to learn English in any form. We checked their self-reported educational backgrounds and involvement in early intervention, as well as their self-assessments of their abilities with ASL and all forms of English (written, spoken, lipreading, cued speech, and signed English). We also checked for evidence of their interest in writing as well as for the encouragement they received from their parents to write.

Our goal was, as explained above, to see if there is evidence that participants have mastered the syntax of English sentences and usage of English words according to the standards of written English. Such evidence would allow a clinician or teacher to build on these skills to enhance a student's writing in a variety of tasks.

Results

Characteristics of the 30 Target Sentences of the Lipreading Screening Test

We first analyzed the stimuli of the LST, the 30 target sentences, with respect to the categories of nouns, verbs, adjectives, and function words in order to answer the following question: "Is the set of 30 target sentences that comprise the LST

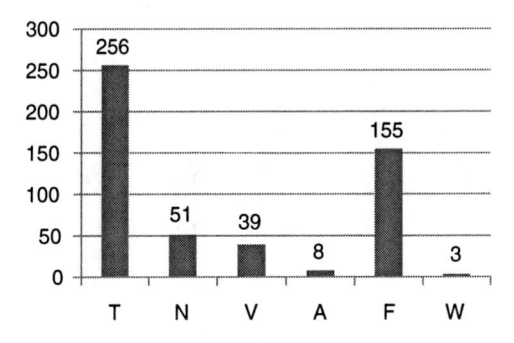

Fig. 12.1 Numbers of total words in the 30 target sentences of the Lipreading Screening Test (T), and nouns (N), verbs (V), adjectives (A), function words (F), and wh-words (W). The categories of word classes follow the definitions in Singleton et al. (2004)

representative of the distribution by syntactic class of English vocabulary known to school-aged students?" We accept the word categories used by Singleton et al. (2004) as a baseline measure of the vocabulary items known to young students. We will interpret a positive answer to our question as a positive answer to the question "Are the sentences in the lipreading test representative of spoken English?" (in the experience of our participants). As clinical researchers, we are interested in answering questions that will guide educational practice and clinical interventions and therefore need to first determine the appropriateness of the materials of any test for our research interests.

Distribution by Word Class of Vocabulary in the Target Sentences

The results of our analysis of the target sentences are included in Fig. 12.1, which shows the numbers of words in each class (nouns, verbs, adjectives, function words, and wh-words) in the set of 30 target sentences. Of particular interest to our study is the class of function words; the preponderance of function words is interesting because the use of English function words has been claimed by some researchers (e.g., Albertini and Schley (2003) as explained in Singleton et al. (2004)) to be difficult for deaf writers to master. Because function words comprise the majority of words used in standard written English, they are an important class of words for writers to master.

Distribution by Word Class of Vocabulary in Sentences Written by Hearing Children

In comparing our analysis of the LST to the responses of the hearing writers reported by Singleton and her colleagues, we found that:

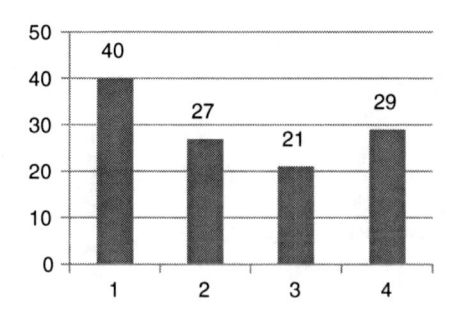

Fig. 12.2 Number of sentences written by each of the 4 single case study participants (Writers 1–4) in response to viewing 30 stimuli sentences. A "sentence" is a string of words that contains at least one subject (possibly implied, as in an imperative sentence) and one verb

- 61% of the words in the sentences of the LST are function words; this test consists of everyday sentences.
- 58% of the words written in response to Singleton et al.'s task were function words. This percentage was reported for hearing monolingual group of elementary school students in grades 1–6 (Singleton et al. 2004); their task was to describe a silent video cartoon (The Hare and The Tortoise).

Although the task of writing a description of a video cartoon is different from the task of writing sentences in response to a lipreading test of everyday sentences, we feel that the description task is a sensible way to collect a sample of descriptive writing. We also feel that the descriptive writing samples provide a baseline for comparing the prevalence of function words to the prevalence of function words in the everyday sentences of the LST. The percentage of function words in the target sentences of the LST (61%) is similar to that reported by Singleton and her colleagues (58%) for their writing task.

Characteristics of Responses to the Lipreading Screening Test

Number of Sentences Written

We first counted the number of sentences that each participant wrote (Fig. 12.2), using the definition of "sentence" as a string of words that consists of at least a subject (perhaps implied, as in the sentence "Come here") and a verb. Only Writer 3 did not respond to all of the stimuli (three of the responses were blank).

We also counted the total number of sentences with standard syntax written by each participant and computed the percentage of grammatically correct sentences for each participant (Fig. 12.3).

Writer 1, who scored only 7% on lipreading accuracy (percentage words correct, i.e., response words that matched a stimulus word), wrote 40 sentences, i.e., 10

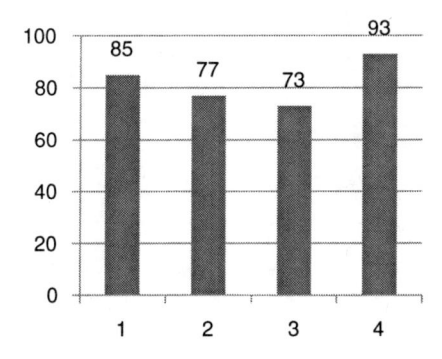

Fig. 12.3 Percentage of grammatically correct sentences written by each of the 4 single case study participants (Writers 1–4) in response to viewing 30 stimuli sentences

more sentences than were presented in the stimuli; sometimes a response of this participant consisted of 2 sentences. Interestingly, 85% of this participant's responses were grammatically correct sentences, even though they did not contain any of the content words in the stimuli sentences (matches on function words and one wh-word account for the 7% accurate score).

Distributions by Word Class of Vocabulary in Sentences Written by Respondents

We next analyzed the words written by each participant (Writers 1–4) according to word class to answer the question: "Are the words written by the four single case study participants representative of the distribution by word class in written English?" We interpreted a positive response to this question as a positive response to the question "Are the responses written by the four single case study participants representative of written English?" The results of our analyses are shown in Figs. 12.4–12.7; each figure shows the numbers of nouns, verbs, adjectives, function words, and wh-words in the sentences written by the participants. When comparing percentages of words in the target sentences to the percentages of words written by the participants, we see similar patterns of preponderance of function words. Each figure shows the total number of words written as well as the number of words in each syntactic class.

In comparing the percentages of words in each syntactic class (noun, verb, adjective, function word, and wh-word) in the target sentences to the sentences written by the participants, it is clear that the patterns are similar: the four participants wrote approximately the same percentages of words in each class as are contained in the target sentences. For all of our case study participants, the most frequently written words were function words, followed by nouns and verbs. Whether or not the writers used these words in patterns that form acceptable written English is analyzed next.

Throughout our discussion of these results runs the theme that writing responses to a lipreading task involves more than just being able to read words on the lips of

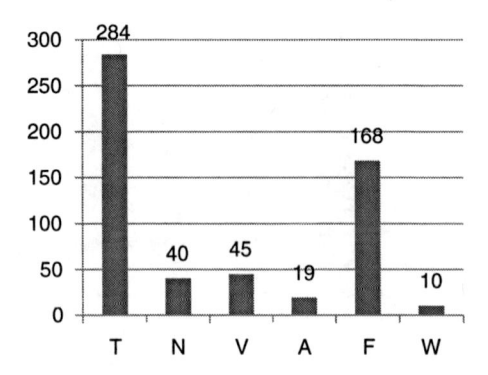

Fig. 12.4 Number of total words written (1), and numbers of nouns (2), verbs (3), adjectives (4), function words (5), and wh-words (6) written in response to viewing the 30 stimuli by Writer 1. Note the preponderance (64% for this writer) of function words. Writer 1 wrote 40 sentences (284 words) in response to viewing 30 stimuli sentences (sometimes this writer wrote 2 sentences in response to viewing 1 spoken sentence, e.g., "How are you doing? Study hard and good luck.")

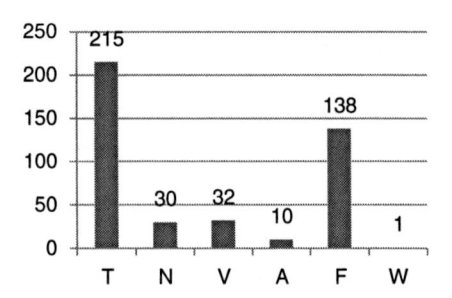

Fig. 12.5 Number of total words written (T), and numbers of nouns (N), verbs (V), adjectives (A), function words (F), and wh-words (W) written in response to viewing the 30 stimuli by Writer 2. Note the preponderance (64% for this writer also) of function words. Writer 2 wrote 30 sentences (191 words), i.e., 1 response sentence for each 1 stimulus sentence

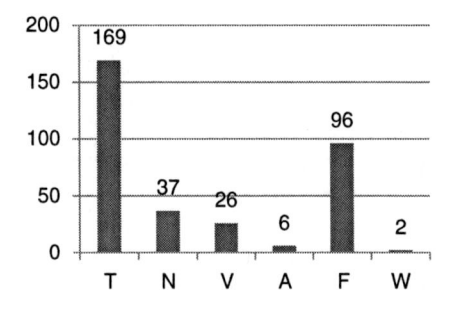

Fig. 12.6 Number of total words written (1), and numbers of nouns (2), verbs (3), adjectives (4), function words (5), and wh-words (6) written in response to viewing the 30 stimuli for Writer 3. Note the preponderance (65%) of function words. Writer 3 wrote 27 sentences (216 words); 3 stimuli received no response

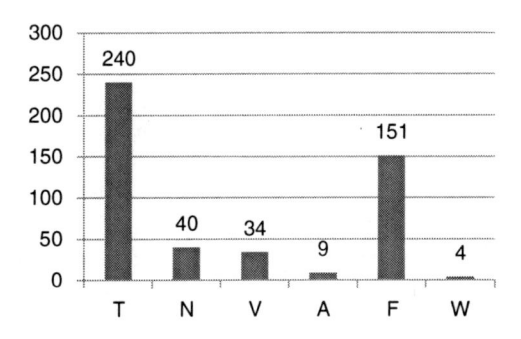

Fig. 12.7 Number of total words written (T), and numbers of nouns (N), verbs (V), adjective (A), function words (F), and wh-words (W) written in response to viewing the 30 stimuli for Writer 4. Note the preponderance (56%) of function words. Writer 4 wrote 25 sentences (169 words); 5 stimuli received no response

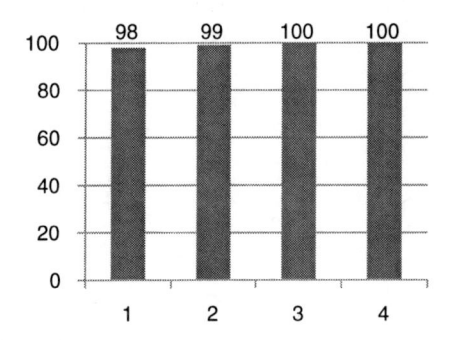

Fig. 12.8 Percentage of function words that were used grammatically; results for each single case study participant are shown ("1" designates Writer 1, "2" for Writer 2, "3" for Writer 3, and "4" for Writer 4)

the speakers because not all spoken words can be distinguished by vision alone. Knowledge of English grammar and awareness of frequency of usage are likely influences on the responses that are written, particularly in the case of words like function words that are often difficult to discern from only lip, tongue, and jaw movements seen on a face. Bernstein and her colleagues (1998) offered similar reasoning in discussing their results of a different lipreading task. In the LST, some words are visually similar to some of the participant's responses, such as "let" (stimulus word) and "get" (response word), "don't" (stimulus word) and "go" (response word), and "new" (stimulus word) and "two" (response word); these similarities are of interest in our study of word choice and sentence patterns as the words in each pair above belong to the same word class.

We also compared the usage of the function words that were written by the participants to the standards of professional written English. We cannot discern what meaning the writers intended to convey, but we can judge the grammaticality of each sentence that was written. The results of this analysis are presented in Fig. 12.8. Two of the writers used all of the function words that they wrote correctly; one other writer only misused one function word and the other misused two function words.

Trends in Syntactic Patterns

Three trends were observed in the patterns of words in the sentences (where "sentence" is defined as a sequence of words that contains at least a subject and a verb) written by the four case study participants. These trends in writing both grammatically correct patterns and also ungrammatical patterns were found. To repeat, our goal is to answer the question "what patterns of words show correct syntax?" in the responses of the four case study participants. We looked at the use of function words, errors in syntax, semantic choices, and syllabic structure in the participants' responses.

Trend 1: Deaf writers use function words correctly, even though they may not lipread accurately.

Listed below are examples from each of the four writers that illustrate Trend 1, i.e., that these four writers use function words in syntactically correct patterns without lipreading every word accurately. The underlined function words do not match any function word in the stimulus sentence.

- Writer 1
  - "You look nice in the outfit today." (in response to "Put that cookie back in the box!")
  - "Do you understand me?" (in response to "Everything's all right.")

- Writer 2
  - "Please put your name in front then initial in the back." (in response to "Put that cookie back in the box!")
  - "Did you realize that you need to get back off?" (in response to "I'll take sugar and cream in my coffee.")

- Writer 3
  - "She will call in a few minutes." (in response to "She'll only be gone a few minutes.")
  - "Wait for me in the car" (in response to "Wait for me at the corner")

- Writer 4
  - "He got lost once again." (in response to "People ought to see a doctor once a year.")
  - "Now that you have all the focus on you, you will lose." (in response to "Call her on the phone and tell her the news.")

Trend 2: In a lipreading task, syntax errors are similar to the syntax errors reported in the literature in other writing tasks.

Listed below are examples from each of the four writers that illustrate Trend 2, i.e., that these four writers make the same kinds of syntax errors in their responses to the lipreading task that researchers have observed in writing samples of deaf students in many previous studies.

- Writer 1
  - "You <u>should done</u> right this time" (auxiliary verb deletion)
  - "Did you get a car ticket after you drove over the speed limit <u>in highway</u>") (missing article)
- Writer 2
  - "<u>Did</u> you <u>knew</u> that we didn't know the answer?" (auxiliary verb error)
  - "we can <u>start clean</u> the house" (missing "to")
- Writer 3
  - "<u>Music</u> always <u>cheer</u> me up" (agreement error)
  - "Everything all right?" (copula deletion)
- Writer 4 (punctuation errors only)
  - "id like some cream in my coffee" (apostrophe missing, capitalization not standard)
  - "its really dark at night so watch for traffic" (apostrophe missing, capitalization not standard)

The writers also did not recognize appropriate syntactic forms on the TSA. For instance:

- Writer 1 made one error on the TSA concerning use of articles ("a meat" selected instead of "the meat") and also failed to include an article in writing the phrase "in highway."
- Writer 2 made several errors on the TSA concerning verb forms, types of errors that are similar to some of the syntactic errors made in writing
  - Incorrect TSA answers selected concerning verb forms were "Mother make a cake?," "When you plant the flowers?," and "What John did see?"
  - Incorrect TSA answers selected concerning use of infinitives were "I showed the little boy how to jumped." and "Dad forgot to made the fire."
- Writer 3 made two errors on the TSA concerning subject–verb agreement, a type of syntactic error also made in writing
  - Incorrect TSA answers selected involving subject–verb agreement were "The laughter of the girl surprise the man." and "The growth of the girl surprise her mother."
  - No incorrect TSA answers involving copula deletion were selected by this writer
- Writer 4 did not take the TSA

Listed below are examples from each of the four writers that illustrate Trend 3, i.e., that these four writers do not always lipread correctly but yet write sentences that are semantically appropriate and plausible.

Trend 3: In a lipreading task, deaf writers choose words that do not match the stimuli but are semantically appropriate in the sentence being written.

- Writer 1: did not write any content words that matched stimulus words; only some function words in responses were also contained in the stimuli sentences
- Writer 2:
  - "<u>Stay</u> there and do not move until I tell you" for "Stand there and don't move until I tell you!")
  - "<u>Please</u> put <u>your name in front then initial</u> in the back" (in response to "Put that cookie back in the box.")
- Writer 3:
  - "Did you forget to <u>turn</u> off the water?" (in response to "Did you forget to shut off the water?")
  - "<u>Go get</u> the dog out of the house." (in response to "Don't let the dog out of the house.")
- Writer 4:
  - "Why don't they make their walls some other color?" (in response to "Why don't they paint their walls some other color?")
  - "If we don't get rich soon we'll have no" (in response to "If we don't get rain soon we'll have no grass.")

Interestingly, in the case of the response of Writer 3 above, both of the word sequences "don't let" and "go get" differ only by constrictions formed in the alveolar, velar, and palatal areas of the vocal tract (difficult to see) and nasalization (nearly impossible to see). The semantic intent of the target sentence, though, can be missed if "Go get the dog out of the house" is understood instead of "Don't let the dog out of the house".

A trend that was unexpected in our analysis of syntactic patterns was the similarity of syllabic structure in some of the response sentences to a corresponding stimulus sentence.

Trend 4: In the lipreading task, deaf writers choose words that match the syllabic structure of the stimulus even though the words do not match the stimulus.

- Writer 1
  - "Know better" (in response to "It's raining.")
  - "You look beautiful outside" (in response to "Music always cheers me up.")
  - "Why do you ruin everything that don't involve you?" (in response to "Wait for me at the corner in front of the drugstore.")
- Writer 2
  - "All this goes for you" (in response to "The phone call's for you.")
  - "Did you knew that we didn't know the answer?" (in response to "If we don't get rain soon, we'll have no grass.")

- Writer 3
  - "let me when to call you" (in response to "Come here when I call you.")
- Writer 4
  - "You can actually brush in the streets" (in response to "You can catch the bus across the street.")

Trends in responses to the Background Questionnaire. We reviewed our four single case study participants' responses to the Background Questionnaire for evidence of language experience and self-perception of mastery of written English. The categories of background information that we have noted below are similar to some of the "personal variables" reported in Table 6 of Bernstein et al. (1998). (As explained previously, these four participants were the VL2 Toolkit participants who wrote the most responses to the LST.) As stated in the Background section, we are interested in comparing the participants' responses concerning their experiences learning the English language with their responses to a test that requires writing English sentences.

Educational backgrounds. All four participants attended mainstream schools (elementary school, junior high school, and high school) and also deaf education elementary schools. In addition, Writer 1 attended a deaf education junior high school, Writers 2 and 3 attended deaf education junior high and high schools, and Writer 3 also attended a deaf education preschool. Writer 4 reported attending a residential high school also.

Family support for language development. The mothers of all four participants and two of their fathers encouraged learning to read and write. Writers 2 and 4 reported that their mothers signed "well enough to communicate with me fully and effectively"; Writer 1's mother signed, using "only basic signs." Writer 3 was encouraged to learn ASL by a mother. Three of the participants (Writers 1–3) reported learning to read and write from their parents.

Access to sound. Writer 1 reported hearing "Only well enough to hear loud sounds, but unable to hear speech"; the other three writers responded "Well enough to hear normal speech, but not quiet sounds."

Learning to write. All of the participants reported learning to write from teachers. Three participants (Writers 1, 3, and 4) included parents as a source for learning to write.

Writing competence and use. All of the participants responded to the questions "How well do you write in English?" and "How often do you currently use written English?" Responses to the competence question varied: Writers 1 and 3 self-assessed being able to write "Very well"; Writer 2, as "Sufficiently", and Writer 4 as "Perfectly."

Learning to lipread. Three Writers (2–4) reported learning to lipread from parents, siblings, friends, and teachers. Writer 4 also reported learning to lipread from a Hearing/Speech Center. Writer 1 reported learning "by myself." All of the participants included friends and others as other sources in their learning to lipread.

Lipreading competence and use. All four writers reported frequent use of lipreading. Interestingly, on the LST, their scores covered a wide range: 7% (Writer 1), 19% (Writer 2), 56% (Writer 3), and 75% (Writer 4) of words correct. This disparity is not surprising in light of the differences between a screening test in which participants had access to no context when viewing the moving faces. In day-to-day use of lipreading, people most likely utilize many communication skills to interact successfully using lipreading.

Discussion

We suggest that written responses to a previously administered test, such as the LST, can be reanalyzed for evidence of knowledge of the rules of written English. For example, a clinician might be interested in knowing whether a deaf student could use English function words correctly; she could review the responses to an existing test, like the LST, for evidence of a student's ability to use English function words correctly. Written responses that contain many function words and particularly those in which the content words do not match stimulus words are particularly useful in answering such a question, as the student writer must be creating the sentences based on internalized rules of English syntax, and not be simply recording the words in the sentences in the lipreading test.

We observed that the four writers in our study used function words with a high degree of accuracy, which contrasts with some previously published results. Our writers are all college students and therefore are expected to be able to write adequately at the college level.

The patterns of syntactic errors made by our writers are ones that have been reported to be commonly found in written English samples. Our writers made similar syntactic errors in producing written sentences as they did in recognizing correctly written English sentences.

Our participants' recognition of the syllabicity of the sentences seen on the screen argues for the importance of watching closely the entire face—jaw lowering, lip rounding, and facial expression—when speech reading. During the lipreading test, the participants were observed to pay close attention to the screen. When using speech reading in actual conversations, listeners are more likely to be able to hear the vowels in each syllable than many of the consonants. Thus, even limited auditory input can support speech reading.

Compared to the larger group of VL2 Toolkit participants who completed the LST, the four writers discussed in this report wrote more sentences than the other participants. We noticed several shared background characteristics of these four writers that might help explain their ability or willingness to write. For instance, all four self-reported that they wrote in English "very well." Although the sentences written by each of the four contained some syntactic errors, these four writers were confident and willing to write. In many cases, they needed to guess at the words they saw on the screen, but almost all of their responses were written in correct English syntax. This sort of willingness to guess is a useful skill in speech reading in which a person who is deaf or hard of hearing converses with a friend who uses oral English.

Another shared characteristic among the four writers in our study was having a mother (or mother and father) who encouraged learning to read and to write. The details of parental support for learning language are not known from the responses to the Background Questionnaire, but it is not surprising that these four writers remembered having received support to learn to write as early intervention has been shown to be important although the type of education has not been shown to matter.

We offer the following recommendations for developing the language skills of deaf and hard-of-hearing students:

- Look for evidence wherever you can find it to avoid excessive testing, i.e., alternative scoring methods can possibly reveal strengths that are not obvious by traditional scoring methods
- Include recognition of the syllabic structure of an utterance as a form of evidence of a student's awareness of the structure of a spoken English sentence
- Build on strengths (Marschark and Hauser 2012; Moseley and Bally 1996) wherever you find them
- Encourage early intervention to promote language development

Acknowledgments We are grateful to Prof. Lynne Bernstein for her advice concerning the setup of the video and data collection equipment that was used for administering the LST. We thank Brittany Burkhardt and Shani Spence for their important contribution in administering the TSA and LST reported here as well as audiometric tests for the VL2 Toolkit Project.

References

Albertini, J. A., & Schley, S. (2003). Writing: Characteristics, instructions, and assessment. In M. Marschark & P. Spencer (Eds.), *Handbook of deaf studies, language, and education* (pp. 123–135). New York: Oxford University Press.

Allen, T., Hwang, Y., & Stansky, A. (2009). *Measuring factors that predict deaf students' reading abilities: The VL2 Toolkit-Project Design and Early Findings.*

Auer, E., & Bernstein, L. E. (2007). Enhanced visual speech perception in individuals with early-onset hearing impairment. *Journal of Speech Hearing Language Research, 50*, 1157–1165.

Bally, S. J. (1996). Communication strategies. In M. J. Moseley & S. J. Bally (Eds.), *Communication therapy: An integrated approach to aural rehabilitation*. Washington, DC: Gallaudet University Press.

Berger, K. W. (1972). *Speechreading: Principles and methods*. Baltimore: National Educational Press, Inc.

Bernstein, L. E., Auer, E. T., Jr., & Jiang, J. (2011). Lipreading, the lexicon, and cued speech. In C. LaSasso, K. L. Crain, & J. Leybaert (Eds.), *Cued speech and cued language for deaf and hard of hearing children*. San Diego: Plural Publishing.

Bernstein, L. E., Demorest, M. D., & Tucker, P. E. (1998). What makes a good speechreader? First you have to find one. In R. Campbell, B. Dodd, & D. Burnham (Eds.), *Hearing by eye (II): The psychology of speechreading and audiovisual speech* (pp. 211–228). East Sussex, United Kingdom: Psychology Press.

Bernstein, L. E., Demorest, M. D., & Tucker, P. E. (2000). Speech perception without hearing. *Perception & Psychophysics, 62*(2), 233–252.

Birnbaum, M., Bickley, C., & Burger, B. (2006). Composition corrector—A computer-based tool to support professional writing by the deaf and hard-of-hearing. In *Lecture notes on computer science (LNCS)*. Berlin: Springer.

Bochner, J. H., Albertini, J. A., Samar, V. J., & Metz, D. E. (1992). External and diagnostic validity of the NTID Writing Test: An investigation using direct magnitude estimation and principal components analysis. *Research in the Teaching of English, 26*(3), 299–313.

Bunger, A. (1932). *Speech reading—Jena method*. Danville, IL: The Interstate.

Carlisle, J. F. (1996). An exploratory study of morphological errors in children's written stories. *Reading and Writing, 8*(1), 61–72. doi:10.1007/BF00423925.

Carrow-Woolfolk, E. (1995). *Oral and Written Language Scales (OWLS)*. Circle Pines, MN: American Guidance Service.

Cheng, S., & Rose, S. (2008). Assessing written expression for students who are deaf or hard of hearing: Curriculum based measurement. In *Progress report #11 of The Research Institute on progress monitoring*. Minneapolis, MN: University of Minnesota.

Craig, H. K., & Washington, J. A. (1994). The complex syntax skills of poor, urban, African-American preschoolers at school entry, *Language, Speech, and Hearing Services in Schools, 25*, 181–190.

Davis, H., & Silverman, S. R. (1970). Central Institute for the deaf everyday sentences. In *Hearing and deafness, appendix*. New York: Holt, Rinehart, and Winston.

DeLand, F., & Montague, H. A. (1968). *The story of lipreading: Its genesis and development*. Washington, DC: Alexander Graham Bell Association for the Deaf, Inc.

Hazard, E. (1971). *Lipreading: For the oral deaf and hard-of-hearing person*. Springfield, IL: Charles C. Thomas.

Kalikow, D., Stevens, K., & Elliott, L. (1977). Development of a test of speech intelligibility in noise using sentence materials with controlled word predictability. *Journal of the Acoustical Society of America, 61*, 1337–1351.

Kaplan, H. (1996). Speechreading. In M. Moseley & S. J. Bally (Eds.), *Communication therapy: An integrated approach to aural rehabilitation*. Washington, DC: Gallaudet University Press.

Marschark, M., & Hauser, P. (2012). *How deaf children learn: What parents and teachers need to know*. New York: Oxford University Press.

Moseley, M. J., & Bally, S. J. (1996). In M. J. Moseley & S. J. Bally (Eds.), *Communication therapy: An integrated approach to aural rehabilitation*. Washington, DC: Gallaudet University Press.

Nichols, M. N., & Moseley, M. J. (1996). Language skills. In M. J. Moseley & S. J. Bally (Eds.), *Communication therapy: An integrated approach to aural rehabilitation*. Washington, DC: Gallaudet University Press.

O'Neill, J. J., & Oyer, H. J. (1961). *Visual communication for the hard of hearing: History, research and methods*. Englewood Cliffs, NJ: Prentice-Hall, Inc.

Paul, P. (2009). *Language and deafness*. Boston: Jones and Bartlett Publishers.

Qi, S., & Mitchell, R. E. (2011). Large-scale academic achievement testing of deaf and hard-of-hearing students: Past, present, and future. *Journal of Deaf Studies and Deaf Education, 17*, 1. doi:10.1093/deafed/enr028.

Quigley, S. P., Steinkamp, M. W., Power, D. J., & Jones, B. W. (1978). *Test of syntactic abilities: A guide to administration and interpretation*. Beaverton, OR: Dormac, Inc.

Singleton, J., Morgan, D., DiGello, E., Wiles, J., & Rivers, R. (2004). Vocabulary use by low, moderate, and high ASL-proficient writers compared to hearing ESL and monolingual speakers. *Journal of Deaf Studies and Deaf Education, 9*, 1. doi:10.1093/deafed/enh011.

Strauss, A., & Corbin, J. (1990). *Basics of qualitative research: Grounded theory procedures and techniques*. Newbury Park, CA: Sage Publications.

Yoshinago-Itano, C. (2003). From screening to early intervention and intervention: Discovering predictors to successful outcomes for children with significant hearing loss. *Journal of Deaf Studies and Deaf Education, 8*(1), 11–30.

Part V
Further Analyses and Translational Implications

This part ties together the threads presented in the preceding chapters and investigates both the interrelationships among the various cognitive, linguistic, and academic measures administered and the relationships between the constructs represented by these variables and background characteristics of the sample. Data are presented, which address two questions: (1) *Can the wide range of measures included in the toolkit be characterized by a reduced set of cohesive factors that can help to clarify underlying cognitive, language, and achievement structures for deaf individuals and their potential role in learning and development?* and (2) *Are levels of performance on the neurocognitive factors in any way determined by the respondents' early communication and language experiences?* The data analyses used to investigate these questions and the answers discovered are reported in this part. Concluding remarks, including the potential translational implications of these outcomes, are discussed.

Chapter 13
Underlying Neurocognitive and Achievement Factors and Their Relationship to Student Background Characteristics

Thomas Allen and Donna A. Morere

The previous chapters in this volume have presented descriptions and analyses of a wide range of individual achievement, language, and neurocognitive measures, as administered to our toolkit sample of deaf college students. As noted in the first chapter, presenting this compendium of individual tools as a guide to help in the selection of instruments for both research and diagnosis represents only part of our goal in designing this Toolkit Project. We are also motivated by a desire to contribute to the growing research literature and emerging theory on cognitive and language development among individuals who are deaf.

The current chapter capitalizes on the fact that many of the tools in the toolkit were administered to the same group of students, allowing us to examine underlying neurocognitive and achievement constructs through factor analysis (FA) of the individual measures. Furthermore, with background data on each participant, we can test hypotheses regarding the impacts of specific early language experiences on student performance on the derived cognitive variates.

These analyses are particularly important for furthering our understanding of the underlying cognitive dispositions for a population almost wholly reliant of visual information for learning. Linking these dispositions to background variables may shed light on critical interconnections among family background, cognitive development, educational, and academic achievement variables.

Understanding deaf individuals' unique patterns of cognitive development, given their visually based perceptual experiences, is a burgeoning area in contemporary

---

T. Allen (✉)
Science of Learning Center on Visual Language and Visual Learning, Gallaudet University,
SLCC 1223, 800 Florida Avenue, NE, Washington, DC 20002, USA
e-mail: thomas.allen@gallaudet.edu

D.A. Morere
Department of Psychology, Gallaudet University,
800 Florida Avenue, NE, Washington, DC 20002, USA
e-mail: Donna.Morere@Gallaudet.edu

research (see the excellent reviews in Marschark and Hauser 2009; Marschark and Spencer 2003). Researchers are increasingly taking a greater interest in examining the nature of cognitive experience for individuals who are deaf. Implicit in these examinations is the belief that improvements in educational outcomes for deaf students require a better understanding of the cognitive foundations of learning. Also implicit in these efforts is the desire to advance a "difference" model, as opposed to a "deficit" model for cognitive development among students who are deaf. A deficit model conceptualizes deaf learners as broken hearing learners and leads to pedagogies that stress "fixing" (or accommodating) the broken aspects of the learners so that they will thrive in learning environments designed for hearing learners. In contrast, a difference model acknowledges that individual differences in learning and cognition must be understood, and pedagogies must be designed that optimally account for those differences. It is presumed that deaf learners may require learning environments that are quite different from those of their hearing counterparts. However, until we have a better understanding of the cognitive foundations of learning for individuals who are deaf, our efforts at reforming educational curricula for deaf students will be hampered (Marschark et al. 2006).

As noted, the Toolkit Project described in this book was, in part, designed to contribute to increasing our understanding of these cognitive underpinnings and to explore the relationship between cognitive development and the early language experiences of young deaf adults. The research was guided by the following questions:

1. *Can the wide range of measures included in the toolkit be characterized by a reduced set of cohesive factors that can help to clarify underlying cognitive, language, and achievement structures for deaf individuals and their potential role in learning and development?* We are particularly interested in learning whether student performances on measures of various aspects of cognition are influenced by the mode of presentation (sign versus print) of the test stimuli. For example, is performance on digit span memory tasks altered depending on whether the stimuli (digits or letters) are presented in print or in ASL? Similarly, is retrieval of lexical items from memory different when respondents are given prompts (i.e., letters) based on spoken language phonology as opposed to prompts (i.e., handshapes) that are based on ASL phonology? (Note: we use the term phonology here to refer to the sublexical structure of linguistic form regardless of modality, and may therefore refer either to the sound-based phonemes of spoken language and their alphabetic representations in print or to the component handshapes that define the internal sublexical structure of signs which have been alternatively labeled cheremes (e.g., Stokoe 1972) due to their manual, rather than acoustic, basis.)

Marschark (2003) suggests that different coding modalities may be under different strategic control and therefore may depend on qualitatively different processing systems. If true, the importance of this for educational curriculum reform cannot be overstated. If learning and memory processes of deaf individuals who rely on visual language for learning are under the control of different processing systems than those for students who rely on auditory processes, then we need to rethink how these systems respond to varying pedagogies and learning environments.

2. *Are levels of performance on the neurocognitive factors in any way determined by the respondents' early communication and language experiences?* Many researchers have pointed to the importance of early language experience for later academic success (e.g., Droop and Verhoeven 2003; Mayberry 2007; Mayberry et al. 2011; Musselman 2000). A major focus within this area of research emphasizes the importance of "sensitive periods" in language development, and an invariant set of milestones in language development that hold for both hearing babies learning a spoken language and deaf babies learning sign (Petitto 1987). Based on this research, it appears that, regardless of the form of the language it is critical that babies be exposed to accessible language at an early age in order for them to demonstrate a typical developmental time frame (Lenneberg 1967; Mayberry and Eichen 1991). Over 90% of deaf children are born to hearing, nonsigning parents (Mitchell 2004; Mitchell and Karchmer 2004; Schein and Delk 1974). There is a clear danger that they will not be adequately exposed to ANY language (signed or spoken) during the sensitive period of acquisition, and this may present serious obstacles to the development of literacy and cognition.

We noted in Chap.2 that the sample for the current project is predominantly comprised of signing students who have elected to attend a bilingual ASL–English university. As has been amply demonstrated in the previous chapters in this volume, students in our sample show considerable variability in their skill levels in both English and ASL, as well as differences in their levels of cognitive functioning in a wide variety of domains. It is reasonable to suppose that these differences can, in part, be explained by differences in their early childhood experiences, especially those that expose them to one or both languages. Here, we examine whether there is evidence in the current toolkit data to support the hypothesis that early language experiences in both English and ASL lead to enhanced cognition and literacy.

In the last decade, a considerable number of studies have pointed to the benefits of bilingualism and bilingual education (for example, Kovelman et al. 2008) for both literacy and cognitive development (Bialystok 1999). Petitto et al. (2001) and others (Johnson and Newport 1989; Sanders et al. 2002) have also demonstrated that bilingual children who are exposed to two languages at an early age during the sensitive period for language development achieve language milestones in both languages at precisely the same sequence and timing as do monolinguals. It is noted that these conclusions are by no means universally accepted in the literature, and others have pointed to alternative explanations for the hypothesized "sensitive" period for bilinguals (e.g., Birdsong and Molis 2001; Snow and Galabudra 2002, as cited in Kovelman et al. 2008). Nevertheless, whether the acquisition of a second language will optimally co-occur with the acquisition of a first language during a bilingual sensitive period for acquisition, or whether a strong native language serves as a scaffold for the acquisition of a second language (Cummins 1991; Pinar et al. 2011)—this is more likely the case for native deaf signers, it is clear that an early age of acquisition for both ASL and English may be critical.

Question 1: Factor Analysis of Toolkit Measures

The toolkit database was evaluated for missing data, as FA requires a full data set for all measures to be included. We made decisions based on excluding subscale scores in favor of total scores, scores where there were significant missing data, and raw scores, whenever standard scores were available. Ultimately, 30 measures were selected for which complete data were collected on 31 respondents.

The means and standard deviations for of the selected scores are presented in Table 13.1. We note that, with the exception of the WJ-III tests, on which this subset performed both at lower levels (5–10 points) and with greater variability and the BVMT, on which this group's performance was approximately half a standard deviation above that of the entire sample, the means of these 30 measures for these 31

Table 13.1 Descriptive statistics for toolkit measures included in factor analysis

	Mean	Standard deviation	Analysis N
BVMT Total Recall T-score	42.29	11.329	31
Mental Rotation Task Raw Score	4.71	2.901	31
PIAT-R Standard Score	77.84	14.828	31
TOSWRF Standard Score	106.71	14.274	31
Tower of Hanoi Total Score	3.71	1.510	31
K-BIT2 Matrices Standard Score	106.19	11.496	31
Tower of London Total Correct Standard Score	101.16	14.365	31
Koo PDT Total Score	93.13	18.108	31
FAS Total Score	31.42	9.570	31
5–1–U Total Score	36.48	9.953	31
Morere SVLT List A Total	55.97	10.124	31
Morere SVLT Recognition # Correct	34.71	4.995	31
Finger Spelling Test Total Correct	53.61	10.333	31
Finger Spelling Test Real Word Correct	34.81	6.685	31
Finger Spelling Test Fake Word Correct	18.87	3.871	31
Print Digit Span FWD Span	5.87	1.310	31
Print Digit Span BWD Span	5.16	1.715	31
Corsi Blocks CPU FWD Span	6.84	1.214	31
Corsi Blocks CPU BWD Span	5.52	1.122	31
ASL Letter FWD Span	5.45	1.312	31
ASL Letter BWD Span	4.97	1.581	31
ASL Digit FWD Span	5.84	1.186	31
ASL Digit BWD Span	5.03	1.169	31
Corsi Blocks MAN FWD Span	6.35	1.170	31
Corsi Blocks MAN BWD Span	6.03	1.048	31
WJ-III Reading Fluency Standard Score	93.90	28.584	31
WJ-III Writing Fluency Standard Score	90.90	29.897	31
WJ-III Academic Knowledge Standard Score	77.29	25.524	31
WJ-III Passage Comprehension Standard Score	80.29	27.414	31
WJ-III Math Fluency Standard Score	86.65	28.153	31

students are very similar to the means reported throughout this book in the reporting of statistics for the individual measures. This indicates that the sample of students for whom we have complete data is highly representative of the full samples of students taking each test individually.

The data were submitted to a Principal Components Factor Analysis (SPSS, version 19) with Varimax rotation to maximize the distinctiveness of each component and aid in interpretation. Only factors with eigenvalues > 1.0 are reported. The initial and rotated sums of the squared factor loadings for each of the factors are presented in Table 13.2.

Table 13.2 indicates that ten factors meet the eigenvalue cut-off criteria. Each of the first two rotated factors accounts for approximately 15% of the combined variance among the measures. 50.7% of the variance is explained by the top four factors, and 86% of the variance overall is explained by the ten factors meeting the eigenvalue cut-off criteria.

The rotated component matrix is presented in Table 13.3. Coefficients < 0.1 are suppressed, and the rows of the matrix are sorted in decreasing order by the magnitude of the coefficients, factor by factor. Coefficients for each factor > 0.5 are clustered for each factor and are highlighted in the table.

The results present very distinct and interpretable factors. Despite the small sample size, relative to the number of measures, there are clear distinctions among Academic Fluency, Letter and Word Knowledge, Linguistic and Visuospatial Memory tasks, Executive Function tasks, and Visuospatial Reasoning tasks.

Table 13.4 summarizes the derived factors by listing the measures that are associated (with loadings above 0.50) with each of the factors. We have assigned names to each of these factors in an attempt to characterize them.

Table 13.2 Eigenvalues and variance explained by ten extracted and rotated factors

Component		Initial eigenvalues			Extraction sums of squared loadings			Rotation sums of squared loadings		
		Total	% of Var	Cum%	Total	% of Var	Cum%	Total	% of Var	Cum%
Dimension 0	1	8.165	27.217	27.217	8.165	27.217	27.217	4.632	15.440	15.440
	2	3.907	13.023	40.240	3.907	13.023	40.240	4.542	15.139	30.579
	3	2.749	9.163	49.403	2.749	9.163	49.403	3.502	11.674	42.253
	4	2.523	8.409	57.812	2.523	8.409	57.812	2.523	8.409	50.662
	5	2.057	6.858	64.670	2.057	6.858	64.670	1.998	6.659	57.321
	6	1.702	5.673	70.343	1.702	5.673	70.343	1.877	6.255	63.576
	7	1.392	4.640	74.983	1.392	4.640	74.983	1.856	6.186	69.762
	8	1.271	4.237	79.220	1.271	4.237	79.220	1.853	6.176	75.938
	9	1.109	3.698	82.918	1.109	3.698	82.918	1.729	5.762	81.700
	10	1.018	3.394	86.312	1.018	3.394	86.312	1.384	4.612	86.312

Extraction method: principal component analysis

Table 13.3 Component matrix for resulting toolkit factor analysis. Rotated component matrix[a]

	Component									
	1	2	3	4	5	6	7	8	9	10
Finger Spelling Test Total Correct	.95	.15								
Finger Spelling Test Fake Word Correct	.94									
Finger Spelling Test Real Word Correct	.93	.18								
TOSWRF Standard Score	.68			−.26	.42	−.22	.19			
PIAT-R Standard Score	.54	.25	.16	.22	.17	.29	.35	.18	−.24	
WJ-III Writing Fluency Standard Score		.95								
WJ-III Academic Knowledge Standard Score		.94		.16						
WJ-III Reading Fluency Standard Score	.26	.91	.18							
WJ-III Math Fluency Standard Score		.86				−.32				
WJ-III Passage Comprehension Standard Score	−.20	.81	.25		.19	.18			.22	−.15
ASL Digit BWD Span	.17	.26	.85							.20
ASL Letter FWD Span	.31		.85					−.23		
ASL Letter BWD Span	.20		.66		.49	.15		.27		
Tower of London Total Correct Standard Score	−.25	.21	.65	.26	−.18	.25	.23			
Print Digit Span BWD Span	.39	.21	.57	.25			−.22		−.51	
FAS Total Score	.41		.50		.18		−.32		.47	
Print Digit Span FWD Span			.36	.81		.18				
Koo PDT Total Score				.80	.25				.21	−.26
ASL Digit FWD Span	.29		.24	.70	.16	−.28	.27			
Morere SVLT List A Total	.19	.26		.16	.83					
Morere SVLT Recognition # Correct	.24	.28			.67	.18		.25		
BVMT Total Recall T-score	.23				.25	.81	.21	−.15		.18
Corsi Blocks MAN BWD Span	.22	.19	.23	−.17	−.20	.57		.41	.36	
K-BIT2 Matrices Standard Score	.40					.33	.68			
Tower of Hanoi Total Score	.20			.25			.61	.26	.22	
Corsi Blocks CPU FWD Span				.28	.16		−.23	.58	−.18	−.47
Corsi Blocks MAN FWD Span						−.16		.90		
Corsi Blocks CPU BWD Span	.18			.44		.32	.26	.65		
5–1–U Total Score	.16			.20		.16			.90	.15
Mental Rotation Task Raw Score										.89

Extraction method: principal component analysis
Rotation method: Varimax with Kaiser normalization
[a]Rotation converged in 17 iterations

Table. 13.4 Summary of toolkits factors

Factor 1: Letter and Word Knowledge
    Finger Spelling Test Total Correct
    Finger Spelling Test Fake Word Correct
    Finger Spelling Test Real Word Correct
    TOSWRF SScore
    PIAT-R SScore

Factor 2: Academic Fluency
    WJ-III Writing Fluency SScore
    WJ-III Academic Knowledge SScore
    WJ-III Reading Fluency SScore
    WJ-III Math Fluency SScore
    WJ-III Passage Comprehension SScore

Factor 3: Working Memory/Executive Function
    ASL Digit BWD Span
    ASL Letter FWD Span
    ASL Letter BWD Span
    Tower of London Total Correct SScore
    Print Digit Span BWD Span
    FAS Total Score

Factor 4: Speech-based Phonology/Linguistic Short-term Memory
    Print Digit Span FWD Span
    Koo PDT Total Score
    ASL Digit FWD Span

Factor 5: Sign-based Verbal Learning and Memory
    Morere SVLT List A Total
    Morere SVLT Recognition # Correct

Factor 6: Visuospatial Short-term Memory
    BVMT Total Recall Tscore
    Corsi Blocks MAN BWD Span

Factor 7: Visuospatial Reasoning
    K-BIT2 Matrices SScore
    Tower of Hanoi Total Score
    Corsi Blocks CPU FWD Span

Factor 8: Visuospatial Short-Term and Working Memory
    Corsi Blocks MAN FWD Span
    Corsi Blocks CPU BWD Span

Factor 9: Sign-based Retrieval
    5–1–U Total Score

Factor 10: Mental Rotation
    Mental Rotation Task Raw Score

Factor 1: Letter and Word Knowledge (Accounting for 15.4% of the Variance)

All of the finger-spelling measures have loadings above 0.9 on this factor, clearly indicating the strong relationship between the participants' ability to recognize the orthographic patterns of letters on fingers (for both real words and fake words) to this factor. Significantly, performance on The Test of Silent Word Reading Fluency has a strong 0.68 loading on this factor, indicating that word and letter pattern recognition constitutes a strong underlying trait, regardless of the modality of presentation. Word and Letter Knowledge is not the full story of this factor, however. Interestingly, the PIAT-R Reading Comprehension Test also loads heavily onto this factor (loading=0.54), in spite of the complete lack of association between this factor and any of the Woodcock-Johnson Reading subtest scores. (This fact suggests that reading, itself, is a multifaceted skill.) The PIAT-R Reading test requires sentence level comprehension of increasingly complex sentences. It should be noted that this reading task differs significantly from the two WJ-III reading tasks in that it both lacks context (thus requiring word knowledge for comprehension) and requires understanding of complex syntax and grammar for higher levels of performance. Additionally, the participant is only allowed to read the sentence once and must retain the meaning of the sentence briefly in memory while the page is turned so that they can select the picture reflecting the correct meaning. While the WJ-III Reading Fluency also lacks context, it involves only very simple sentence structures. In contrast, while the WJ-III Passage Comprehension involves increasing levels of sentence complexity, it is context rich and has no time constraints, allowing the reader to reread the passage and discern the meaning of component words based on the overall meaning of the paragraph. Thus, while other skills are clearly required for success, basic word knowledge would be expected to have a greater impact on the PIAT-R Reading Comprehension than on the WJ-III reading measures. Consistent with the above noted involvement of multiple aspects of linguistic and literacy functioning on this task, unlike the Woodcock-Johnson, the PIAT-R loadings are distributed more significantly (with loadings greater than .1) across nine of the ten derived factors, indicating that the PIAT-R taps into a wider variety of traits than do the subscales of the Woodcock-Johnson. It is noteworthy that both the overall sample and this subset of participants had a difficult time with the PIAT-R: the average scaled score on the PIAT-R for the 31 participants in the Factor Analysis Sample was 77.8 and that of the entire sample 74.48 (compared to the hearing norm of 100.)

Beyond the top five tests loading on Factor 1, which have loadings of 0.54 and above, Factor 1 shows common variance (loadings greater than 0.1) with quite a few of the other measures. Among these, the FAS lexical retrieval test (loading=0.41), a task which correlates significantly with vocabulary (Tombaugh et al. 1999), and the Print Backward Digit Span (loading=0.39) are among the highest, and it is noteworthy that both of these measures also require facility in the mental manipulation of letters and words. Interestingly, the K-BIT Matrices also load 0.40 on this factor. While this test is not at all dependent on facility with words and letters, it does measure an individual's ability to perceive relationships among visual images. This may emphasize the importance of visual reasoning in decoding letter sequences for deaf individuals, presented either in print or as fingerspelled words.

Factor 2: Academic Fluency (Accounting for 15.1% of the Variance)

This factor is stunning in the degree of cohesion observed from all of the subtests of the Woodcock-Johnson III, all of which load greater than 0.80 on the factor. No other measure in the study loads greater than 0.28 on this factor, and only one of the Woodcock-Johnson-III subtests loads higher than 0.26 on any factor (a negative 0.32 loading of Math Fluency with Factor 6: Visuospatial Short-Term Memory).

Clearly, this factor reflects an aspect of academic skill that is not reflected by the other factors. This achievement factor is represented by skills measured by the subtests selected from the WJ-III of Reading Fluency, Writing Fluency, Math Fluency, Academic Knowledge, and Passage Comprehension. This factor may be defined as a basic Academic Fluency factor; students scoring the highest on this factor will be those who possess a range of basic academic skills which they can perform quickly and accurately.

Factor 3: Working Memory/Executive Functioning (Accounting for 11.7% of the Variance)

Measures of Working Memory and Executive Functioning load highly on the third factor. Working Memory, employing backward span tasks for both print and ASL digits, as well as ASL Letter Forward and Backward Spans, the FAS retrieval task, which requires the production of English words using letter prompts (F, A, and S), and the Tower of London test of problem solving and executive function all load greater than 0.5 on this factor. The print digit and the ASL digit forward spans load 0.36 and 0.24 on this factor, respectively, indicating some correlation with this factor, but both of these tasks load much more highly on Factor 4. WJ-III Passage Comprehension also loads 0.25 on this factor, likely reflecting the use of Working Memory (to hold the incomplete passage while analyzing it for meaning) and executive functioning (reasoning through likely meanings of the paragraph as a whole, determining the nature of the missing information, and selecting the desired word to fill in the blank through an effective lexical search similar to that used for FAS).

Factor 4: Speech-based Phonology/Short-Term Memory (Accounting for 8.4% of the Variance)

Factor 4 combines speech-based phonological awareness (measured by the Koo Phoneme Detection Test (Koo PDT)) with Short-Term Memory for forward digit spans in both ASL (Fingerspelling) and print. The clustering of these measures along this factor is consistent with previous research showing the relationship between speech-based phonological awareness and the processing of sequential information in short-term memory (Baddeley and Wilson 1985; Madigan 1971). Interestingly, in the current project, the stimuli for both print and ASL digit sequences were presented visually; yet higher levels of performance on the measure of sound-based phonology corresponded with longer spans on both tasks. Also, the mean levels of performance for ASL and print digit span were virtually identical (5.87 for forward print digit span and 5.84 for forward ASL digit span, see Table 13.1). Equally interesting is the finding that this factor holds for digits only (both print and fingerspelling), but not for ASL Letters (loadings for both ASL Letter Forward and Backward Span load less than 0.1 on this factor). Performance on memory tasks for letter spans is more closely aligned with measures of executive functioning (Factor 3). This differential loading of the digit and letter spans may relate partially to the fact that the set of options for the digits is much more limited (the numbers 1–9), while the potential set for the letters is significantly larger. While only nine letters were used, the participant was not informed of the subset of letters involved, and therefore was confronted with a larger set of potential responses. This likely placed a greater load on the executive processes during the letter-based tasks.

Factor 5: Sign-Based Linguistic (Verbal) Learning and Memory (Accounting for 6.7% of the Variance)

Memory tasks based on signs rather than letters or digits load on Factor 5. The two Morere SVLT scores included in this analysis loaded most heavily on this factor (0.83 and 0.67), suggesting that this represents a unique reflection of linguistic memory and learning. It is not surprising that these measures load separately from those reflecting linguistic sequential memory, as previous research has indicated that while deaf individuals performance on the latter tasks differ from those of hearing individuals, when retention of order is not required, deaf and hearing individuals perform in a consistent manner on linguistic recall tasks (Hanson 1982). Two other tests had loadings greater than 0.4: The Test of Silent Word Reading Fluency (0.42) and the ASL Letter Backward Span. These loadings support the existence of an underlying verbal learning factor for words that may include both ASL and English verbal tasks. Similarly, the BVMT loading of .25 suggests a more general memory component regardless of modality.

Factor 6: Visuospatial Short-Term Memory (Accounting for 6.3% of the Variance)

Factor 6 entails measures of visual memory for nonlinguistic items (geometric forms and tapping sequences). The Brief Visuospatial Memory Test (BVMT) loads heavily on this factor (0.81), as does the Corsi Block Backward Span (manually presented, 0.57). This analysis demonstrates a disassociation between verbal and Visuospatial Working Memory consistent with the work of Baddeley (1992, 2000, 2003). This suggests that, as with hearing individuals, Visuospatial Working Memory may be processed using Baddeley's visuospatial sketchpad while linguistic working memory is managed using some type of linguistic loop, be it an English-based phonological loop (as suggested by the association of the digit spans with the Koo PDT) or a sign-based loop as proposed by Wilson and Emmorey (1997). It is noteworthy that among the toolkit measures, three other tools that loaded more heavily on other factors showed loadings on Factor 6 greater than 0.3: the Corsi Blocks Backward Span (computer-presented, 0.32); the Kaufman Brief Intelligence Test Matrices (0.33); and (with a surprising negative loading) the Woodcock-Johnson III Math Fluency Subtest (−0.32).

Factor 7: Visuospatial Reasoning/Nonverbal Intelligence (Accounting for 6.2% of the Variance)

The tests loading most heavily on this factor are the Kaufman Brief Intelligence Test Matrices (0.68), the Tower of Hanoi (0.61), and the Corsi Blocks Forward Span (manual presentation, 0.58). This factor taps into an underlying visuospatial intelligence trait in a variety of measures. Interestingly, the PIAT-R Reading Comprehension Test correlates with this factor (0.35), possibly reflecting the individuals' use of visualization of possible interpretations of the sentence, particularly as the response involves selecting a picture which best reflects the intended meaning of the sentence. Thus there are components of this test that require translating both visual and verbal representations to internal representations of meaning before making a response.

Factor 8: Visuospatial Working Memory (Accounting for 6.2% of the Variance)

Two of the Corsi Blocks tests, the forward span manual presentation and the backward span computer presentation, load highly on this factor (with loadings of 0.90 and 0.65, respectively). It is perplexing why these two versions of the Corsi Blocks tests define a unique factor in this data set, and do not align themselves with either Factor 6 (also defined a Visuospatial Working Memory factor), or with Factor 7, a more general nonverbal IQ and Visuospatial Reasoning factor. Perhaps, the skills involved with memory for temporal sequencing of nonlinguistic items represent a complex multidimensional trait that both share trait structures with other aspects of visuospatial cognitive functioning and possess unique characteristics not associated with these other structures.

Factor 9: ASL-Based Retrieval (Accounting for 5.7% of the Variance)

The 5-1-U test, which requires test-takers to retrieve ASL signs containing specific handshapes corresponding to the 5, 1, and U handshapes defines this factor very strongly with a loading = 0.90. The FAS test, which required retrieval of words that begin with particular letters, loaded 0.47 on this factor, indicating that this factor taps into underlying retrieval processes that are independent of the phonological requirements of the task. (The participants in the study, who were predominantly signing deaf adults, retrieved an average of five elements more on the 5-1-U task compared to the FAS task.) However, the results also point to different processes involved, as well, in the memory and retrieval of lexical items in different modalities. For example, the Print Backward Digit Span working memory test showed a moderate negative loading with this factor (−0.51), while the Corsi Blocks Backward Span (manual presentation) showed a moderate positive loading with the factor (0.36). We noted above, under the discussion of Factor 6, a disassociation between verbal and nonverbal working memory performance. Here, we note the competing influences of these disparate cognitive factors on performance of lexical retrieval tasks that require a conscious focus on the visuospatial elements of ALS phonology.

Factor 10: Mental Rotation (Accounting for 4.6% of the Variance)

The Mental Rotation task used in the Toolkit Project loaded only on this one factor (0.89). It showed very little commonality with any of the other factors derived in the current analysis. Significantly, however, the Koo PDT showed a negative loading (−0.26) with this factor, as did the Corsi Block forward span test (computer presentation, −0.47). This may suggest an inverse relationship between capacities for sequential and spatial processing. One additional possibility is that higher scores on the Koo PDT may correspond to a history of greater emphasis on speech and speechreading, while enhanced Mental Rotation performance may reflect a greater reliance on ASL, since a history of ASL use is associated with enhanced functioning on Mental Rotation tasks compared to hearing peers (Emmorey 2002; Emmorey et al. 1998; Marschark 2003).

Summary of Factor Analysis of Toolkit Measures

The current data, while representing a relatively limited sample that addresses the performance of students in a unique population, provide a number of valuable insights into the associations among various aspects of cognitive processing in this population. Through the FA, a strong first factor was observed, which represents a range of assessments having to do with English Word and Letter Knowledge. This factor included reflection of this knowledge based on both print and manual (fingerspelled) forms, indicating that the modality in which the letters and words are represented is not a critical aspect of this factor. It would have been valuable to have a measure of ASL vocabulary to see if it also fell within this factor. Had that been the case, it would suggest that this represents a more general underlying vocabulary function rather than a unique reflection of English skills. This would be an important area for future research as a broader range of well-developed and validated measures of ASL skills become available.

The second factor generated appeared to reflect general academic fluency and facility with basic academic skills. The majority of these measures reflect the ability to quickly and accurately perform basic reading, writing, and math skills rather than representing a depth of knowledge; however, two of the measures did require more advanced skills or knowledge, suggesting that in addition to representing fluency of basic academic skills, this factor does indeed represent a broader aspect of academic achievement. It was interesting that this represented a separate factor from the participants' letter and word skills. It is possible that facility with English vocabulary, while important for the rapid performance of basic reading and writing tasks, may represent only one route to success on these types of measures. It may be that multiple routes—ASL, English, or bilingual —can be used to access the cognitive processes and information required for the performance of the tasks in the second factor which represent general skills/knowledge and fluency rather than facility with and depth of English vocabulary.

The third factor generated reflected multiple aspects of executive functioning, including linguistic short-term/working memory and word retrieval based on English letters as well as reasoning and problem solving. These are all aspects of executive functioning which are critical for functioning in a broad range of environments—social, vocational, and emotional, as well as academic. The discrete nature of this factor compared to the above two linguistic and academic factors is likely related to the fact that while this area of functioning is important for academic and linguistic success, it represents a more general capacity, and in itself is not sufficient for success in specific areas of functioning. Rather, it represents a fundamental set of abilities which allow the individual to best benefit from access to linguistic and academic stimulation and programming, as well as opportunities to develop social, vocational, and other skills.

One of the more interesting outcomes of the FA is the fourth factor generated, which appears to represent awareness of English phonology and verbal/linguistic sequential memory. As discussed above, previous research has supported this association in the general population (e.g., Hansen and Bowey 1994; Mann and Liberman 1984), but results with deaf samples have been less consistent (e.g., Hamilton 2011; Koo et al. 2008). In general, this association is presumed to represent the use of a speech-based rehearsal strategy using a "phonological loop" for the short-term retention of linguistic sequential information. While, as discussed in Chap.5 of this volume, there has been significant controversy as to the use of a speech-based code versus a sign-based code or other means of processing this type of information in deaf individuals (e.g., Wilson and Emmorey 1997), the current data suggest that, as in research with hearing populations (and as suggested by Hamilton), those deaf individuals in this sample who were best able to access Speech-based Phonology appeared to benefit from that when performing the forward digit span tasks whether presented in print or using signed numbers. Thus, while this relationship represents a continued area of controversy, for this sample there appears to be corroboration of the connection between STM for digits and phonological awareness, suggesting that knowledge of phonology helps to facilitate memory of sequential linguistic information.

As in Baddeley's (1992, 2000, 2003) model of working memory, we observed a disassociation between verbal and Visuospatial Working Memory. This suggests that despite having both linguistic and nonverbal information received through the visual modality, deaf individuals process these two types of information in discrete ways. This is consistent with the contention that while nonverbal visuospatial information may be processed using Baddeley's visuospatial sketchpad, as with their hearing peers, deaf individuals use some type of linguistic rehearsal loop, whether it is the speech-based phonological loop proposed by Baddeley, the sign-based loop suggested by Wilson and Emmorey (1997), or involves some other form of linguistic coding.

Interestingly, again consistent with research in hearing populations, not only is there a disassociation between visual and verbal STM in our sample, a dissociation was observed between linguistic memory involving ordered recall and that for unordered recall. The scores associated with the sign-based list learning task produced a unique factor, and the component scores had minimal association with the factor involving English phonology and linguistic working memory. These data suggest that although the modality may differ, similar underlying processes are consistent across the hearing and deaf populations.

Despite the overlapping of cognitive processes between the two populations, we also have aspects of difference, such as the unique loading of the handshape-based sign retrieval task which represents the use of ASL phonology as a prompt for recalling lexical items. In this case, we see that while, not unexpectedly, the English-based verbal fluency task loads with other measures of executive functioning, this task, which should in most ways be analogous to its speech-based form, apparently taps a separate set of skills in addition to those involved in the speech-based task. On the other hand, the two tasks clearly do involve an underlying linguistic search and retrieval process, as the speech-based task loads nearly as strongly on this factor as it does on the executive functioning factor (0.47 compared to 0.50). Thus, we again see consistency between both the languages/modalities and the research on hearing individuals and this population.

Question 2: Multivariate Analyses of the Impact of Background Characteristics on Factor Score Performance

We now turn to Question 2: Are levels of performance on the neurocognitive factors (derived from the above FA) in any way determined by the participants' early communication and language experiences? The analyses designed to answer this ques-

Table 13.5 Is the participant's language preference EXCLUSIVELY ASL?

	Full sample		Factor analysis sample	
	N	%	N	%
Yes	56	87.5	21	87.5
No	8	12.5	3	12.5
Total	64	100	24	100.0

Table 13.6 How do the participants characterize their degree of hearing loss?

	Full sample		Factor analysis sample	
	N	%	N	%
Profound	35	45.5	13	44.8
Not profound—some hearing	42	54.5	16	55.2
Total	77	100	29	100

tion derive from two bodies of research: the first focuses on the strong relationship that has been demonstrated between early language experience (independent of modality) and later academic success. The second focuses on whether there is evidence to support the benefits of early bilingualism on subsequent cognitive development and academic success.

Data for these questions come from a background questionnaire that was administered to study participants at the time of testing which probed a variety of areas pertaining to the participants' family, communication, and education backgrounds. We have selected a range of variables that we hypothesize will have an impact on cognitive development and literacy. Our analytic strategy is to use the top four toolkit factors ((1) Letter and Word Knowledge; (2) Academic Fluency; (3) Working Memory and Executive Function; and (4) Speech-based Phonology/Short-Term Memory) as dependent measures in a MANOVA design for each variable selected, and to examine the univariate F-tests for those analyses that have demonstrated over-all MANOVA p-values <0.15.

Additionally, we have chosen to dichotomize each of our independent variables in the analysis for two reasons: first, again, we have relatively small sample sizes; therefore dichotomizing our categorical variables keeps acceptable sample sizes in each of our comparison groups. Second, dichotomization allows us to focus the statistical analysis around two-group comparisons for groups that are hypothesized to differ.

The Variables Included in the MANOVA

Tables 13.5–13.15 present the variables we have chosen to analyze, the labels for each level of the dichotomies associated with each variable, and frequency information for

Table 13.7 What is the participant's parents' deaf–hearing status

	Full sample N	Full sample %	Factor analysis sample N	Factor analysis sample %
Both parents are hearing	38	55.9	12	46.2
Either or both parents are deaf or hard of hearing	30	44.1	14	53.8
Total	68	100	26	100

Table 13.8 Are BOTH of the participant's parents of European-American heritage?

	Full sample N	Full sample %	Factor analysis sample N	Factor analysis sample %
Yes	38	48.1	17	56.7
No, one, or both parents are from a non-European-American heritage	41	51.9	13	43.3
Total	79	100	30	100

Table 13.9 Did the participant's mother encourage the participant to speak English growing up?

	Full sample N	Full sample %	Factor analysis sample N	Factor analysis sample %
Yes	54	62.1	19	61.3
No, either she did not care or actively discouraged the respondent from speaking English	33	37.9	12	38.7
Total	87	100	31	100

Table 13.10 What is the mother's level of education?

	Full sample N	Full sample %	Factor analysis sample N	Factor analysis sample %
Less than a BA	49	63.6	21	70
BA or above	28	36.4	9	30
Total	77	100	30	100

Table 13.11 How well does the participant know spoken English (self-report)?

	Full sample N	Full sample %	Factor analysis sample N	Factor analysis sample %
Less than very well	19	32.8	6	26.1
Very or perfectly well	39	67.2	17	73.9
Total	58	100	23	100

Table 13.12 How fluent was the mother's sign when the participant was growing up?

	Full sample		Factor analysis sample	
	N	%	N	%
She did not sign or she only knew basic signs	38	43.7	13	41.9
She signed well enough to carry on conversation	49	56.3	18	58.1
Total	87	100	31	100

Table 13.13 When did the participant start to learn spoken English?

	Full sample		Factor analysis sample	
	N	%	N	%
Before starting school	35	60.3	14	60.9
After starting school	23	39.7	9	30.1
Total	58	100	23	100

Table 13.14 When did the participant start to learn ASL?

	Full sample		Factor analysis sample	
	N	%	N	%
Before starting school (age 4 or earlier)	33	42.3	12	38.7
After starting school (age 5 or later)	45	57.7	19	61.3
Total	78	100	31	100

Table 13.15 Did the participant begin learning BOTH English and ASL before starting school?

	Full sample		Factor analysis sample	
	N	%	N	%
Yes	10	18.5	5	18.5
No	44	81.5	22	81.5
Total	54	100	27	100

both the full toolkit sample, and the FA sample of toolkit participants with complete test data.

Table 13.5: Is the participant's language preference EXCLUSIVELY ASL? Participants were given a set of language options (ASL, spoken English, English with sign support, cueing, and other language) and asked to identify their language preferences. They were permitted multiple responses. For the current purposes, the set of responses were dichotomized into those that indicated a sole preference for ASL versus those that indicated other language preferences (whether or not ASL was also selected). This split identified a group of participants who were immersed in ASL as a language with no stated preference for English. The numbers in Table 13.5 show that the toolkit participant sample was overwhelmingly made up of individuals who reported ASL as their sole language preference. In both the full toolkit sample and the FA sample, 87.5% of the participants reported ASL as their sole language preference. It is noteworthy that relative frequencies of both the full sample and the FA sample are identical, suggesting that the FA sample is highly representative of the larger group of participants.

Table 13.6: How do the participants characterize their degree of hearing loss? Participants were asked to characterize their own level of hearing loss using standard categories (mild, moderate, severe, and profound). Here, we have collapsed the bottom three categories to create a dichotomy that divides the sample into those who self-characterize their hearing loss as profound versus those who report that they have some level of hearing. As shown in Table 13.5, the participants are fairly evenly distributed across the two groups. In the FA sample, 44.8% characterize their hearing loss in the profound range. This percentage is similar to that reported by the full sample (45.5%), again attesting to how well the FA sample represents the full sample.

Table 13.7: What is the participant's parents' deaf–hearing status? Participants were asked to report separately whether their mother and father were deaf, hard of hearing, or hearing. For the current analysis, we split the sample into those who reported both their parents were hearing versus those who reported that either or both their parents were deaf or hard of hearing. In the FA sample, 46.2% of the sample came from families with both hearing parents, and 53.8% came from families where one or both parents were deaf or hard of hearing. In the full sample, a lower percentage (41.1%) of the participants reported that one or both their parents were deaf or hard of hearing; however, this is still a significantly greater proportion than expectations, considering that over 90% of deaf individuals are born to hearing parents.

Table 13.8: Are both of the participant's parents of European-American heritage? This dichotomy combines race and ethnicity into a single heritage question, splitting the sample into those for whom both parents are reported to come from a European-American heritage versus those for whom one or both parents come from different heritage. This other category is comprised of those who reported that either or both parents came from African-American, Asian-American, Latino/Hispanic, Middle Eastern, Native American, Pacific Islander, or Other heritages. (The breakdowns for these other categories are presented in Chap. 1.) The FA sample was comprised of 56.7% having both parents from European-American heritage. This compares to 48.1% of the full sample.

Table 13.9: Did the participant's mother encourage the participant to speak English growing up? We asked participants to indicate which of three statements best characterized whether their mothers encouraged them to "learn to speak English growing up" (Yes; No, she didn't care if I learned to speak English or not; No, she discouraged me from speaking English). Here, we collapsed the two "No" responses into a single category. In the FA sample, 61.3% of the respondents reported that their mothers encouraged them to speak English growing up, while 38.7% reported that their mothers either did not care if they spoke English or not or actively discouraged them from speaking English growing up. These compare to 62.1% and 37.9%, respectively for the full sample, indicating that the FA sample was highly representative of the full sample on this variable.

13 Underlying Neurocognitive and Achievement Factors and Their Relationship... 249

Table 13.10: What is the Mother's level of education? Participants were asked to indicate their Mother's level of education using eight categories that ranged from "Some high school, but no diploma" to "Doctorate". For the purpose of this analysis, participants were split into two groups: those whose mothers earned less than a BA versus those whose mothers earned a BA or higher. In the FA sample 70% of the participants reported that their mothers earned less than a BA and 30% reported that their mothers earned more than a BA. These percentages were 63.6% and 36.4% for the full sample, respectively.

Table 13.11: How well does the participant know spoken English? Toolkit participants were asked to self-evaluate how well they used spoken English, using four anchors: (perfectly, very well, sufficiently, hardly at all). Here, we collapsed the top two and the bottom two categories forming a dichotomy of "less than very well" and "very well or perfectly." In the FA sample, 26.1% were reported in the less than very well categories, and 73.9% in the very well or perfectly category. These percentages were 32.8% and 67.2%, respectively, in the full sample.

Table 13.12: How fluent was the mother's sign when the participant was growing up? Toolkit participants were asked, "Did your mother know and use sign when you were growing up?" They were given three response categories: "Yes, well enough to communicate with me fully and effectively"; "Yes, but only basic signs"; and "No". We dichotomized the sample into those whose mothers signed well enough to communicate fully and effectively versus those whose mothers either did not sign or who only knew basic signs. In the FA sample, 41.9% were reported in the "No use or only basic signs" category, and 58.1% in the "well enough to communicate fully and effectively". The percentages for the full sample were 43.7% and 56.3%, respectively.

Table 13.13: When did the participant start to learn spoken English? Participants were asked "How long have you known or been using spoken English?" and were given five response options: "Since before I started school", "Since Elementary school", "Since middle or junior high school", "Since high school", and "Since I left school". As we are primarily interested in understanding the effects of early exposure to language, the sample was dichotomized into those who reported knowing or using spoken English since before starting school versus those who have been using spoken English only since starting school. In the FA sample, 60.9% reported using spoken English before starting school. This compares to 60.3% in the full sample.

Table 13.14: When did the participant start to learn ASL? The parallel question to the question about the age of acquisition of spoken language asked the respondent to report the actual age at which they first began learning ASL. To make the dichotomy comparable, participants reporting age 4 or earlier were categorized as having started using ASL before starting school, and those starting at age 5 or above were reported as having started using ASL after starting school. In the FA sample, 38.7% reported that they started using sign before starting school (with 61.3% starting after starting school). The comparative percentages from the full sample are 42.3% and 57.7% respectively.

Table 13.16 MANOVA: impact of language preference on neurocognitive and achievement factors

Is the participant's language preference EXCLUSIVELY ASL?
Wilke's Lamda—.580, $F(4,19) = 3.435$, $p = .028$
Univariate tests

	N	Mean	SD	F-statistic	Prob.
Letter and Word Knowledge					
Yes	21	−0.01	0.93		
No	3	−0.98	0.79	$F(1,22) = 2.924$	0.101
Academic Fluency					
Yes	21	−0.11	1.19		
No	3	0.27	0.26	$F(1,22) = .300$	0.590
Working Memory/Executive Function					
Yes	21	0.21	0.99		
No	3	0.01	0.94	$F(1,22) = .112$	0.740
Speech-based Phonology/STM					
Yes	21	−0.14	0.83		
No	3	1.60	1.57	$F(1,22) = 9.391$	0.006

Table 13.15: Did the participant begin learning BOTH English and ASL before starting school? Answers to the two questions about the age when the participants acquired English and ASL were combined to form a single variable that split the sample into those participants who began using BOTH English and ASL before starting school versus those who began using one or both languages after starting school. This new variable identified the subgroup of participants who were in bilingual family environments before starting school. In the FA sample, only 18.5% (five participants) reported using both English and ASL before starting school. This is identical to the 18.5% of the full sample who reported using both languages before starting school.

MANOVAs

Each of the 11 dichotomized background variables described above was entered into a MANOVA with performance on the derived scores for the first 4 factors from the FA as the dependent variables. The factor scores are standard scores of the factor variates (means of 0 and SD = 1) derived from the linear combinations of the 30 Toolkit tests, weighted by the factor loadings on each factor.

Table 13.16 shows the results for the first variable: whether or not the participants' reported language preference was exclusively ASL. The MANOVA resulted in a significant Wilke's Lamda ($F(4,19) = 3.435$, $p = 0.028$). The significance of the F is tempered by the fact that there were only three participants who reported that their language of preference was not exclusively ASL. Obviously this makes any conclusion from this finding extremely tenuous. Looking at the univariate tests, only Factor

Table 13.17 MANOVA: impact of participant's characterization of their degree of hearing loss on neurocognitive and achievement factors

How do respondents characterize their degree of hearing loss?
Wilke's Lamda = .945, F(4,24) = .394, p = .81

Univariate statistics not presented

Table 13.18 MANOVA: impact of parents' deaf–hearing status on neurocognitive and achievement factors

What are the participants' parent's deaf–hearing status?
Wilke's Lamda = .621, F(4,21) = 3.344, p = .029
Univariate tests

	N	Mean	SD	F-statistic	Prob.
Letter and Word Knowledge					
Both parents hearing	12	−0.28	0.89		
Either or both parents deaf or hard of hearing	14	0.34	0.96	$F(1,24)=2.912$	0.101
Academic Fluency					
Both parents hearing	12	0.27	0.28		
Either or both parents deaf or hard of hearing	14	−0.01	1.26	$F(1,24)=.578$	0.455
Working Memory/Executive Function					
Both parents hearing	12	−0.37	1.07		
Either or both parents deaf or hard of hearing	14	0.38	0.98	$F(1,24)=3.483$	0.074
Speech-based Phonology/STM					
Both parents hearing	12	−0.41	0.63		
Either or both parents deaf or hard of hearing	14	0.40	1.21	$F(1,24)=4.282$	0.047

4 (speech-based phonological awareness/short-term memory for digit spans) showed a significant F-test. The three participants who expressed language preferences other than ASL outperformed their counterparts by 1.74 standard deviations (the difference between the means in both groups, $F(1,22)=9.391$, $p=0.006$). These three participants showed much higher scores on this factor, indicating that their language preferences for English was associated with higher levels of phonological knowledge and memory for digit spans. It is noteworthy that the two groups in this analysis did not differ in performance on the other three factors, although they demonstrated poorer performance on the Letter and Word Knowledge factor at a level that approached statistical significance ($p=0.101$).

Table 13.17 shows the results for the second variable: whether the participants self-reported their level of hearing loss to be profound or less than profound. For this variable, the Wilke's Lambda was not significant ($F(4,24)=0.394$, $p=0.81$). Univariate tests were not performed.

Table 13.18 shows the results for the third variable: whether or not the participants had one or both deaf or hard-of-hearing parents. This analysis resulted in a significant Wilkes Lambda ($F(4,21)=3.344$, $p=0.029$). Univariate tests revealed a significant difference in Factor 4 (Phonological Awareness/Short-Term Memory, $F(1,24)=4.282$, $p=0.047$), with participants having one or both deaf or hard-of-hearing parents outscoring their counterparts with both hearing parents by 0.81

Table 13.19 MANOVA: impact of parents' race–ethnic heritage on neurocognitive and achievement factors

Are BOTH parents of European-American Heritage?
Wilke's Lamda = .754, $F(4,25) = 2.041$, $p = .119$
Univariate tests

	N	Mean	SD	F-statistic	Prob.
Letter and Word Knowledge					
Yes	17	0.38	0.80		
No, one, or both parents from non-European-American heritage	13	−0.50	1.08	$F(1,28) = 6.645$	*0.015*
Academic Fluency					
Yes	17	0.22	0.90		
No, one, or both parents from non-European-American heritage	13	−0.07	0.84	$F(1,28) = .854$	*0.363*
Working Memory/Executive Function					
Yes	17	0.13	1.10		
No, one, or both parents from non-European-American heritage	13	−0.09	0.89	$F(1,28) = .346$	*0.561*
Speech-based Phonology/STM					
Yes	17	0.07	1.05		
No, one, or both parents from non-European-American heritage	13	−0.15	0.97	$F(1,28) = .364$	*0.551*

standard deviations. While this was the only univariate test significant at the 0.05 level, two other tests approached significance at the 0.1 level: participants with deaf or hard-of-hearing parents outperformed participants with both hearing parents in Letter and Word Knowledge by 0.62 SDs ($F(1,24) = 2.912$, $p = 0.101$) and in Working Memory/Executive Function by 0.75 SDs ($F(1,24) = 3.483$, $p = 0.074$). In Academic Fluency, these two groups differed by only 0.28 SDs (a slight advantage for the group with both hearing parents, $F(1,24) = 0.578$, $p = 0.455$).

Table 13.19 shows the results for the fourth variable: whether the participants' parents were both from European-American heritages. The analysis resulted in a Wilke's Lambda that approached significance ($F(4,25) = 2.041$, $p = 0.119$). Examining the univariate tests shows a significant difference between those participants with both parents from European-American backgrounds and those with one or both parents from non-European heritages only for the Letter and Word Knowledge factor ($F(1,28) = 6.645$, $p = 0.015$). Participants with both parents having European-American heritages outperformed participants with parents from non-European heritages by 0.88 SDs. The groups did not differ on the Academic Fluency Memory/Executive Function, or Speech-based Phonology/STM factors.

Table 13.20 shows the results of the MANOVA for the comparison between those participants whose mothers encouraged them to use spoken English growing up versus those whose mothers either did not care or actively discouraged their use of spoken English growing up. For this comparison, across the four neurocognitive factors, the Wilke's Lambda was not significant ($F(4,26) = 0.885$, $p = 0.487$). Univariate tests are not presented.

Table 13.20 MANOVA: impact of mother's encouragement of spoken language use on neurocognitive and achievement factors

Did the participant's mother encourage the participant to speak English growing up?
Wilke's Lamda = .880, F(4,26) = .885, p = .487

Univariate tests not presented

Table 13.21 MANOVA: impact of mother's level of education on neurocognitive and achievement factors

What is the mother's level of education?
Wilke's Lamda = .904, F(4,25)=,904, p = .625

Univariate tests are not presented

Table 13.22 MANOVA: impact of participant's self-rating of English skill on neurocognitive and achievement factors

How well does participant know spoken English (self-report)?
Wilke's Lamda = .821, F(4,18) = .981, p = .442

Table 13.21 shows the results of the MANOVA for the comparison between those participants whose mothers' level of education was less than a BA versus those whose mothers' level of education was a BA or above. For this comparison, the Wilke's Lambda was not significant ($F(4,25)=0.904$, $p=0.625$). Univariate tests are not presented.

Table 13.22 presents the MANOVA for comparing the participants who self-rated their ability to use English skill perfectly or very well versus those who rated their English use as less than perfectly well. The Wilke's Lambda for this comparison was not significant ($F(4,18)=0.981$, $p=0.442$). Univariate tests are not presented.

Table 13.23 shows that the comparison between participants whose mothers were reported as being able to sign fluently enough to carry on conversations with them during childhood to those whose mothers could, at best, sign only a few words, produced a significant Wilke's Lambda ($F(4,26)=4.121$, $p=0.010$). Univariate tests reveal significance for only the Word and Letter Knowledge Factor where the two groups differed by more than a full SD ($F(1,29)=12.462$, $p=0.001$). The magnitude of this difference is noteworthy, as it emphasizes the strong effect of early communication with the mother on the development of the broad array of skills that define this factor. Furthermore, it should be reiterated that this factor represents knowledge of English words and letters; thus, the impact of the mother's sign skills on this factor further supports the importance of early language access, regardless of the modality, on later literacy skills.

Table 13.24 shows the results of the MANOVA comparing those participants who reported that they began using spoken English before starting school versus those who reported that they began using spoken English after they started school. The Wilke's Lambda for this MANOVA approached statistical significance ($F(4,18)=2.344$, $p=0.094$), so the univariate comparisons were evaluated. They

Table 13.23 MANOVA: impact of mother's sign fluency on neurocognitive and achievement factors

How fluent was the mother's sign when the participant was growing up?
Wilke's Lamda = .612, F(4,26) = 4.121, p = .010
Univariate tests

	N	Mean	SD	F-statistic	Prob.
Letter and Word Knowledge					
None, or only basic signs	13	−0.64	1.00		
Fluent enough to carry on conversations	18	0.46	0.72	$F(1,29)=12.462$	0.001
Academic Fluency					
None, or only basic signs	13	−0.109	0.828		
Fluent enough to carry on conversations	18	0.079	1.12	$F(1,29)=.261$	0.614
Working Memory/Executive Function					
None, or only basic signs	13	−0.288	0.77		
Fluent enough to carry on conversations	18	0.208	1.11	$F(1,29)=1.910$	0.178
Speech-based Phonology/STM					
None, or only basic signs	13	0.150	1.21		
Fluent enough to carry on conversations	18	−0.108	0.83	$F(1,29)=.494$	0.488

Table 13.24 MANOVA: impact of when the participant began to learn spoken English on neurocognitive and achievement factors

When did the participant start to learn spoken English?
Wilke's Lamda = .657, F(4,18) = 2.344, p = .094
Univariate tests

	N	Mean	SD	F-statistic	Prob.
Letter and Word Knowledge					
Before starting school	14	−0.116	1.19		
After starting school	9	0.090	0.93	$F(1,21)=.194$	0.664
Academic Fluency					
Before starting school	14	0.309	0.37		
After starting school	9	−0.751	1.59	$F(1,21)=5.897$	0.024
Working Memory/Executive Function					
Before starting school	14	0.321	1.01		
After starting school	9	−0.405	1.07	$F(1,21)=2.716$	0.114
Speech-based Phonology/STM					
Before starting school	14	0.110	1.19		
After starting school	9	0.275	0.83	$F(1,21)=.131$	0.721

reveal a significant difference between these two groups of participants only for the Academic Fluency factor: those who began using English before starting school out performed their counterparts by more than 1 SD ($F(1,21)=5.897, p=0.024$). While the data are not available on the students' access to early intervention programs, this difference may reflect the impact of participation in early intervention (where oral skills were then, and continue to be commonly emphasized for young deaf children) compared to those who did not have access to early intervention programs. Although significance was not achieved, the differences between the two groups approached

Table 13.25 MANOVA: impact of when the participant began to learn ASL on neurocognitive and achievement factors

When did the participant start to learn ASL?
Wilke's Lamda = .518, F(4,26) = 6.048, p = .001
Univariate tests

	N	Mean	SD	F-statistic	Prob.
Letter and Word Knowledge					
Before starting school	12	0.70	0.56		
After starting school	19	−0.44	0.97	F(1,29)=13.765	0.001
Academic Fluency					
Before starting school	12	−0.11	1.35		
After starting school	19	0.07	0.74	F(1,29)=.213	0.648
Working Memory/Executive Function					
Before starting school	12	0.47	0.97		
After starting school	19	−0.30	0.92	F(1,29)=4.870	0.035
Speech-based Phonology/STM					
Before starting school	12	0.12	0.83		
After starting school	19	−0.07	1.11	F(1,29)=.264	0.611

the 0.1 level for Working Memory/Executive Functioning factor. Considering the relationships observed between components of this factor and phonological processing, as well as both English and Reading skills, early English skills are likely supportive of this factor. Data with a larger set of participants could clarify this relationship.

Table 13.25 presents the comparisons of those who reported that they began using ASL before starting school with those who reported that they began using ASL after starting school. The Wilke's Lambda for this comparison was highly significant ($F(4,26)=6.048$, $p=0.001$). Univariate tests revealed statistical significance for two of the factors: Word and Letter Knowledge (mean scores differed by 1.14 SDs, favoring participants who began signing before starting school, $F(1,29)=13.765$, $p=0.001$), and Working Memory/Executive Function (mean scores differed by .77 SDs, also favoring participants who began signing before starting school, $F(1,29)=4.870$, $p=0.035$). This may again reflect impacts of early intervention, in this case possibly combined with parental hearing status. Regardless, the results of these two sets of analyses again emphasize the importance of early language access for literacy and academic success, as well as WM functioning.

Table 13.26 shows the comparisons of those participants who began using both English and ASL before starting school to those who began using one or both languages after starting school. The MANOVA yielded a significant Wilke's Lambda ($F(4,22)=4.343$, $p=0.010$). Univariate tests revealed significance only for the Letter and Word Knowledge factor: participants who were bilingual before starting school outperformed those who were not bilingual until after starting school on this factor by 1.1 SDs ($F(1,25)=5.415$, $p=0.028$). Unfortunately, in the current sample, only five participants reported beginning to use both languages before starting school (this is unfortunate for statistical reasons in the context of the current analysis, and also for educational reasons as well, given the mounting evidence for the benefits of

Table 13.26 MANOVA: impact of whether participant began learning BOTH English and ASL before starting school on neurocognitive and achievement factors

Did the participant begin learning BOTH English and ASL before starting school?
Wilke's Lamda = .559, $F(4,22) = 4.343$, $p = .010$
Univariate tests

	N	Mean	SD	F-statistic	Prob.
Letter and Word Knowledge					
Yes, bilingual before starting school	5	0.82	0.76		
No, one, or both languages learned after starting school	22	−0.28	0.98	$F(1,25) = 5.415$	*0.028*
Academic Fluency					
Yes, bilingual before starting school	5	0.64	0.31		
No, one, or both languages learned after starting school	22	−0.21	1.10	$F(1,25) = 2.80$	*0.107*
Working Memory/Executive Function					
Yes, bilingual before starting school	5	0.53	1.44		
No, one, or both languages learned after starting school	22	−0.18	0.92	$F(1,25) = 2.002$	*0.169*
Speech-based Phonology/STM					
Yes, bilingual before starting school	5	0.47	1.15		
No, one, or both languages learned after starting school	22	−0.07	1.03	$F(1,25) = 1.119$	*0.300*

both early language experience AND early bilingualism); thus the results are tentative. However, given the lack of statistical power associated with this small N, it is instructive to note that the results for two other factors yielded *p*-values under 0.17: academic achievement (showing a 0.85 SD advantage for the early bilingual group, $F(1,25) = 2.80$, $p = 0.107$), and Working Memory/Executive Function (showing a 0.71 SD advantage for the early bilingual group, $F(1,25) = 2.002$, $p = 0.169$).

Summary of the MANOVA Analysis

Factors that Showed No Multivariate Significance

Self-reported level of hearing loss. Given the relative homogeneity of the participant sample (most were in the severe to profound level of hearing loss), and the potential for inaccuracies in self-reporting on this variable, it is not surprising that this variable failed to show overall statistical significance across the four factors included in the analysis.

Mother's encouragement of spoken language use growing up. Participants who reported that their mothers actively encouraged them to use spoken language when they were growing up did not differ appreciably from those who reported that their mothers either did not care or actively discouraged the use of spoken language. This may indicate that the use of spoken language growing up, per se, does not have an impact on cognitive or academic development, or it may be due to other factors. Given the advantages noted for participants with deaf parents (who may be less likely to encourage the use of spoken), this is clearly an issue that would merit further research.

Mother's level of education. The level of mother's education did not result in significant differences in factor scores for the current sample. It should be noted that this variable was defined as a dichotomy (those participants whose mothers had a BA or higher versus those whose mothers did not have a BA), and this may have obscured any differences that may have been observed had we used finer distinctions among categories, which was not possible given the sample size.

Self-reported rating of how well the participant knew spoken English. Those participants who self-rated their knowledge of spoken English as "very well" or "perfectly well" did not differ significantly on the Toolkit factor scores from those who rated their skills as less than very well. It should be noted that there was a significant amount of missing data for this variable (only 23 of the 31 participants who had complete data on the FA measures provided an answer to this question, indicating a reluctance to self-rate in this area among participants).

Factors That Showed Multivariate Significance

Preference for ASL. The Toolkit Project participants were overwhelmingly ASL users. It might be noted that, at Gallaudet University, where there is a strong culture of ASL use, the expression of this preference would be expected. Even so, those few individuals (only three in the FA Sample) who did not express an exclusive preference for ASL demonstrated far higher scores on the Speech-based Phonology/Short-Term Memory factor, but for none of the other factors. However, they scored more poorly—at a level that approached significance—on the Letter and Word Knowledge factor. These individuals had strong oral preferences, were practiced and knowledgeable about the phonemic properties of words, and had good sequential memory for linguistic sequences, but these advantages did not translate to elevated factor scores on the other factors. We note that the small number of students in this category and the likelihood that they are not representative of orally trained deaf students nationwide lead us to be cautious about over interpreting these findings.

Parental hearing–deaf status. Participants who indicated that one or both of their parents were deaf or hard of hearing showed a significant *advantage* in the Speech-based Phonology/Short-Term Memory factor, and advantages that approached significance in the Letter and Word Knowledge factor and the Working Memory/Executive Function factor. This finding is consistent with previous research demonstrating a number cognitive and achievement advantages for deaf children of deaf parents. Parsing the reasons for this will require additional research. To be sure, there may be self-selection bias in the Gallaudet student body such that the deaf participants with hearing parents may not be representative of their non-Gallaudet counterparts. Clearly, though, study participants from deaf families may be expected to have enriched early language experiences, but this may not be the only reason for the advantages noted in research findings. Coming from a deaf family may correlate with other important variables, such as socioeconomic status, a diminished likelihood of having a learning disability, and other factors.

Race–ethnic heritage. Although the multivariate F for this variable only approached significance, the univariate tests were examined, revealing a significant advantage only in the Letter and Word Knowledge factor for participants coming from families where both parents were of European-American heritage.

Mother's use of sign when the participant was growing up. Participants who reported that their mothers were fluent enough in sign to carry on conversations outperformed participants whose mothers either did not sign or who knew only basic signs in the Letter and Word Knowledge factor. It is likely that this variable correlates with the deaf–hearing status variable (deaf mothers are also likely to use fluent signing with their children); however this again provides support for the benefits of early signing and language in developing later literacy.

When participants began to learn spoken English. This variable produced a multivariate F that approached significance. The univariate tests revealed significant advantages for those reporting exposure to spoken English before starting school for the Academic Fluency factor, and near-significant advantages for these participants for the Working Memory/Executive Function factor. It is noteworthy that the reported early exposure to spoken English is the only variable that had a significant effect on Academic Fluency. Given the impact of early sign language exposure to elevations in Word and Letter Knowledge, this finding suggests the importance of early language training in both English and ASL to ensure full gains in literacy skills.

When participants began to learn ASL. Reported early exposure to ASL yielded significant elevations in both the Letter and Word Knowledge and Working Memory/Executive Function. This evidence supports the hypothesis that early exposure to ASL contributes to academic gains throughout childhood.

Whether the participants began learning both English and ASL before starting school. Participants who reported learning both English and ASL before starting school displayed higher factor scores on Letter and Word Knowledge. They displayed higher scores (with differences that approached significance) for Academic Fluency and Working Memory/Executive Function as well. One disheartening factor in the present data is the low number of participants reporting early exposure to both languages. Only five participants were in this group. Given the importance of early exposure in both languages, the findings here may have considerable significance in focusing efforts on early bilingual training for students who are deaf.

Concluding Observations

This chapter began by posing two questions: 1. *Can the wide range of measures included in the toolkit be characterized by a reduced set of cohesive factors that can help to clarify underlying cognitive, language, and achievement structures for deaf individuals and their potential role in learning and development?* And, 2. *Are levels of performance on the neurocognitive factors in any way determined by the respondents' early communication and language experiences?*

The answer to the first question is a resounding, "Yes". The FA described here presents a clear set of cohesive factors, whose content presents rich information for improving our understanding of the underlying cognitive structures of signing deaf college students. Whether this set of factors generalizes to a broader population of deaf individuals is an important consideration for future research. Most interesting to us are the findings of similarities in underlying constructs regarding the manipulation and processing of linguistic information, regardless of modality. At the same time, the separation of visuospatial processing from linguistic processing is very clearly indicated in the data. Finally, the strong factor associations between sound-based phonemic knowledge and the short-term recall of digit spans in both print and fingerspelling provides support for existing theories about the importance of phonemic knowledge for this kind of sequential memory task (although the failure of letter span tasks to load on this factor was quite intriguing and suggests the increased importance of Working Memory and Executive Function for letter recall, especially in the case of signed letters).

Regarding Question 2, the answer, again is a resounding "Yes". Differences in background characteristics did affect the levels of performance on the derived factors despite the small sample and use of retrospective self-report for the background data. The resulting impacts emphasize both the importance of early visual language and the early exposure to both ASL and English to ensure successful development in both cognition and literacy.

References

Baddeley, A. D. (1992). Working memory. *Science, 255*, 556–559.
Baddeley, A. (2000). The episodic buffer: A new component of working memory? *Trends in Cognitive Sciences, 4*, 417–423.
Baddeley, A. (2003). Working memory: Looking back and looking forward. *Nature Reviews Neuroscience, 4*, 829–839.
Baddeley, A., & Wilson, B. (1985). Phonological coding and short-term memory in patients without speech. *Journal of Memory and Language, 24*(4), 490–502.
Bialystok, A. (1999). Cognitive complexity and attentional control in the bilingual mind. *Child Development, 70*(3), 636–644.
Birdsong, D., & Molis, M. (2001). On the evidence for maturational constraints in second-language acquisition. *Journal of Memory and Language, 44*, 235–249.
Cummins, R. (1991). *Meaning and mental representation*. Cambridge, MA: MIT Press.
Droop, M., & Verhoeven, L. (2003). Language proficiency and reading ability in first and second language learners. *Reading Research Quarterly, 38*, 78–103.
Emmorey, K. (2002). *Language, cognition and the brain: Insights from sign language research*. Mahwah, NJ: Lawrence Erlbaum Associates.
Emmorey, K., Klima, E., & Hickok, G. (1998). Mental rotation within linguistic and non-linguistic domains in users of American sign language. *Cognition, 68*(3), 221–246.
Hamilton, H. (2011). Memory skills of deaf learners: Implications and applications. *American Annals of the Deaf, 156*(4), 402–423.

Hansen, J., & Bowey, J. A. (1994). Phonological analysis skills, verbal working memory, and reading ability in second-grade children. *Child Development, 65*(3), 938–950.

Hanson, V. L. (1982). Short-term recall by deaf signers of American Sign Language: Implications of encoding strategy for order recall. *Journal of Experimental Psychology: Learning, Memory, and Cognition, 8*(6), 572–583.

Johnson, J. S., & Newport, E. L. (1989). Critical period effects in second language learning: The influence of maturational state on the acquisition of English as a second language. *Cognitive Psychology, 21*(1), 60–99.

Koo, D., Crain, K., LaSasso, C., & Eden, G. (2008). Phonological awareness and short-term memory in hearing and deaf individuals of different communication backgrounds. *Annals of the New York Academy of Sciences, 1145*, 83–99.

Kovelman, I., Baker, S., & Petitto, L. (2008). Bilingual and monolingual brains compared: A functional magnetic resonance imaging investigation of syntactic processing and a possible "Neural Signature" of bilingualism. *Journal of Cognitive Neuroscience, 20*(1), 153–169.

Lenneberg, E. H. (1967). *Biological foundations of language*. Oxford, England: Wiley.

Madigan, S. A. (1971). Modality and recall order interactions in short-term memory for serial order. *Journal of Experimental Psychology, 87*, 294–296.

Mann, V. A., & Liberman, I. Y. (1984). Phonological awareness and verbal short-term memory: Can they presage early reading problems? *Journal of Learning Disabilities, 17*, 592–599.

Marschark, M. (2003). Cognitive functioning in deaf adults and children. In M. Marschark & P. Spencer (Eds.), *Oxford handbook of deaf studies, language and education* (pp. 464–477). New York: Oxford University Press.

Marschark, M., Convertino, C., & LaRock, D. (2006). Optimizing academic performance of deaf students: Access, opportunities, and outcomes. In D. F. Moores & D. S. Martin (Eds.), *Deaf learners: Developments in curriculum and instruction* (pp. 179–199). Washington, DC: Gallaudet University Press.

Marschark, M., & Hauser, P. (2009). *Deaf cognition: Foundations and outcomes*. New York: Oxford University Press.

Marschark, M., & Spencer, P. (2003). *Oxford handbook of deaf studies, language, and education*. New York: Oxford University Press.

Mayberry, R. I. (2007). When timing is everything: Age of first language acquisition effects on second language learning. *Applied linguistics, 28*, 537–549.

Mayberry, R. I., del Guidice, A. A., & Lieberman, A. (2011). Reading achievement in relation to phonological coding and awareness: A meta-analysis. *Journal of Deaf Studies and Deaf Education, 16*(2), 164–188.

Mayberry, R., & Eichen, E. (1991). The long-lasting advantage of learning sign language in childhood: Another look at the critical period for language acquisition. *Journal of Memory and Language, 30*(4), 486–512.

Mitchell, R. E. (2004). National profile of deaf and hard of hearing students in special education from weighted survey results. *American Annals of the Deaf, 149*(4), 336–349.

Mitchell, R. E., & Karchmer, M. A. (2004). Chasing the mythical ten percent: Parental hearing status of deaf and hard of hearing students in the United States. *Sign Language Studies, 4*(2), 138–163.

Musselman, C. (2000). How do children who can't hear learn to read an alphabetic script? A review of the literature on reading and deafness. *Journal of Deaf Studies and Deaf Education, 5*, 9–31.

Petitto, L. (1987). Theoretical and methodological issues in the study of sign language babbling: Preliminary evidence from American Sign Language (ASL) and Langue des Signes Québécoise (LSQ). Paper presented at the Fourth International Symposium on Sign Language Research. Lappeenranta, Finland.

Petitto, L., Katerelos, M., Levy, B., Gauna, K., & Ferraro, V. (2001). Bilingual signed and spoken language acquisition from birth: Implications for the mechanisms underlying early bilingual language acquisition. *Journal of Child Language, 28*, 453–496.

Pinar, P., Dussias, P., & Morford, J. (2011). Deaf readers as bilinguals: An examination of deaf readers' print comprehension in light of current advances in bilingualism and second language processing. *Language and Linguistics Compass, 5*(10), 691–704.

Sanders, L., Neville, H., & Woldorff, M. (2002). Speech segmentation by native and non-native speakers: The use of lexical, syntactic, and stress-pattern cues. *Journal of Speech, Language, and Hearing Research, 45*, 519–530.

Schein, J. D., & Delk, M. T., Jr. (1974). *The deaf population of the United States*. Silver Spring, MD: National Association of the Deaf.

Snow, C., & Galabudra, A. (2002). Second language learners and understanding the brain. In A. Galaburda, S. Kosslyn, & Y. Christen (Eds.), *The languages of the brain* (pp. 151–165). Cambridge, MA: Harvard University Press.

Stokoe, W. (1972). *Semiotics and human sign language*. The Hague, Netherlands: Moulton & Company N.V., Publishers.

Tombaugh, T. N., Kozak, J., & Rees, L. (1999). Normative data stratified by age and education for two measures of verbal fluency: FAS and animal naming. *Archives of Clinical Neuropsychology, 14*(2), 167–177.

Wilson, M., & Emmorey, K. (1997). Working memory for sign language: A window into the architecture of the working memory system. *Journal of Deaf Studies and Deaf Education, 2*(3), 121–130.

Index

A
Academic achievement
   and Japanese students, 135
   general academic knowledge, WJ-III, 131–135
   long term memory, 136
   math skills, 129–131
   reading achievement
      critical factor, 108
      Peabody Individual Achievement Test-Revised, 117–122
      phonological awareness, 108
      reading comprehension data, 107
      test of silent word reading fluency, 122–124
      Woodcock-Johnson III (WJ-III) tests of achievement, 109–116
   second language skills, 135
   short term memory, 136
   standardized measures, 127
   working memory capacity, 135–136
   writing fluency subtest, 128–129
Animal based linguistic fluency, 151–153

B
Bilingualism, 143
Brief Visuospatial Memory Test-Revised (BVMT-R)
   delayed recall correlations, 63
   discrimination index, 64
   results, 61–64
   test characteristics, 60–61
   total recall correlations, 62

C
Cognitive function
   executive functions, 44–55
   intellectual functions, 39–44
   linguistic learning and memory
      instrument design and administration, 93–94
      M-SVLT correlations, 94–101
      M-SVLT descriptive data, 94, 95
      Morere signed verbal learning test, 92–101
   visuospatial ability
      Brief Visuospatial Memory Test-Revised (BVMT-R), 60–64
      mental rotation ability, 65–70
   working memory
      Corsi Blocks manual and computer version, 89–92
      linguistic spans
         measure, 77–79
      phonological similarity, 76–77
      print and ASL digit/letter spans, 80–89
      reciprocal interaction of, 76
      tasks focused, 75
      visual/spatial spans, 79–80
Constructs
   academic achievement, 12–13
   general cognitive functioning, 10–11
   linguistic ability, 13–15
   short term memory, 11–12
   visuospatial ability, 11
   working memory, 11–12

D

Deafness
  cochlear implant usage, 27–28
  hearing aid, 27, 28
  language preference, 26–27
  onset age, 26, 27
  pure tone average, 26

E

English phonological knowledge
  demographic characteristics, 168
  lipreading screening test, 169
  phoneme detection test, 167–168
  reading skills, 168–169
  strategies, 167
English syntax knowledge
  and working memory, 171–172
  correlations, 172–173
  descriptive statistics, 171
  pronominalization score, 172
  readers ability, 168–169
  syntactic ability test, 169
  TSA scores, 170–171
Ethical standards, 6–8
Executive function
  component processes, 44–45
  Corsi Blocks, 56
  deaf individuals, 45–47
  Tower of Hanoi, 51–52
  Tower of London, 53–55
  WCST, 47–50
Expressive language
  bilingualism effects, 143
  correlational relationships, 148–154
  descriptive statistics, 147–148
  phonemic fluency, 144–146
  semantic fluency, 146–147
  tasks associated, 141–142
  verbal fluency, 142–143

F

Fingerspelling
  academic knowledge correlation, 164
  American Sign Language, 180–181
  ASL manual alphabet, 181–182
  descriptive statistics, 163
  error codes, 187
  history, 179
  linguistic fluency correlation, 164–165
  literacy bridge, 183–184
  manual alphabet systems, 179–180
  measurement, 185–186
  omissions, 187–188
  pseudo-words, 186
  pseudo-words effects, 163
  real word substitutions, 188
  reception and expression, 184–185
  reverse digit span task, 166
  skill development, 182–183
  test of, 163
  words and signs, 162
Fingerspelling Test, 15
Food-based linguistic fluency, 153–155

G

General Academic Knowledge, WJ-III
  descriptive statistics, 132
  rasch analysis, 133–135
  significant correlations, 131–132
  strategy, 131

H

Hopkins Verbal Learning Test-Revised
  (HVLT-R), 62

I

Intellectual function
  K-BIT2 Results, 44
  Kaufman brief intelligence test, 39–40
  Rasch Analysis
    advantages, 40–41
    person and item reliability analysis, 42–44

K

Kaufman Brief Intelligence Test (K-BIT), 10, 39–40
Koo Phoneme Detection Test (Koo PDT)
  descriptive statistics, 168
  participants activity, 167–168
  results, 168–169

L

Legal implications, 6–8
Linguistic fluency
  bilingualism effects, 143
  correlational relationships
    5-1-U-significant correlations, 149–151
    animal fluency tasks, 151–153
    F-A-S-significant correlations, 148–149
    food-based tasks, 153–155
  descriptive statistics, 147–148

Index

phonemic fluency, 144–146
semantic fluency, 146–147
tasks associated, 141–142
verbal fluency, 142–143
Linguistic function
  expressive language, 141–155
  receptive language
    American Sign Language, 159–162
    English phonological knowledge, 166–169
    English syntax knowledge, 169–173
    fingerspelling, 162–166
    (*see also* Fingerspelling)
    visual reception, spoken language, 173–176
Linguistic learning and memory
  instrument design and administration, 93–94
  M-SVLT correlations, 94–101
  M-SVLT descriptive data, 94, 95
  Morere Signed Verbal Learning Test, 92–101
Lipreading
  Background Questionnaire Trends, 223–224
  early intervention role, 209–210
  lipreading screening test, 210–212
  materials, 212–213
  parental support, 225
  participants, 212
  procedures, 213–214
  responses characteristics
    number of sentences written, 216–217
    word class of vocabulary written, 217–219
  syntactic patterns trends
    function words usage, 220
    mismatched stimulus words, 222
    syllabic structure matching words, 222–223
    syntax errors, 220–221
  target sentences
    characteristics, LST, 214–215
    word class of vocabulary, 215–216
  Test of Syntactic Abilities, 210
Lipreading Screening Test (LST)
  definition, 173–174
  descriptive statistics, 175
  results correlations, 174–176
  strategy, 174
Literacy, 8–10

M

Math skills
  descriptive statistics, 130
  source, 129
  WJ-III math fluency subtest, 130–131
Memory
  academic achievement, 135–136
  constructs, 11–12
  English syntax knowledge, 171–172
  linguistic learning, 92–101
  psychometric analyses, 11–12
  short-term memory (STM), 75–92
  working memory
    (*see* Working memory (WM))
Mental Rotation
  definition, 65
  English skills, 65–66
  math reasoning skills, 65
  rasch analysis, 68–70
  results, 66–68
  test characteristics, 66
Mental Rotation Test (MRT), 40
Morere Signed Verbal Learning Test (M-SVLT)
  correlations, 94–101
  descriptive data, 94
  instrument design and administration, 93–94
  long-delay cued recall correlations, 99, 100
  long-delay free recall correlations, 98–99
  recall correlations, 95–96, 97
  recognition correct responses correlations, 99–101
  short-delay cued recall correlations, 97–98
  short-delay free recall correlations, 96–97
  total recall correlations, 95, 96

N

Neurocognitive measurement, factor analysis (FA)
  academic fluency, 239
  academic skills, 243
  ASL usage, before *vs.* after school, 255–256
  ASL-based retrieval, 242
  coding modalities, 232–233
  descriptive statistics, 234
  early language experience, 233
  educational outcomes, 232
  eigenvalues factor, 235
  executive functioning, 239
  importance, 231–232
  letter and word knowledge, 237–238
  mental rotation, 242
  mother's impact, 253–254
  multivariate analyses, 244–250
  multivariate significant factors, 257–258

Neurocognitive measurement (*cont.*)
  no multivariate significant factors, 256–257
  nonverbal intelligence, 241
  parent impact, 250–252
  participant impact, 250–251
  phonological loop, 243
  principal components factor analysis, 235
  rotated component matrix, 235–236
  short-term memory, 239–240
  sign-based linguistic learning and memory, 240
  speech-based phonology, 239–240
  visuospatial reasoning, 241
  visuospatial short-term memory, 240–241
  visuospatial working memory, 241
  working memory, 239
Nonverbal intelligence tests, 4

P
Peabody Individual Achievement Test-Revised (PIAT-R), 12–13
  Rasch Analysis, 120–122
  results, 117–120
  test characteristics, 117
Phoneme Detection Test (PDT), 14
Phonemic fluency
  5-1-U task
    development, 144
    English translation instruction, 145
    scoring method, 146
  correlational relationships, 148–154
  descriptive statistics, 147–148
  F-A-S task, 144
Phonological processing skills, 9
Pintner non-language test, 5–6
Proficiency interviews
  common understanding, 200
  disagreements, 200–201
  scoring criteria, 199–200
  standardized form, 200
Psychometric analyses
  academic achievement, 12–13
  constructs and instruments, toolkits, 10–15
  critical measurement issues, 4–5
  ethical standards, 6–8
  general cognitive functioning, 10–11
  history, deaf individuals, 5–6
  legal implications, 6–7
  limitations, 3–4
  linguistic ability, 13–15
  linguistic list memory, 12
  literacy and cognitive development, 8–10
  short-term memory, 11
  test scores purposes, 3
  visuospatial ability, 11
  working memory, 11–12

R
Rasch Analysis
  academic knowledge, 133–135
  intellectual functioning, 40–44
  mental rotation, 68–70
  reading achievement, 115–116, 120–122
Reading achievement
  critical factor, 108
  Peabody Individual Achievement Test-Revised, 117–122
  phonological awareness, 108
  reading comprehension data, 107
  Test of Silent Word Reading Fluency, 122–124
  Woodcock-Johnson III (WJ-III) Tests of Achievement, 109–116
    Passage Comprehension, 112–116
    Reading Fluency, 109–112
Receptive language
  American Sign Language
    computer-administered signed sentences, 159–160
    moderate to large correlations, 160–162
    scoring crteria, 160
  English phonological knowledge, 166–169
  English syntax knowledge, 169–173
  fingerspelling, 162–166
  visual reception, spoken language, 173–176
Recruitment, 22–23

S
Semantic fluency, 146–47
Short-term memory (STM)
  Corsi Blocks manual and computer version, 89–92
  linguistic spans measure, 77–79
  phonological similarity, 76–77
  print and ASL digit/letter spans, 80–89
  reciprocal interaction of, 76
  tasks focused, 75
  visual/spatial spans, 79–80
Sign language assessment
  5C's, 205
  arbitrary decisions, 194–195
  backward design model, 204
  behavior checklists, 201

Index

British *vs.* American language, 192
crosslinguistic activation, 192
depicting and nondepicting verbs, 194
importance, 191
multiple viewing modes, 194
numbers and space usage, 195
objective tests, 203–204
Peabody Picture Vocabulary Test, 193–194
performance-based tests, 201–203
proficiency interviews, 199–201
spoken and signed languages, 193
standardization, 204–205
Standards Collaborative Board, 205
tests
    design and format, 199–204
    item development, selection and piloting, 196–199
word frequencies disparity, 193–194

T

Test of Silent Word Reading Fluency (TOSWRF), 12–13, 84
    results, 122–124
    test characteristics, 122
Test of Syntactic Ability (TSA), 14
Tower of London (TOL), 10–11
Towers of Hanoi (TOH), 10–11
    definition, 51
    results, 51–52
Towers of London (TOL)
    defintion, 53
    results, 53–55

V

Vandenberg mental rotation test, 66
Visual language, 8–9
Visual Language and Visual Learning (VL2) Toolkit Psychometric Study
assistive device usage, 26–28
background questionnaire, 24–34
communication history, 32–34
database development, 24
deafness and language usage, 26–28
demographics, 24–26
language history, 30–32
parents and family members, 28–30
protocol development and design, 21–22
sample recruitment, 22–23
scoring procedures, 24
Visual reception, spoken language
lipreading screening test, 173–176
speechreading skills, 173

Visuospatial ability
brief visuospatial memory test-revised (BVMT-R), 60–64
mental rotation ability, 65–70
Visuospatial skills
constructs, 11
neurocognitive measurement, 241
psychometric analyses, 11

W

Wisconsin Card Sorting Test (WCST), 10–11
Wisconsin card sorting test-64 card version (WCST)
categories completed, 50
perseverative errors, 50
results, 48
strategy, 47–48
test manual, 47
total score, Pearson correlations, 49
Woodcock Johnson Test of Academic Achievement (WJ-III), 12–13
Woodcock-Johnson III (WJ-III) Tests of Achievement
General Academic Knowledge, 131–135
Passage Comprehension
    Rasch Analysis, 115–116
    results, 112–115
    test characteristics, 112
Reading Fluency
    results, 110–112
    test characteristics, 109–110
WJ-III Math Fluency Subtest, 130–131
Writing Fluency subtest, 128–129
Working memory (WM)
ASL digits backward, 88
ASL digits forward, 87–88
ASL letters backward, 89
ASL letters forward, 88
Corsi Blocks manual and computer version, 89–92
Cued Speech, 76
descriptive statistics, 81
linguistic spans, 78–79
phonological similarity, 76–77
print and ASL digit/letter spans, 80–89
print digits backward, 85
print digits forward, 81–85
print letters backward, 86–87
print letters forward, 85–86
sign length effect, 76
significant correlations, 81–84
tasks focused, 75
visual/spatial spans, 79–80

Writing ability
- background questionnaire trends, 223–224
- early intervention role, 209–210
- lipreading screening test, 210–212
- materials, 212–213
- parental support, 225
- participants, 212
- procedures, 213–214
- responses characteristics, 216–219
- syntactic patterns trends, 220–223
- target sentences, 214–216
- test of syntactic abilities, 210

Writing Fluency, 128–129